Moral Challenges in a Pandemic Age

The COVID-19 pandemic, whose consequences will be felt in the long term, can be interpreted as a signal that we have been living in a pandemic age. A pandemic is humanity's common ground, so the moral problems inherent in it are of interest to everyone from now on. It brought a set of moral challenges that cannot be ignored.

This book – which emerged amid the novel coronavirus crisis – is designed to fill the gap in the current literature on the topic, offering an original approach to its moral implications. It can be taken as a guide in the face of these pandemic-age challenges for human relations.

The pandemic is a multifaceted phenomenon, and its debate involves a wide variety of practical philosophical concerns. All the chapters of this book, divided into four sections, aim to clarify its central aspects, while each chapter provides an original approach to the debate's leading issues and relies on each most significant collaborator's expertise. Also, they reflect their unique pandemic experiences under the scrutiny of philosophical unrest.

Since the pandemic is an ongoing event, *Moral Challenges in a Pandemic Age* will be of interest to professors, students, and researchers engaged in understanding the ethical dimension of the age we are experiencing. The problems addressed in this collection transcend the boundaries of the philosophical field, offering an innovative approach to individuals keen on discussing the pandemic from a moral point of view. Such a discussion encompasses the philosophical inquiry but is not restricted to it. Those interested in related areas such as psychology, sociology, biology, public health, education, anthropology, and cultural studies – to name a few – will find connections with parallel themes in this book. In addition, the collection brings a theoretically supported approach to several related debates in a language accessible to anyone who wants to know more about the topic.

Evandro Barbosa is an Associate Professor of Philosophy at the Federal University of Pelotas, Brazil, and a visiting scholar in the Department of Philosophy at the University of North Carolina at Chapel Hill. He is a Brazilian National Research Council (CNPq) Fellow, leading the project *Pandemic and Human Relations: Moral Considerations in the Time of COVID-19*. He also has received financial support from Brazilian research funding agencies to develop pandemic ethics-related projects (www.pandemiclives.com).

Routledge Research in Applied Ethics

For more information about this series, please visit: https://www.routledge.com/Routledge-Research-in-Applied-Ethics/book-series/RRAES

Moral Challenges in a Pandemic Age

Edited by Evandro Barbosa

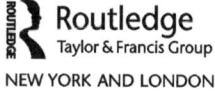
Routledge
Taylor & Francis Group

NEW YORK AND LONDON

First published 2023
by Routledge
605 Third Avenue, New York, NY 10158

and by Routledge
4 Park Square, Milton Park, Abingdon, Oxon, OX14 4RN

*Routledge is an imprint of the Taylor & Francis Group, an
informa business*

Library of Congress Cataloging-in-Publication Data
Names: Barbosa, Evandro, editor.
Title: Moral challenges in a pandemic age / edited by Evandro Barbosa.
Description: New York, NY : Routledge, 2023. | Series: Routledge research
in applied ethics | Includes bibliographical references and index.
Identifiers: LCCN 2022061289 (print) | LCCN 2022061290 (ebook) | ISBN
9781032315201 (hbk) | ISBN 9781032315195 (pbk) | ISBN 9781003310129 (ebk)
Subjects: LCSH: COVID-19 Pandemic, 2020---Moral and ethical aspects.
Classification: LCC RA644.C67 M683 2023 (print) | LCC RA644.C67 (ebook) |
DDC 362.1962/4144--dc23/eng/20230428
LC record available at https://lccn.loc.gov/2022061289
LC ebook record available at https://lccn.loc.gov/2022061290

ISBN: 978-1-032-31520-1 (hbk)
ISBN: 978-1-032-31519-5 (pbk)
ISBN: 978-1-003-31012-9 (ebk)

DOI: 10.4324/9781003310129

Typeset in Sabon
by SPi Technologies India Pvt Ltd (Straive)

Contents

vi   *Contents*

Notes on contributors

Peter R. Anstey is Professor of Philosophy at the University of Sydney. He specializes in early modern philosophy and also works on contemporary moral philosophy and the philosophy of mind. He is the author (with Alberto Vanzo) of *Experimental Philosophy and the Origins of Empiricism* (2023).

Marcelo de Araujo is Professor of Philosophy of Law at the Federal University of Rio de Janeiro and Professor of Ethics at the State University of Rio de Janeiro. He is also Ambassador Scientist of the Alexander-von-Humboldt Foundation in Brazil. PhD in Philosophy from the University of Konstanz, 2002.

Alcino Eduardo Bonella is Full Professor at Federal University Of Uberlândia (Ufu) and member of the Internacional Association of Bioethics (Iab).

Lisa Bortolotti is Professor of Philosophy at the University of Birmingham, affiliated with the Department of Philosophy and the Institute for Mental Health. Lisa is a philosopher of the cognitive sciences, interested in rationality, belief, self-knowledge, agency, and mental health. She is the author of *Delusions and Other Irrational Beliefs* (2009), *Irrationality* (2014), and *The Epistemic Innocence of Irrational Beliefs* (2020). She is also the Editor of *Philosophical Psychology* (Taylor & Francis).

Thaís Alves Costa is a Lawyer in Brazil and Visiting Scholar at the Department of Philosophy at the University of North Carolina, Chapel Hill. Her main research areas are Smithian political philosophy, moral psychology, and human rights, especially the intersection of these areas. She is the author of *Between Morality and Evolution: Naturalizing the Sentiment of Sympathy* (2022), *In Search of a Sympathetic Liberalism in Adam Smith.* (2021), and *Adam Smith's Tripartite Theory: The Possibility of Sympathetic Engagement* (2021).

Denis Coitinho is an associate professor of philosophy at the University of Vale do Rio dos Sinos.

Ryan Doody is an assistant professor of philosophy and political economy at Brown University. He works on issues at the intersection of decision theory, epistemology, ethics, and the philosophy of economics, in particular, on issues regarding rationality, value, and risk.

Simone Gubler is an Assistant Professor of Philosophy at the University of Nevada, Reno.

Anneli Jefferson is Lecturer in Philosophy at Cardiff University. Anneli works in the areas of moral philosophy and philosophy of psychology and psychiatry and is interested in moral psychology, moral responsibility, cognitive biases, and issues surrounding mental health. She is author of *Are Mental Disorders Brain Disorders?* (Routledge 2022).

Leonardo de Mello Ribeiro is currently Professor of Philosophy at the Federal University of Minas Gerais, Brazil. He holds a PhD in philosophy from the University of Sheffield (United Kingdom) and works mainly in ethics, metaethics, moral psychology, and the philosophy of action.

Matheus de Mesquita Silveira is Professor at the Graduate Program in Philosophy of Caxias do Sul University and lead researcher at X-Lab: Philosophy, Ethology and Neurosciences.

Martina Orlandi is Assistant Professor of Philosophy at Trent University.

Joshua Preiss is Professor of Philosophy and Director of the Program in Philosophy, Politics, and Economics at Minnesota State University-Mankato. His recent monograph *Just Work for All: The American Dream in the 21st Century*, was published by Routledge in 2021.

Jana S. Rošker is a Professor of Sinology at the University of Ljubljana in Slovenia.

Mauro Rossi is Full Professor in the Department of Philosophy at the Université du Québec à Montréal. His main research interests are in value theory and prudential psychology. He is currently working with Christine Tappolet on a monograph on the relationship between well-being and psychological happiness, under contract with Oxford University Press.

Maxwell J. Smith is an Assistant Professor and Western Research Chair in Public Health Ethics in the Faculty of Health Sciences and Associate Director of the Rotman Institute of Philosophy at Western University in London, Ontario, Canada. He serves as a member and rapporteur of the World Health Organization's COVID-19 Ethics and Governance Expert Working Group.

Flavio Will(ges is Associate Professor at the Department of Philosophy at the Federal University of Santa Maria (Brazil) and has edited with Marcelo Fischborn and David Copp the book "O lugar das emoções na ética e na metaética" [The Place of Emotions in Ethics and Metaethics].

Foreword

Maxwell J. Smith

In many ways, the world's response to the COVID-19 pandemic represents a triumph of science but a failure of humanity. Safe and effective vaccines were developed, manufactured, and distributed at astonishing speed, saving millions of lives,[1] yet their global rollout was – and continues to be – profoundly inequitable. The same can be said for diagnostics (e.g., tests), prophylactics (e.g., personal protective equipment), and therapeutics (e.g., monoclonal antibodies). Even when we had the tools, we often chose not to use them, especially when society's most privileged no longer felt COVID-19 posed a significant threat. Nonpharmaceutical interventions (e.g., isolation, quarantine) were effectively introduced to interrupt the spread of disease, yet insufficient attention was paid to mitigating their unintended impacts on people's livelihoods and well-being.[2] Decision-makers claimed they understood that collective threats require collective action, yet often eschewed collective responsibility in favor of personal responsibility. We said, "We're all in this together," but didn't act like it. These reflect *moral* failures, not failures of innovation or ingenuity.[3] Consequently, progress in pandemic preparedness and response is predicated on recognizing our *moral*, not just technical or scientific, shortcomings, committing to making decisions that are *ethics-informed* in addition to being evidenced-informed, and appreciating the inextricably moral dimensions of the ways in which we stand in relation to one another.[4]

The ethics of how we stand in relation to one another animates concerns central to solidarity and justice.[5, 6] It's therefore unsurprising that solidarity and justice figured prominently in the rhetoric of political leaders in response to COVID-19.[7] And yet, this infrequently translated into more ethical actions, policies, or outcomes; the COVID-19 pandemic continues to be marked by stark injustice and a conspicuous absence of solidarity. Hence, important questions remain regarding the *desiderata* and requirements of solidarity and justice during public health emergencies – for individuals, for private, public, and nongovernmental organizations, and for states – and how these can be effectively translated into policy and realized in practice.

The COVID-19 pandemic has resulted in an increased scholarly and lay interest in these questions. Indeed, the COVID-19 pandemic has served as the first occasion for many to meaningfully reflect upon the relationship between one's behaviors and the health of others, and, conversely, the relationship between the behaviors of others and one's health. It raised new questions for some, including about one's responsibilities toward one's neighbors, co-workers, and even those living on the other side of the world. It highlighted questions about the sacrifices one can reasonably be expected to make in the name of protecting the health of the public, and more specifically, the health of those most at risk and least advantaged. It also provided the first occasion for many to reflect upon the appropriate relationship between the state and the public *vis-à-vis* the pursuit of public health objectives. Some ended up forming very firm views about what these relationships ought to look like. At the same time, some who had given serious thought to these relationships prior to COVID-19 no doubt shifted their views after witnessing the behaviors and actions taken, or not taken, in response to the pandemic. Hence, we're at a key inflection point where societal norms, values, and virtues related to the management of infectious diseases are being scrutinized and shaped for the future.

An important opportunity, therefore, exists to contribute to and shape this exercise. But care must be taken when doing so. Pandemic preparedness and response are key functions of *public health*. Accordingly, if the key features of public health – an emphasis on populations and communities rather than individuals, prevention rather than treatment, and collective action rather than individual intervention – are overlooked, ethical analyses are more likely to be inept and lead to specious conclusions. As Angus Dawson observes, if one were to approach questions in public health from the perspective of, say, medicine and contemporary medical ethics, "many public health policies and activities are likely to be viewed as ethically dubious."[8] This point is worth emphasizing given the increased attention pandemic ethics is enjoying as a result of COVID-19, where some may be keen to proffer ethical judgments without first appreciating the contours, features, functions, activities, limitations, histories, concepts, and values that inform and constitute the practice of public health.

This brings me to the importance of *public health ethics*, an established field of scholarship and practice that has long interrogated ethical questions in relation to the activities of public health,[9] including in relation to epidemics and pandemics like HIV/AIDS, SARS, H1N1 influenza, MERS-CoV, Zika, tuberculosis, Ebola, and now COVID-19.[10] Since the turn of the millennium, public health ethics guidance has been promulgated to inform pandemic preparedness and response, including via seminal publications by health authorities like the World Health Organization.[11] Much thought has gone into, for example, the fair allocation of scarce resources during pandemics, vaccination mandates, challenge trials, the use of restrictive measures like quarantine and isolation, and other issues. Significant scholarship, particularly in feminist public health ethics, has interrogated the relational dimensions of key issues and concepts in public health, like autonomy, justice, and solidarity.[12] With an explosion of interest in pandemic ethics and public health ethics as a result of the COVID-19 pandemic, it will be important that future work recognize, engage with, and build upon the extant scholarship, experiences, and lessons in these areas. Much work remains, particularly in ensuring issues in pandemic ethics are understood and that resulting knowledge is effectively integrated into policy and practice, and this volume helps significantly to advance these aims.

References

1. Watson OJ, Barnsley G, Toor J, Hogan AB, Winskill P, Chani AC. (2022). Global impact of the first year of COVID-19 vaccination: a mathematical modelling study. *The Lancet Infectious Diseases*, 22(9): 1293–1302.
2. Silva DS, Smith MJ. (2022). Is the cure worse than the disease? The ethics of imposing risk in public health. *Asian Bioethics Review*. doi: 10.1007/s41649-022-00218-1.
3. Smith MJ, Upshur REG. (2020). Learning lessons from COVID-19 requires recognizing moral failures. *Journal of Bioethical Inquiry*, 17(4): 563–566.
4. Emanuel EJ, Upshur REG, Smith MJ. (2022). What COVID has taught the world about ethics. *New England Journal of Medicine*, 387(17): 1542–1545.
5. Dawson A, Jennings B. (2012). The place of solidarity in public health ethics. *Public Health Reviews*, 34: 65–79.
6. Smith MJ. (2022). Social justice and public health. In Routledge Handbook of Philosophy of Public Health (pgs. 333–346), eds. Venkatapuram S, Broadbent A. Routledge.
7. Silva DS, Jackson C, Smith MJ. (2021). Mere rhetoric? Using solidarity as a moral guide for deliberations on border closures, border re-openings, and travel restrictions in the age of COVID-19. *BMJ Global Health*, 6: e006701.
8. Dawson A. (2011). Resetting the parameters: public health as the foundation for public health ethics. In Public Health Ethics: Key Concepts and Issues in Policy and Practice (pgs. 1–19), ed. Dawson A. New York: Cambridge University Press.
9. Smith MJ, Nixon S, Upshur R, Benatar SR, Thompson AK. (2019). Public health ethics. In Public Health Law and Policy in Canada (pgs. 43–66) (4th Edition), ed. Bailey TM, Sheldon CT, Shelley JJ. Markham, ON: LexisNexis.
10. Smith MJ, Upshur REG. (2019). Pandemic disease, public health, and ethics. In Oxford Handbook of Public Health Ethics, ed. Mastroianni AC, Kahn JP, Kass NE. New York, NY: Oxford University Press.
11. World Health Organization. (2016). Guidance for managing ethical issues in infectious disease outbreaks. Geneva: World Health Organization.
12. Baylis F, Kenny N, Sherwin S. (2008). A relational account of public health ethics. *Public Health Ethics*, 1(3): 196–209.

Acknowledgments

This compendium appears in an unexpected way, somewhat like the COVID-19 pandemic. My wife and I were working as visiting scholars at the University of North Carolina (UNC) – Chapel Hill in 2020 when the pandemic hit. At that time, I was studying Hume's theory of moral sentiments. Among the themes, the problem of justice intrigued me during a Jennifer Morton seminar to the point that I decided to write about the pandemic, justice, and conditions of scarcity. This was the spark I needed to get interested in the subject.

I thank Geoffrey Sayre-Mccord for receiving me at UNC and encouraging a project like this, even though I was moving away from the research subject that took me to Chapel Hill. This project would only go ahead with his support.

This project matured and took shape throughout the "Symposium – Pandemic Relations" sponsored by the Department of Philosophy at the Federal University of Pelotas (UFPEL) – Brazil, with colleagues Denis Coitinho, Leonardo Ribeiro, Flavio Williges, Matheus Mesquita, and Sérgio Tenenbaum. I am grateful to these colleagues and partnerships. I am also grateful to the students and colleagues in my pandemic seminars at UFPEL for their excellent questions.

Some colleagues have contributed to shaping this book through comments, suggestions, or criticisms. My warmest thanks to Gigi Taylor, Warren, Thaís, Lan, Cati, and Masa.

Also, this book would only have surfaced with the proper financial support. I gratefully acknowledge the Brazilian research funding agencies Coordination for the Improvement of Higher Education Personnel (CAPES) for the scholarship to work as a visiting scholar at the UNC and National Council for Scientific and Technological Development (CNPq) for supporting the project on Ethics and Pandemic Relations. During the initial year, UNC provided an ideal research place, combining a wonderful setting with an open and friendly academic atmosphere.

I want to acknowledge the continuous support and warm encouragement I received throughout this book's gestation process from the editor Andrew Weckenmann. Also, Rosaleah Stammler, Suba Ramya, and

Melissa Brown Levine did an excellent job. I am indebted to all on the Routledge team for their dedication and support throughout the project.

I especially thank Vicki for her always careful and insightful reading of my work. I owe a non-negotiable debt of gratitude to you, who has become an inseparable academic friend over the last few years, both for friendship and for being a discerning reviewer in this process. Her insightful observations made everything more evident to me.

Thanks to all contributors to this project for agreeing to build their knowledge in the pages ahead.

A project like this has the price of absence many times, so my most significant debt is to my family. First, I thank my wife, Thaís Alves Costa, for her editorial and academic help. You have been so patient and caring with me in treating this project as "ours" – it is, indeed! The pandemic has locked us at home, and this companion portrays our pandemic life in so many different ways: you, me, our adorable cat, and our son, who is arriving in a defiant world. Finally, I would like to acknowledge my family – Keti, Ignes, and Paulo – by encouraging my musings about the pandemic and patiently enduring my absences from my hometown.

1 The pandemic age

An overview

Evandro Barbosa

*What is not good for the hive
cannot be good for the bee.*

Marcus Aurelius

1.1 Between pandemics and morality

We are in a pandemic age. One way to explain this statement involves briefly telling the story of this project. When we began this work in 2020, one of the questions we asked to understand the impact of the novel coronavirus on people was the following: When was your "pandemic day"[1] – the day you realized that COVID had finally arrived in your own life and would change the course of human history? This question invited people to focus on the pandemic's beginning more than its effects. Each response we received was unique, but all agreed that COVID would have a lasting impact on humanity.

At that time, we expected to be asking another question at the end of the project: When was your "post-pandemic day" – the day you realized the pandemic was behind you and life would soon get back on track? Soon we recognized, however, that the closing question would remain unanswered. We couldn't talk about post-pandemic life because, as of this writing, COVID has not ended and humanity has into a pandemic age.

An age can be understood as a chronological period beginning with a specific fact or event whose characteristics or events shape a subsequent stretch of time. We have had the information age and the age of globalization. Now we have embarked upon an age of pandemics, and there are some reasons to believe this.

First, take the novel coronavirus as a pandemic sample. The COVID-19 pandemic officially started in March 2020, and three years later, several sanitary control measures are in place to prevent a new outbreak. Second, data indicates the high probability of a pandemic occurring in the near future. A recent study of novel disease outbreaks coordinated by Marani, Katul, Pan, and Parolari (2021) indicates that the risk of a new

DOI: 10.4324/9781003310129-1

pandemic similar to COVID-19 could be three times greater in the coming decades and the chance of facing a COVID-19-like pandemic is 2% per year or 38% over our lifetime. The third element is the expression of our concern with this scenario. The increased risk of a new pandemic has raised awareness and prompted efforts on avoiding or reducing such risks. For that, there is a global effort to track and prevent or mitigate the effects of the next pandemic. These initiatives require worldwide mobilization and involve the engagement of several international agents (World Health Organization – WHO, United Nations, States, and relevant global social agents). Some attempts to coordinate efforts are present in the projects such as those coordinated by the WHO,[2] the *Pandemic Preparedness and Response* (*PANDEM* and *PANDEM 2*) of the European Commission,[3] the *Pandemic Prevention Initiative*,[4] or the *Global Epidemic Response and Mobilization Team* – to monitor the pandemic scenario.[5]

We also need to explain the moral meaning of the term pandemic, as the objective of this book is not limited to interpreting it as a global public health emergency. Instead, we seek to read the pandemic as a moral phenomenon. A pandemic is not an individual problem but a collective one, as the quote attributed to Marcus Aurelius illustrates; this is true even though its consequences may affect each person distinctively. And yet moral inquiry into pandemics is still at an early stage. When we consider a pandemic as simply a fact of human life, we have little to say about it from the point of view of morality. Instead, we view it primarily through the lens of science, and our discussions take place as if within a scientific echo chamber in which moral considerations cannot penetrate with any force or intensity.

However, when we view the COVID pandemic through the lens of morality, we find features that moral theorists can scrutinize. A wide range of ethical discussions is embedded in it, which allows us to study the ethical roles agents play in preparing for, combating, and eradicating pandemics. A Pandemics needs to be understood as nonpure moral phenomena, as they involve several areas of discussion – health, economics, science, and politics, to name a few. Moral philosophers have primarily addressed questions of bioethics related to the pandemic, such as assigning priority for ICU beds or respirators or the ethics of testing vaccines. While the focus on bioethics is valuable, it can lead us to overlook some relevant moral features.

Consider, by analogy, the ethical controversies surrounding war. Some critics question how justifiable it is to wage a war, evaluating the morality of war itself – what they call *jus ad bellum*. Others ask what methods of waging war are acceptable, considering issues like the tactics of targeting civilians or breaking an armistice – an area well-known as *jus in bello*. When we set up criteria for assessing the moral features of war, we are taking it as a phenomenon worthy of moral discussion.

The same happens with the pandemic when we recognize how it is shaping our moral landscape. It interests us as an object of scrutiny in itself, and the attempt to systematize the discussion by some theorists has laid the foundations for this way of thinking about it. Terms like pandethics (Selgelid, 2009), pandemic ethics (Araujo, 2021), or similar indicate that moral considerations are inherent in the pandemic phenomenon.

But pandemics also function to generate phenomena worthy of moral consideration, as in the discussion of *jus in bello*. Many concrete aspects of the pandemic may require our ethical gaze, including our priorities in assigning limited ICU beds, lockdowns, vaccine queues, and using masks and other protective devices. These issues can serve as a gateway to the broader moral discussion. Whether we focus on the pandemic itself or the pandemic as a generator of moral phenomena, there is room for discussing its moral challenges.

As philosophers, we are interested in the moral challenges that the pandemic has posed for discussions in ethics. The works in this compendium aim to do the work of the moral anatomist – following Hume's suggestion – to lay bare the truths hidden within the depths of human moral relationships during the pandemic. Our initial assumption is that the pandemic has altered our human relationships on many levels.

Literature enthusiasts may recall how Camus, in his work *The Plague*, portrays the impact of a pandemic through a dialogue between a night watchman and Jean Tarrou, one of the major characters, as they discuss the pandemic's effects on the population.

> Ah, if only it had been an earthquake! A good bad shock, and there you are! You count the dead and living, and that's an end of it. But this here damned disease – even them who haven't got it can't think of anything else.
>
> (Camus, 1974, 94)

This passage provides a clue by clarifying that the pandemic has forced its way into current discussions. Our question about the post-pandemic day may never be answered, but the debates presented here will echo through time. The insights offered by the contributors in this book – each playing the role of the anatomist – throw light on pivotal moral issues that seem more relevant and more likely to be perennial than ever before. After all, we all are in a pandemic age.

1.2 Book summary

Our compendium's guiding question is this: *Could the COVID-19 pandemic be (re)forging new kinds of moral bonds among humans?* Living in pandemic times is like having the sword of Damocles hanging over our necks each day. A host of significant changes have shaped and strained our family, work, and social relationships. Although a wide range of philosophical discussions have mapped out some of the ethical issues related to the pandemic, one crucial aspect that seems to have been over-looked is that these human relationships should be an object of study for ethicists. Our intention in this companion is to bring into focus novel questions about how relations during pandemic times shape and are shaped by our moral behavior, attitudes, and judgments. The contributors have all been experiencing this global crisis in widely varying contexts across the planet. Their explorations of the moral content at the heart of our relationships can help us all to unfold and to understand in depth the implications of this new (provisional or not) social dynamic for morality.

The book is organized into four main parts: I – Rationality and Moral Emotions, II – Virtues and Traits of Character, III – Social Arrangements and Moral Conflicts, and IV – After COVID-19 Life: Some Moral Issues. Although there are intersections between the points covered, each contributor to this volume offers an original approach to the initial question raised.

Part I could be seen as examining two sides of the same coin. The first relevant question concerns the level of rationality of agents in threatening contexts. Would they be in the best position (rationally and epistemically speaking) to make a moral decision? To answer this question, Anneli Jefferson and Lisa Bortolotti offer their considerations on the moral psychology of the pandemic agent. Since this agent could not be in the best position to make a decision, the sole responsibility of citizens must be questioned. Recent surveys have offered a view of how extreme conditions, such as those found during a pandemic, act as triggers for certain emotions. For instance, the emotion of loneliness is often present in contexts that overwhelm individuals. Flavio Williges advocates that loneliness can offer a transforming epistemic experience. Other feelings, however, are less generous to individuals and may undermine their thought structure and agency. This is the case with the emotions of fear and anger analyzed by Matheus de Mesquita Silveira, which can interfere with choices and lead to biased attitudes. Similarly, the rationality conditions of agents are also affected by strenuous situations, especially regarding risks. Indeed, the novel coronavirus has tested people's resilience at a more acute level. In response, Martina Orlandi suggests questioning the limits of an individualist conception of resilience while offering a relational proposal for its interpretation.

Part II considers the role that virtues and character traits play in shaping the moral quality of our relationships during pandemic times. The context of a pandemic complicates the use of core virtues and challenges us to transcend our own secluded point of view – to step out of our safety zone and put ourselves in each other's shoes. For instance, consider this question: in harsh settings, do we need to develop new habits and ways of assessing the correctness of our actions? In such conditions, we may find those essential virtues like honesty, prudence, and self-control take second place. Denis Coitinho inquires whether we should maintain our moral integrity in this particular setting and whether we should lower or raise the moral standards to which we hold other members of society. Of course, even a pandemic cannot wholly undermine the moral relevance of key virtues, but it is clear that hostile environments make these virtues more challenging to apply.

Scenarios like these are also an opportunity to apply different ethical approaches. Jana S. Rošker put forward for consideration Confucian relationism as a relevant alternative to understand the aspects of solidarity and cooperation between different cultures worldwide facing struggling times such as the coronavirus outbreak. It is also relevant to explore the discussion presented by Simone Gubler on the idea behind onlooker morality to understand how we should behave in the face of other people's tragedies under these circumstances. And despite many of the shifts in relationships that the pandemic has produced being negative, genuine values related to the well-being of others can emerge in social interactions, even in the presence of suffering and anguish. Based on the happiness theory of well-being, Mauro Rossi shows how the pandemic brought up happiness and certain pleasures relevant to developing certain moral values and virtues.

Part III points out the ethical challenges of the pandemic in social dynamics. Leonardo de Mello Ribeiro explores in detail the case of the COVID "denier," a figure who emerges amid the chaos and best represents the difficulty of assessing risks rationally. A quick glance at the news is enough to realize that deniers' existence is not mere fiction. They are everywhere, engaged in the anti-vaccine movement or even rejecting the very existence of the virus. Deniers usually underestimate situations and generate doubts about what should be done. While we may be tempted to label such people irrational, Ribeiro will say that it is not so simple.

The COVID-19 pandemic was also a terrain of endless debate about individual rights in the face of health measures, namely a lockdown. As a result, advocates of an alleged inalienable right to my freedom as opposed to the right not to be exposed to unnecessary risk came face-to-face in the debate. Peter R. Anstey examines three specific types of this group in detail through the lens of the social contract: the conspiracy theorist, the so-called generic dissenter (who rises up against the state), and a well-known philosophical character, the sensible knave.

During the harshest phase of the pandemic, individuals were at a crossroads. Some people became very concerned with the possible loss of enshrined rights. Others began to question the legitimacy of the moral and political authority of prominent groups or persons on crucial pandemic issues, confirming that our social fabric was at risk of falling apart. Ryan Doody presents elements to explain why there is no legitimacy in breaking through a block such as a lockdown without violating certain relevant rights. Finally, the relationship between the scarcity of medical resources and high patient demand in the new coronavirus pandemic left uncertainties regarding the criteria for determining priority in ICU beds and the use of ventilators. After examining how the age criteria must be taken into account in these cases, Alcino Eduardo Bonella argues that some arguments count in favor of using this criterion without incurring any ageism.

Part IV increases the book's scope by addressing relevant issues after the coronavirus pandemic. Evandro Barbosa and Thaís Alves Costa present the big picture of duties and types of agents in a pandemic. Beyond outlining the parameters of the discussion, they discuss the degree of responsibility individual agents have concerning pandemic duties. In another relevant approach, Joshua Preiss identifies the pandemic as a catalyst that accelerated changes in the world of work. Because such changes are challenging for workers to enjoy certain relational goods, namely community, care, and social recognition, the author analyzes these transformations, presenting arguments to mitigate their adverse effects in a fairer post-COVID world. Finally, Marcelo de Araújo captures the discussions by proposing pandemic ethics as an emerging field in which moral theorists and the like should be interested. As mentioned earlier, we are in a pandemic age, and its morally relevant issues open the floor for this new field of debate.

The set of issues presented here focuses on the moral implications of the relationships established during the 21st century's first devastating pandemic. Humanity will almost certainly be subject to similar situations in the future. We hope this book will shed light on issues of lasting relevance while also proving valuable to those who are, as we write, still confronting the challenges of the ongoing pandemic. Before we can (re)create our disrupted social bonds, we must pause to understand how they have been altered. The coronavirus viral spread has inspired us to think back to what life was like before it began, reflect on what happened during its most acute phase, and consider what future pandemics may bring. While the authors wrote the pieces in this book during the COVID-19 outbreak and draw examples from our recent experiences, we aim to articulate more general questions and principles that will remain relevant as humans might confront new pandemics. Any remarks about "the pandemic" can be taken as referring to the coronavirus crisis, but we hope future readers will consider how our thoughts might apply to their own circumstances.

Notes

1 You may find testimonials worldwide answering this question at www. pandemiclives.com.
2 See https://www.who.int.

3　See https://cordis.europa.eu/project/id/883285.
4　See https://www.rockefellerfoundation.org/pandemicpreventioninitiative/.
5　See https://www.gatesnotes.com/Health/Meet-the-GERM-team.

References

Araujo, M. D. 2021. "The nascent field of pandemic ethics: Prevention, mitigation, responsibility, and adaptation." *SSRN*. https://doi.org/10.2139/ssrn.3984756

Camus, Albert 1974 [1947]. *The Plague*. Translated from the French by Stuart Gilbert. New York: Vintage International.

Gates, B. [n.d.]. "Meet the GERM team." *gatesnotes.com*. Available at https://www.gatesnotes.com/Health/Meet-the-GERM-team. Accessed in December 5, 2022.

Hodson, R. 2022. "Preparing the world for the next pandemic." *Nature*, 610(7933), S33–S33. https://doi.org/10.1038/d41586-022-03353-9

Marani, M., Katul, G. G., Pan, W. K., & Parolari, A. J. 2021. "Intensity and frequency of extreme novel epidemics." *Proceedings of the National Academy of Sciences*, 118(35), e2105482118. https://doi.org/10.1073/pnas.2105482118

"PANDEM." [n.d.] *European Commission*. Available at https://cordis.europa.eu/project/id/883285.

"Pandemic prevention initiative." [n.d.]. *The Rockefeller Foundation*. Available at https://www.rockefellerfoundation.org/pandemicpreventioninitiative/.

Selgelid, M. J. 2009. "Pandethics." *Public Health*, 123(3), 255–259. https://doi.org/10.1016/j.puhe.2008.12.005

World Health Organization (WHO). [n.d.]. Available at https://www.who.int.

Part I
Rationality and moral emotions

2 On the moral psychology of the pandemic agent

Anneli Jefferson and Lisa Bortolotti

2.1 Introduction

Extreme events such as pandemics bring out the best and the worst in people. During the COVID-19 pandemic, there have been outpourings of help, as well as mad scrambles to secure the last roll of toilet paper for oneself. In the early stages of the pandemic, we realised how challenging it is for individual agents and governments to make good decisions under extreme uncertainty. Individual agents had to decide what risks were acceptable for them to take, and governments had to decide whether and when to lock down. In this context, we witnessed risk-taking behaviour by political leaders and citizens alike, which was subsequently justified as being acceptable under the circumstances.

Due to some facets of human psychology, it is particularly difficult for agents to make good decisions in situations of uncertainty. These facets include the mere unpredictability of the events, difficulties in assessing unexpected threats, knowledge gaps among laypeople and experts, challenges in regulating emotions (particularly in managing anxiety and stress), and time pressures. In this chapter, we consider some of the challenges for good decision-making in an uncertain world, using the COVID-19 pandemic as our test case. In particular, we discuss psychological and epistemic factors affecting decision-making. We examine the tendency to avoid uncertainty by confidently adopting an explanation of the events before all the relevant evidence is available, letting that explanation guide choice and action. We also consider the tendency to believe that one's future will be either better than it is likely to be or better than that of one's peers, behaving as if potentially threatening events are more likely to affect others than oneself.

Here, we focus on how individual agents' decisions and policy decisions are influenced by a number of cognitive biases and motivational factors. Whilst there are no easy answers to the question of how rational agents should behave in a pandemic, we close by making some recommendations that might help mitigate the threats and uncertainties affecting human psychology at a time of crisis.

DOI: 10.4324/9781003310129-3

2.2 Decision-making in an uncertain world

At the start of the COVID-19 pandemic and for large parts of 2020 and 2021, many countries found themselves in various stages of lockdown. Both at the government policy level and at that of personal conduct, people disagreed, sometimes quite radically, about the severity of the threat and the best course of action to contain the effects of the pandemic. Western countries reduced COVID restrictions significantly earlier than some Eastern countries, where a zero COVID strategy was pursued for far longer. Not just at the policy level, but at the personal level, too, people's appetite for risk, their perception of risk, and their view of what constituted morally acceptable behaviour in the face of significant health risks varied significantly. In the face of so much disagreement, we consider two questions: (1) What factors influence decision-making in a period of uncertainty and anxiety such as during a pandemic? (2) In the light of those factors, how should individual agents and political leaders decide what the rational and moral course of action is at the time of a major crisis?

The early stages of the pandemic were marked by extreme uncertainty about the risks countries and individual citizens were facing. How lethal was the virus? How was it transmitted? Would face coverings be effective in reducing infection? How quickly would the virus spread? Who was most at risk from it? Would it be possible to achieve herd immunity? When (if ever) would there be a vaccine, and how effective would it be? Were there any long-term health effects to worry about? Different answers led to different decisions being made, and sometimes decisions were diametrically opposed.

Some people stopped all unnecessary social interactions, working from home and refraining from seeing even family and friends. When it was necessary to go out, they used face masks and gloves, frequently washing their hands and keeping their distance from others. They were also cautious in what they considered acceptable risk imposition on others, self-isolating for long periods of time and wearing face coverings even when it was no longer required. Other people denied the devastating effects of the virus and acted in ways that were almost indistinguishable from how they had acted prior to the pandemic. They refused to comply with safety recommendations and even actively protested against such measures. One common attitude was to claim that the restrictions imposed by governments undermined their personal freedom (Murphy-Hollies and Bortolotti 2021). Some citizens broke COVID regulations, for example by socialising with others when it was not allowed or by going to work as usual, or travelling after having tested positive for COVID. One prominent case was that of the UK Prime Minister at the time, Boris Johnson, who participated in a birthday party for himself in Downing Street (BBC News January 24, 2022b). Another notorious case is that of Scottish MP

Margaret Ferrier, who took the train from London to Glasgow after learning that she had tested positive for COVID because she did not want to self-isolate for two weeks in London (BBC News August 18, 2022a). Similar disagreements applied to attitudes towards vaccination. People disagreed not only about whether it was in their own interest to get vaccinated and receive boosters of the COVID vaccine to avoid infection but also about whether they had a duty to be up to date with COVID vaccination as a way of helping to reduce the spread of COVID through the community.

At the level of national policy, a range of responses was witnessed, with leaders in countries such as the UK, the US, and Brazil openly prioritising personal freedom – at least in early 2020 – and expressing a more optimistic outlook towards the possible outcomes of the pandemic than their colleagues in other countries. Policies in countries such as China, Korea, New Zealand, and Italy were more heavily influenced by a desire to reduce the risk of death for the elderly population and less inclined to prioritise the values of personal freedom and freedom of the markets. Other countries were unique in their responses, generating curiosity and a lively debate about the likely success of their policies. For instance, in 2020, Sweden pursued a policy that has been defined by commentators as "light-touch" or "anti-lockdown" and was at least partially motivated by the hope that herd immunity could be achieved (Rice 2022). So, in Sweden, very few restrictions on public life were imposed compared to other countries, in line with the emphasis on safeguarding citizens' autonomy and on trusting citizens to adopt safety behaviours without the need for mandates. Over time, it emerged that, with new variants and reinfections, herd immunity wasn't really a viable strategy, even if one was prepared to bear the cost of lost lives. Indeed, as of August 2022, the number of lives lost to COVID-19 in Sweden has greatly exceeded the number of lives lost in other Scandinavian countries (Stewart 2022).

The uncertainty surrounding an event like the pandemic is in some respects different from other situations where the outcome of agents' decisions and actions is difficult to predict. As Nicholas Shackel (2022) argues, events like the COVID-19 pandemic involve uncertainty which is *irresolvable* in the short term because it can only be resolved once we have a considerable amount of data to feed into models and predictions. Ioannidis and colleagues (2022) list some of the failed predictions in the early stages of modelling the pandemic; one of their examples is the Massachusetts General Hospital News predicting far more deaths on reopening than in fact occurred. Similarly, reopening in the summer of 2021 in the UK was often predicted to lead to 100,000 cases in the short term, but case numbers peaked at around 50,000 in the summer and only rose steeply with the omicron wave. Of course, estimates didn't always err on the side of being overly pessimistic, there were many predictions that were rosier than actual events turned out to be.

These mismatches between predictions and outcomes do not suggest that modelling was bad or even that predictions were faulty. Predictions can only ever give a probabilistic estimate of a range of outcomes, and it is the most spectacular, worst-case scenario ones which will be picked up in the media but also in contingency planning and decision-making. Rather, the important lesson here is that the early pandemic was a point in time when *it was impossible to tell* what the probabilities of each possible outcome were. All decisions had to be made based on insufficient evidence, but nevertheless, decisions needed to be made. Furthermore, these decisions were morally important and had significant implications because they could make a huge difference in terms of lives saved or lost.

In the following two sections, we consider agents' epistemic and psychological needs in the context of an uncertain event that is likely to cause distress and anxiety. When people form beliefs about the future and have to make decisions based on such beliefs in scenarios fraught with uncertainty, their thinking and decision-making are especially vulnerable to a host of biases and motivational factors. We focus on two main factors. First, people have *a need for certainty*. People need to come to certain expectations about what is going to happen so that their decisions can be grounded in their perceived knowledge of reality, and they have a psychological need to think of themselves as having an equally good or better idea of what is going on as their peers to restore their sense of control in a volatile situation. Second, and relatedly, people have *a need to feel good about themselves and their prospects*. This often manifests in a sense of being unique and superior to others, which gives rise to forms of exceptionalism in a crisis and is not just manifested in people's claim to have knowledge about a critical situation but also in their tendency to see themselves as better than average at avoiding threats. Similarly, people see their own future as rosier than that of other people, predicting that the weeks, months, and years to come will not hold major crises and failures.

2.3 Filling gaps and resolving uncertainty

Human agents are notoriously bad at tolerating uncertainty, as shown by the copious evidence that people need to resolve uncertain situations to feel less anxious. Shackel (2022) diagnoses something he calls *uncertainty phobia* when people make predictions in situations characterised by uncertainty that is irresolvable at the time. This results in people treating a given prediction as having a certainty that is not evidentially warranted. When people are confident without good reason, this may be costly to them in terms of rushing to the wrong course of action prematurely. It also typically means that people are irresponsive to changes in the evidence that should undermine their conviction in a given belief.

As Shackel concedes, there are situations where it is good to be more certain than the evidence warrants:

[I]magine that you must leap over a yawning chasm to save your life, and we know that you are more likely to succeed if you act with certainty that you will succeed. In such a case, it may be practically wise to become (however temporarily) uncertainty phobic so that you can acquire the certainty you need to succeed, despite this being theoretically irrational. That people have this ability may even be an evolved tendency. That being said, a lot of the time uncertainty phobia is badly irrational.

(Shackel 2022, 286)

Although Shackel may be right about the theoretical irrationality of being more certain than the evidence warrants, the case of the pandemic, like the case where we need to leap over a chasm to save our lives, is one where making a decision before all the relevant evidence is available may be a necessity and even the rational course of action. Furthermore, when policymakers are trying to persuade others to abide by their decisions, as was the case when leaders had to adjust COVID regulations on the hoof, the appearance of certainty in the knowledge underlying their decisions might have helped justify these decisions. Interestingly, in science communication, a recent study found that disclosing uncertainty did not affect the credibility of the news, the trustworthiness of the experts, or the objectivity of the scientists' information (Ratcliff and Wicke 2022). However, in a political context where a crisis is unfolding, acknowledging uncertainty can undermine trust and authoritativeness.

Decision-makers were caught in a bind. They needed to be prepared to change their minds and be responsive to evidence in order to make decisions that were well justified. But they also needed to convince themselves and others of the rationality of the decisions they were making and to sustain their and other people's motivation for acting accordingly. Underplaying uncertainty is particularly tempting when decisions require significant sacrifices and may be difficult for other people to accept. But to consider the decision sufficiently grounded in the current evidence means that the decision-maker becomes less sensitive to potentially conflicting evidence that may emerge at a later stage. In recent studies on risk taking in financial investments, researchers found that "high rather than low need for cognitive closure can lead to a lack of openness to new information": people are less likely to update the beliefs they feel they have already established as true (Disatnik and Steinhart 2015).

2.3.1 Need for cognitive closure

The need for cognitive closure (NFCC) is described as "a desire for a quick and unambiguous answer to a question and an aversion to uncertainty" that "may indeed act as a motivational factor that determines successful coping with uncertainty" (see Czernatowicz-Kukuczka et al. 2014, based on the classic work by Kruglanski 1989). The effect of NFCC is that agents exit critical situations faster and thus better manage their anxiety: taking a stance about the situation in order to remove the uncertainty reduces people's sense of risk and increases their estimation of the correctness of their predictions. NFCC is tightly linked to the uncertainty phobia we described earlier.

The NFCC can be both a stable personal characteristic and a situational phenomenon that depends on the circumstances (for instance, it manifests more strongly when there is a time pressure on decision-making). There is empirical support for the view that people who are more prone to stress and anxiety exhibit NFCC to a higher degree: in a recent study on college students during the pandemic (White 2022), those who manifested a greater NFCC were also those who suffered greater distress as a result of unpredictable situations.

What are the consequences of NFCC?

> [H]eightened levels of this need foster cognitive activities aimed at the attainment of certainty. This need promotes "seizing" on information that promises closure quickly and "freezing" one's own judgment once it has been formed. By contrast, lower levels of this need promote thorough information processing in order to arrive at accurate judgments.
>
> (Pica et al. 2021, 691)

The NFCC has an important connection with doxastic conservatism, that is, with the common tendency not to revise or give up a belief that has already been adopted, even when the belief seems to be disconfirmed by new evidence. What does this mean? If agents arrive at some conclusion about a problem without waiting for all the relevant evidence to become available, they will be less open to questioning that conclusion on the basis of new information (see Pica et al. 2021).

2.3.2 Need for uniqueness

The need for uniqueness (NFU) is defined by Snyder and Fromkin (1977) as "a positive striving for abnormality relative to other people." Agents have contrasting needs. They need an affiliation, so they want to belong to a group and feel like they resemble their peers (leading to a sense of conformity), but they also need to stand out and reaffirm their identity (leading to the sense that they are special and unique). Just like the NFCC, the NFU, too, is a personality trait that some people exhibit more than others and a trait that becomes more accentuated when the environmental circumstances change. One situation that increases the NFU is the presence of a threat characterised by uncertainty (Tilner et al. 2022).

When nobody really knows what is going to happen and what the best course of action is (often not even the experts), one way to restore control and reduce anxiety is to claim superior knowledge or a privileged access to the truth. This explains why conspiracy theories emerge in moments of crisis: such theories are often used to justify agents' failure to accept official explanations for the threatening events and their failure to follow the rules imposed by the authorities. It is not a coincidence that the NFU is associated not only with conspiratorial thinking but also with violent forms of non-conformity such as extremism (Rottweiler and Gill 2022).

In general terms, people with a high NFU value independence, anti-conformity, and present themselves as inventive and high achieving. Usually, the NFU is manifested in consumer choices: people who need to feel unique are more likely to choose unusual items that set them apart from others and express their identity – brands exploit this tendency in advertising. But the same need can be manifested in other ways too – for instance, by having unusual beliefs. While beliefs are not strictly speaking things that people consume and (materially) possess, they do express identity. In its cognitive dimension, the NFU is manifested as a unique way of understanding the world and has been correlated with the adoption of non-official explanations for significant events (Lantian et al. 2017; Imhoff and Lamberty 2017). Especially when the information available is scarce, people with a higher NFU are more likely to endorse conspiracy theories. As Lantian et al. (2017, 161) put it, "people who cultivate original views about the world convey to others the special nature of their personality."

When we examined the need for closure, we saw that believing that one's decisions are well supported by relevant evidence helps justify those decisions to others. Another way for decisions to look well-grounded is for the agent to appear confident about their decision-making process, even when the choice made differs significantly from choices made by other agents dealing with similar circumstances. People like the idea that their ideas and decisions are different from other people's: they often convey this by saying that they are less gullible and better informed than their peers. The NFU is problematic when the person who acts on it is not in the superior epistemic position they claim for themselves, and thus their sense of superiority is illusory – as when someone with no formal qualifications and limited experience in the knowledge domain claims that they know better than epistemically authoritative sources such as government advisors and other experts. Illusory or not, claims to epistemic superiority can influence risk perception.

A problem for national policy at a time of a crisis is that, when NFU and NFCC are combined, the decision-maker is less likely to listen to advice that diverges from their own view, something researchers have called *egocentric advice discounting* (Yaniv and Kleinberger 2000). In general, agents are more likely to value their own view than a conflicting view held by other agents because they are better acquainted with the justification for their view than with the justification for other agents' views. But in addition to that understandable asymmetry, when making decisions, people tend to discount advice from others if the advice conflicts with the course of action they want to take. This seems to be influenced by two factors: how confident they are that they are right, and how trustworthy they judge the advisors to be (Wang and Du 2018). Even people who are convinced of their own uniqueness and act accordingly maintain some level of trust in some individuals, groups, and institutions. As Neil Levy (2019) aptly observes, endorsing something like a conspiracy theory requires a low-trust condition (low trust towards authorities who promote the official theory) and a high-trust condition (high trust towards oneself and members of the non-mainstream group responsible for spreading the alternative theory).

Conservatism with respect to one's beliefs and theories also applies to collective decision-making (Larson et al. 2020): when a group has discussed different possible courses of action and settled on a consensus, it is extremely resistant to external advice that conflicts with the achieved consensus. Governments at the time of the pandemic were facing similar challenges: they had to make decisions that appeared to be justified by the available evidence, and they needed such decisions to be accepted by the majority of the population to be effective at changing collective behaviour. Once an initial course of action had been agreed on, changing that in the light of new information or medical advice proved extremely hard.

2.4 Unrealistic optimism

Aversion to uncertainty at a time of crisis is not the only factor that affects belief formation in situations where people lack sufficient evidence to be sure of an outcome. It interacts with numerous other biases and affective influences on cognition. For example, confirmation bias may interact with NFCC to amplify irrational certainty. Another factor that affects our predictions of risk is unrealistic optimism.

2.4.1 *What is unrealistic optimism?*

A *Guardian* article from 2020 cites Johnson's optimistic assessment of the likely trajectory of the pandemic:

> The next 12 weeks could "turn the tide of this disease", Johnson told the daily Downing Street press conference on the pandemic, saying it was possible to "send coronavirus packing in this country, but only if we all take the steps we have outlined."
>
> (Walker 2020)

It is of course difficult to discern to what extent Boris Johnson's statements reflected his actual beliefs. But this was almost certainly a statement partly driven by what he wanted to believe and by what he felt the country wanted to hear. What we see in Johnson's statement (if we take it at face value as a statement of belief), is an overly optimistic prediction for the future.

When we talk about predictions being unrealistically optimistic, some clarification is in order: a prediction can be *optimistic* (in the sense that it anticipates a good outcome) without being *unrealistic*, even if that good outcome does not come to pass. If one thinks that a good outcome was the most likely one, one might be correct, even if the bad outcome then occurs. So, for example, if Jenny gets breast cancer and the chances of full recovery are 90%, she is justified in thinking that most likely, she will make a full recovery, even if she ends up being one of the 10% who doesn't. Of course, there are complicating factors, for example, there may be further evidence specific to Jenny's case, e.g., family history or other risk factors that suggest she is more likely to be one of the 10%. But if all she knows is the recovery rate statistic, an optimistic prediction is warranted by the evidence, even though she cannot be *certain* of a positive outcome (Jefferson et al. 2017).

What is called the *optimism bias* or *unrealistic optimism* in the literature is the tendency to adopt and maintain a specific kind of optimistic belief, whereby an agent thinks that their own future will be better than it is objectively likely to be or better than that of comparable others (Shepperd et al. 2013). This is also known as self-specific optimism. In order to establish how a positive belief about the future compares to the objective likelihood of an event happening, people need information that frequently isn't available. It is easier to tell when people are being optimistic in the comparative sense, thinking they will have better outcomes than a similar other. This kind of bias seems to be underwritten by asymmetrical belief updating, where people are more likely to take on board positive information (information that makes a good outcome appear more likely) and ignore negative information (information that makes a bad outcome appear more likely) for themselves than for others (Sharot, Korn, and Dolan 2011; Kuzmanovic, Jefferson, and Vogeley 2015; Kuzmanovic and Rigoux 2017). Importantly, this is different from the kind of confirmation bias we see in NFCC; rather than discounting new evidence altogether, evidence that makes a desirable outcome appear more likely is taken on board, whereas evidence that makes an undesirable outcome appear more likely is ignored.

Tom might be unrealistically optimistic about the COVID pandemic, thinking that it will be over soon. While this belief may be unrealistic and optimistic, it isn't one where Tom has more optimistic expectations for himself than for others. By contrast, in self-specific optimism, Tom might think that he is less likely to get infected than a person of the same age, sex, and demographics. The latter is what is normally known as unrealistic optimism, and it is part of a set of other self-enhancing beliefs called *positive illusions*, such as the illusion of control (whereby one overestimates the control one has over outcomes) or the better-than-average effect (where one has an unrealistically rosy view of one's own abilities and personality traits). These different forms of optimism are not always carefully separated in the literature: for example, Eshel et al. (2022) do not distinguish between general unrealistically positive expectations and self-specific optimism when talking about unrealistic optimism.

2.4.2 Reasons for unrealistic optimism

Unrealistic optimism is a form of motivated cognition, where agents are prone to attending more to information that supports subjectively desirable beliefs. There is some evidence that positively biased information updating activates brain areas associated with reward (Kuzmanovic, Jefferson, and Vogeley 2016). A cognitive factor that appears to underlie unrealistic optimism is the *representativeness heuristic.*

> People judge their likelihood of experiencing an event based on how well they match their stereotype of the people who experience the event. For example, when asked to estimate their risk of getting in an automobile accident relative to the average driver, the question itself seems to prompt thinking about someone who drives too fast, mixes alcohol and driving, and is inattentive to other drivers (Perloff & Fetzer, 1986). In comparison to this prototype, people naturally conclude that their risk is lower.
>
> (Shepperd et al. 2015, 234)

When agents assess the likelihood of an event happening, they envision the kind of person to which that sort of thing typically happens to. If they don't fit that stereotype, they think that the event is less likely to happen to them. Both motivational factors such as the desire for a positive outlook and cognitive factors such as the representative heuristic contribute to unrealistically optimistic explanations.

2.4.3 Unrealistic optimism in the pandemic

Unrealistic optimism is a commonly observed phenomenon in the pandemic (Salgado and Berntsen 2021; Kuper-Smith et al. 2021). In a recent study by Salgado and colleagues, people thought that they and those close to them (e.g., a partner or a family member) were less likely to be infected with COVID-19 than a comparable acquaintance of the same age, sex, and geographical location. They also found that people who exhibited that kind of self-specific optimism believed they were more likely to engage in protective measures such as hand-washing and wearing face masks. The authors hypothesise that there might be a causal link between optimism and the belief that one is more likely to engage in protective behaviour. People might think they are less likely to get infected *because* they believe they are more likely to take precautions.

An even more pronounced self-specific optimism bias was found in people's predictions as to whether they would pass the disease on to others, but no self-specific optimism was found in people's prediction of the likelihood of getting severe COVID if they did get infected. (Kuper-Smith et al. 2021). One plausible hypothesis is that unrealistic optimism is affected by perceived control. If a person does get infected, it is under their control whether they isolate, whereas the severity of the disease once the infection is contracted is not under their control.

This is consistent with the finding that, by increasing people's sense of control, optimism contributes to their sense that they can do something meaningful to avoid threats or respond to setbacks, resulting in more marked changes in behaviour and consequently to better outcomes (Bortolotti et al. 2019). Even when the sense of control is excessive and illusory, it does seem to have a positive effect on motivation. A sense of helplessness, instead, may lead people to think that they are powerless and unable to change how the events impact on their lives. Applied to the pandemic, if people think it is in their power to avoid infection by adopting certain preventative behaviours, then they will be more likely to follow the health and safety recommendations than if they thought that infection is inevitable.

One might object that if belief in control means that one is more likely to do things that will in fact reduce risk of infection, then optimism is not *unrealistic*. There are two ways to interpret the relationship between beliefs about avoiding infection and engaging in health-promoting behaviours. One is that engaging in health-promoting behaviours supports beliefs about likelihood of avoiding infection. No obvious bias in there. The other is that beliefs about likelihood of avoiding infection lead to and support health-promoting behaviour. That is one claim made in the literature on unrealistic optimism. It is because one believes that they can avoid infection that one engages in health-promoting behaviour in the first place. Now in this case, the prediction becomes a more realistic one over time as self-fulfilling prophecies do.

However, there are two further caveats. First of all, people might be unrealistically optimistic about the level of control they have. The illusion of control is a well-established bias. Furthermore, the fact that people believe that they are more likely to take precautions doesn't mean that they actually will. Instead, this belief may be another instance of unrealistic optimism, this time optimism about their capacity to turn good intentions into good actions that have significant costs. For instance, there is evidence that people are likely to overpredict their likelihood of engaging in socially desirable behaviour (Epley and Dunning 2000). So, whilst it makes sense to think that one is less likely to avoid infection if the behaviour that results in infection is under one's control, one can be unduly optimistic in one's perception of control or in one's expectations regarding one's own future behaviour.

What was the effect of unrealistic optimism on risk taking in the pandemic? We as authors of this chapter differ in our levels of optimism about the effects of unrealistic optimism. Bortolotti has stressed the positive features of unrealistic optimism for motivation and agency (Bortolotti 2018), whereas Jefferson has highlighted the danger that optimism can lead to complacency and inaction (Jefferson 2017). Clearly, there is a case to be made that optimism supports motivation and action by presenting certain desirable goals as more easily attainable than is the case. Agents need to believe that there is some likelihood of success in order to consider the pursuit of their goals worth the effort. However, there is a risk here that people are exhibiting compounded unrealistic optimism: they are unrealistically optimistic about their own future behaviour, which then has knock-on effects on their optimism about specific outcomes.

Overall, the data on the connection between unrealistic optimism and risky behaviour are very noisy – there are studies showing no link between unrealistic optimism and protective behaviour (Kuper-Smith et al. 2021), as all participants in the study reported that they adhered closely to protective measures against COVID. Some studies show a positive association between optimism and intention to engage in protective behaviour (Salgado and Berntsen 2021) and others a negative association between optimism and intention to engage in protective behaviour (or, in other words, a positive association between optimism and risky behaviour) (Pivovar et al. 2022; Shukla, Mishra, and Rai 2021).

2.5   Effects of biases in the pandemic – the good and the bad

Two things emerge from the previous discussion. First, biases should not automatically be seen as negative features of human cognition because they often enable individuals to cope with uncertainty, retain a sense of agency, and consequently, preserve the motivation to act. Second, the biases described earlier flourish in times of extreme uncertainty and threat, such as a pandemic, and they can mutually reinforce each other: In an interview on the *European Science Media Hub*, Arie Kruglanski explains the link between NFCC and the pandemic:

> Our place in society depended on us being able to take care of ourselves, economically and physically, and all of a sudden, we are weakened, and our freedom is reduced. That is the main impact of the pandemic; the fragility, the vulnerability, the susceptibility, and the fear that this uncertain situation raises because it contains very bad

possibilities. Now, what does it do to people? When you have that kind of uncertainty, you have a "need for closure" and you want certainty – but not just any certainty, you want a certainty that will promise good outcomes and will tell you what you can do in order to improve your outcomes. So, when you feel threatened, frightened, or vulnerable because of the pandemic, then you want a certainty that things will be good. This quest for specific certainty – as a promising and optimistic certainty – is a major consequence of the pandemic.

(Photopoulos 2021)

There is further empirical confirmation that the pandemic leads to increased NFCC: Sachdeva (2022) finds that "perceived risk is the most important construct for predicting cognitive closure." It is not just the unpredictability of the situation that increases NFCC but also its threatening nature. So, we would be justified in believing that people experienced a higher need for closure during the pandemic and that the need for comforting certainty was one of the motivational aspects driving the optimism bias. Clearly, if the goal of reasoning is accurate beliefs and risk estimates, then the need for closure and the tendency to believe what is reassuring to believe are bad news. However, such tendencies have psychological benefits in terms of reduced anxiety.

How the tendency to settle for a fixed and positive outlook affects behaviour and decision-making depends on further factors. When agents consider what is likely to happen, they settle for an explanation that supports their risk estimate. How they behave depends on the details of that explanation. An interesting study confirms this:

Whereas conspiracy beliefs describing the pandemic as a hoax were more strongly associated with reduced containment-related behavior, conspiracy beliefs about sinister forces purposefully creating the virus related to an increase in self-centered prepping behaviour.

(Imhoff and Lamberty 2020, 1110)

As Imhoff and Lamberty argue, when people recognised the risks but attributed the pandemic to malevolent others, they took more precautions, but they did not listen to the sources that they believed were involved in creating or spreading COVID-19. Rather, they chose to come up with their own measures to be safe. So, if they thought that COVID was due to the Chinese creating a virus in a lab in Wuhan, they acted to protect themselves from infection but did not listen to the wisdom coming from China (e.g., they did not trust face masks to reduce transmission).

The NFCC in the context of responses to the pandemic was combined with another need, the NFU. Buzzell and Rini (2022) argue that in the presence of an overwhelming amount of information from more and less reliable sources, and in a context that is both threatening and uncertain, people are drawn to "epistemic superheroics":

> Some people are unwilling to wait for the authorities – scientific experts and health officials – to handle the situation. They feel a need to draw on their inner power and solve the epistemic problem through sheer force of cognitive will. They hunt for data in obscure journals (despite having no background in medicine) and recalculate the statistics offered by public authorities (despite not understanding sampling correction techniques). Most of all, they brave the sneering of "sheeple" who simply accept conventional wisdom. They seek to become an epistemic superhero, a person who can single-mindedly unravel conspiracies and rescue the truth.
>
> (Buzzell and Rini 2022)

Instances of "epistemic superheroics" were evident in the justification of national responses to COVID-19 by some political leaders. One striking case was the then-president of the US Donald Trump, who clearly underestimated the impact of coronavirus, despite being advised differently, and expressed overly optimistic predictions about the development of the pandemic (see e.g., Mangan 2020; Beer 2020). The attitude we recognise in Trump's 2020 speeches, which we can summarise with the sentences "We know more and can do better," is a direct outcome of the NFU.

The NFU did not only affect political leaders. In March 2020, self-declared "expert" in holistic health Kelly Brogan was filmed stating that she "personally didn't believe in germ-based contagion" and that belief led her to deny the existence of all viral infections, including those attributed to COVID-19, and to the conviction that the deaths attributed to the virus were instead caused by fear. She claimed that germ-based infection did not fit her conceptual framework and did not drive her to act in ways suited to prevent transmission of germs. For instance, she mentioned that when one of her children has a runny nose, she is not less likely to drink from their glass because she is not afraid of catching anything. This is a clear case where presumed expert knowledge is linked to decisions that imply a certain perception of risk: as for Brogan, viruses do not make us ill; there is no need to avoid them. However, she thought fear could kill people, so she advised people to stop being afraid of COVID.

When people underestimated the risks, they were often motivated by denialism or the belief that COVID-19 was not as big a threat as the authorities were suggesting. As a result, they did not engage in behaviour that would have reduced their chances of being infected or passing on the infection. We can see that this is particularly likely when optimism, NFCC, and NFU come together in such a way that people come to believe that scientific authorities and the media are presenting an overblown estimate of health risks. Eshel et al. (2022) state that discounting the risks is one factor that helps psychological coping in the pandemic but supports vaccine hesitancy. Claims such as "[t]he physicians' reports on the danger of the COVID-19 pandemic are exaggerated" appear to be motivationally driven and are also associated with decreased anxiety (Eshel et al. 2022). It's plausible that thinking that the risk of COVID has been exaggerated by the authorities fulfils both the need to believe in a positive future and the desire to feel that one is "in the know" and not just blindly following instructions.

However, this attitude facilitates risky behaviour with ensuing health costs, both for the individuals themselves and for others. Furthermore, it means people do not have the flexibility which is needed in the ever-shifting landscape of the pandemic because they do not easily revise their beliefs in the face of new evidence. This can be seen in everyday cases where people's risk assessments and the decisions based on them are adversely affected by the way our cognition interacts with a situation like the pandemic. The fact that citizens were first advised not to wear face masks and advice then changed led to initial resistance in some and refusal in others. Because of their NFCC, having settled on the belief that "face masks don't work" or "face masks are not needed," it was difficult at a later stage to revise that belief. In addition to these everyday cases, the combination of biases and uncertainty is a breeding ground for conspiracy theories and extreme responses, especially when combined with a desire for uniqueness.

2.6 Moral decision-making in times of crisis

Especially at the start of the pandemic, rational decision-making became a minefield, both at the level of policy and at the individual level. At the level of policy, political leaders had to decide between lives and livelihoods. Should there be a national lockdown to protect the vulnerable, or should businesses and schools be kept open in order to protect livelihoods and children's education? Should countries pursue a zero-COVID strategy or accept that the virus will become endemic? More recently, countries had to decide whether to implement mandatory vaccinations, either for the whole society (as initially planned in Austria) or for specific professions, such as medicine and social care.

Governments faced two problems: they had to balance different goods (e.g., education versus health) but also estimate the likelihood of specific outcomes given specific policies. In other words, even if a government had decided how many lives it was willing to sacrifice in order to keep schools and businesses open, it also needed to be able to come up with a good estimate of what measures would achieve that outcome. If it got those estimates wrong, it would not be able to achieve the trade-off of costs and benefits it was aiming for. Consequently, there was disagreement about what should be achieved or traded off but also about whether the measures taken would achieve what they set out to achieve. Our discussion of cognitive biases and behavioural tendencies at times of crisis addresses the question of whether people can make good decisions if they are badly placed to estimate the likelihood of certain events. Which goals should be prioritised in rational decision-making during a pandemic is a further question we did not cover here. However, it is worth noting that disagreement about likely outcomes and disagreement about desirable goals for action interact. If there is disagreement about risks, one side can argue that trade-offs between personal liberty and public health are not necessary because risks have been overstated.

Individuals, too, had to decide which risks in their personal conduct were acceptable and which ones were not. Our survey of cognitive biases and behavioural tendencies suggests that people are generally not well-placed to make realistic risk estimates. Problems with uncertainty mean that agents' confidence in risk estimates is not justified, and their risk estimates are likely to be coloured by biases in numerous ways: they are influenced by motivated reasoning, but also by the way information is presented to them and by their experiences, be these their own direct experiences, or those they encounter in anecdotes and stories. How can individuals make better decisions in the context of pandemics? It seems that doing a risk-benefit analysis and assessing the likely results of their actions every time they decide whether to wear a mask in the shop, get vaccinated, or meet with friends is not a promising strategy due to the many factors that bias risk estimates. Even though agents have the best intentions and aim to achieve a positive result (stop infection), this result may not be best achieved by trying to work out by themselves how likely they are to infect someone or get infected if today they go shopping without a mask. Paraphrasing Buzzell and Rini, agents should not approach their epistemic environments as superheroes and leave the superheroics to fictional characters.

We argue that individuals are better off following general rules that are aimed at avoiding spreading the virus, rather than making their own risk assessments. However, following the rules that, for example, a country sets is only a good strategy if that country is getting it right. As we have discussed, countries have disagreed about what the right course of action was. This is because the problem of making decisions under risk iterates. Political leaders and scientists may have access to more reliable information than ordinary citizens in some contexts, but in the unexpected COVID-19 pandemic, they faced radical uncertainty as well. They were also subject to biases when making decisions: as discussed earlier, they were often prone to optimism and an NFU and such biases affected their risk estimates. Although members of the scientific community may be better trained at evaluating certain forms of evidence than other citizens, we witnessed a lot of epistemic superheroics by well-established intellectuals and renowned scientists who expressed views about how the pandemic would evolve when they lacked the required disciplinary background. A common observation on social media exchanges during the pandemic was that overnight everybody had become an epidemiologist.

Given the high level of uncertainty, there was quite a lot of disagreement between scientists. As political leaders, scientists, and other citizens have to deal with biases and uncertainties when assessing risks and making decisions, steps must be taken to control and counteract the effects of those biases and the effects of uncertainty on decision-making. Government officials have far more resources available to them than ordinary citizens, and they are expected to legislate for a whole population, meaning that their decisions are more impactful than those of other citizens. The need to include structural measures to counteract biases in their prediction and decision-making is thus even greater for people invested with responsibility.

Openness to new evidence can, to an extent, be structurally enforced by having regular reviews of new evidence and also by having different voices at the table which represent more and less conservative modelling of possible outcomes. It is important that political leaders do not surround themselves with people who have the same agenda or tell them only what they want to hear. Diversity of views and scheduled stock-taking to allow adjustment of predictions and actions are crucial for good political decision-making – indeed having diverse views has been shown to counteract biased information search and biased decision-making in groups (Schulz-Hardt, Jochims, and Frey 2002). The advice to policymakers for decision-making in crisis is to explicitly acknowledge the possible impact of biases, have diverse groups working on projects, welcome dissenting views, and do some of the initial policy analysis separately to cut down on the danger of too quickly settling on a group view (Cash 2022).

This kind of labour-intensive monitoring of the evidence is not feasible for ordinary citizens. It is much harder for agents who do not have access to the latest science briefings to put in place measures to counterbalance their biases in such a way as to allow them to improve their own risk/ benefit analysis. The idea that calculating the likely outcome of individual actions is often not conducive to achieving the best outcomes is familiar from discussions of utilitarianism and from Hume's discussion of artificial virtues (Hume 1998). Outcomes of individual actions are famously hard to assess, and this kind of uncertainty allows scope for rationalisation of problematic behaviour. Given these factors, agents are better served by adopting a higher-order rule such as "follow the scientific advice and guidelines in your own country," rather than trying to work out whether a certain action is beneficial in a certain situation. Clearly, this requires a certain level of trust in the probity and well-informedness of one's own government, which cannot always be taken for granted. If this is not guaranteed, one might follow the advice of other epistemically authoritative sources, such as established scientists. Lack of trust in political or scientific authorities can have serious effects on behaviour, leading to conspiracy theories and extremism.

However, no public health rule is perfect, and following what one's government recommends will not always be conducive to desirable effects due to a lack of consistency. In the summer of 2022, mask wearing was legally mandated in public transport in Germany but not in Belgium. Consequently, passengers travelling from Brussels to Frankfurt were asked to put on masks after crossing the border, having sat maskless in a crowded train for 45 minutes. Recommendations that are not evidence-based or that are inconsistent are not recommendations that it is desirable to follow.

Nevertheless, public health measures depend on widespread observance. Attempts to flatten the curve early in the pandemic depended on populations largely observing the rules. Vaccinations, too, depend on widespread uptake for their effectiveness. Therefore, the majority of people need to observe rules consistently to achieve the desired outcome. Hume identified a similar problem for the observation of property rules. Hume called the disposition to obey and respect laws of property the *artificial virtue* of justice. He thought that observance of property laws was justified by the overall good effect for society and that in order to stop second guessing those rules in the rare instances where they weren't beneficial, people should think of the observance of property rules (justice) as intrinsically valuable, rather than focusing on the consequences of the observance of each individual rule in a specific case. We thus have an artificial virtue, justice, for which it is acceptable, even desirable, to disregard its ultimate, consequentialist justification (Hume 1998).

Would this solution benefit the decision-making of pandemic agents? Should we imbue the guidelines with a more absolute status that is divorced from the calculation of their actual consequences? Unfortunately, the strategy of divorcing the value of rules for behaviour from consequences is not likely to work in the case of COVID-related health recommendations. There is too much variation between government advice in different countries for presenting mask wearing as an intrinsically good action. Even within the same country, advice changed frequently depending on new evidence becoming available. In order to be able to adjust to changing circumstances and new information, we *need* to think of COVID-related health recommendations as justified by their public health consequences. Which means that psychologically, a results-oriented justification cannot drop out of the picture, even if ordinary citizens leave the best strategy for achieving those results up to the experts.

Adjusting to new evidence and guidelines will involve some discomfort, as people need to work against tendencies such as the NFCC and the NFU. Closure will only ever be temporary. People can gain some stability and motivational power by thinking that following the science or government guidelines is a stable virtue or rule for action. But conforming to such a high-level rule will still require significant flexibility in the face of change. For example, it required a switch from not wearing masks to wearing masks when government advice changed.

Adherence to these rules can be reinforced by making their observance part of one's identity and group membership. You can think of yourself as one of the responsible people who follow government advice. This would provide some stability, which is sorely needed given the changing content of the rules. However, it will not resolve cases of synchronous conflict where different countries have rules of varying strictness. In the train example, no sensible risk estimate would recommend putting on a mask halfway through a long journey on a crowded train, nor would it make sense to take the mask off halfway through. As there is no consistently applied rationale for wearing masks across the whole journey, individual agents still have to make a decision based on their own risk estimates in these kinds of situations.

2.7 Conclusions

To conclude, the pandemic poses significant challenges to agents' ability to make realistic risk estimates and remain sensitive to new evidence about risks when making decisions. While biases don't necessarily lead to bad outcomes and can support a sense of agency, the risky behaviour and insensitivity to new evidence that result from these biases pose problems for decision-making.

We suggested a division of labour. Structural measures should be put in place to prevent political leaders and government officials from developing undue confidence in policies that are based on incomplete evidence and to enable them to rely on advice from diverse groups of experts and advisors. This should also help avoid overly optimistic predictions by ensuring that policymakers remain sensitive and responsive to new evidence. It is important for other citizens, too, to become aware of potential biases and behavioural tendencies triggered by threats and uncertain situations, but they should not be expected to bear the burden of making challenging risk estimates and potentially life-saving decisions without support. Rather, citizens should be able to trust the advice of epistemically credible authorities, either their own government or (if their government is in the grip of exceptionalism and unrealistic optimism) the next available authoritative source that is epistemically credible (such as the relevant scientific community).

Acknowledgements

The authors would like to thank Leonardo Ribeiro, Nils Kürbis, Jonathan Webber, Rosa Ritunnano, and Kathleen Murphy-Hollies for very helpful comments on a previous version of the chapter.

References

BBC News. 2022a. "MP Margaret Ferrier pleads guilty to exposing public to Covid" August 01 (2022). Available at: https://www.bbc.co.uk/news/uk-scotland-62589375 (accessed November 2022).

BBC News. 2022b. "PM birthday event was held in No 10 during lockdown" January 01 (2022). Available at: https://www.bbc.co.uk/news/uk-politics-60114812 (accessed November 2022).

Beer, Tommy. 2020. "All the times Trump compared Covid-19 to the flu, even after he knew Covid-19 was far more deadly." *Forbes*, September 10 (2020). Available at: https://www.forbes.com/sites/tommybeer/2020/09/10/all-the-times-trump-compared-covid-19-to-the-flu-even-after-he-knew-covid-19-was-far-more-deadly/?sh=672450cdf9d2 (accessed November 2022).

Bortolotti, Lisa. 2018. "Optimism, agency, and success." *Ethical Theory and Moral Practice* 21 (3): 521–535. doi: 10.1007/s10677-018-9894-6

Bortolotti, Lisa, and Kathleen Murphy-Hollies. 2022. "Exceptionalism at the time of Covid-19: Where nationalism meets irrationality." *Danish Yearbook of Philosophy* 55 (2), 90–111. doi: 10.1163/24689300-bja10025.

Bortolotti, Lisa, Ema Sullivan-Bissett, and Magdalena Antrobus. 2019. "The epistemic innocence of optimistically biased beliefs." In *Reasoning: Essays on Theoretical and Practical Thinking*, ed. By Magdalena Balcerak Jackson and Brandon Balcerak Jackson (Oxford, Oxford University Press), chapter 12.

Buzzell, Andrew, and Regina Rini. 2022. "Doing your own research and other impossible acts of epistemic superheroism." *Philosophical Psychology*. doi: 10.1080/09515089.2022.2138019.

Cash, Tony. 2022. "Three biases that policymakers must avoid in crises – and how to do it." *Global Government Forum*, February 27 (2022). Available at: https://www.globalgovernmentforum.com/three-biases-that-policymakers-must-avoid-in-crises-and-how-to-do-it/ (accessed November 2022).

Czernatowicz-Kukuczka, Aneta, Katarzyna Jaśko, and Małgorzata Kossowska. 2014. "Need for closure and dealing with uncertainty in decision making context: The role of the behavioral inhibition system and working memory capacity." *Personality and Individual Differences* 70: 126–130. ISSN 0191-8869. doi: 10.1016/j.paid.2014.06.013.

Disatnik, David, and Yael Steinhart. 2015. "Need for cognitive closure, risk aversion, uncertainty changes, and their effects on investment decisions." *Journal of Marketing Research* 52 (3): 349–359. http://www.jstor.org/stable/43832364

Epley, Nicholas, and David Dunning. 2000. "Feeling "holier than thou": Are self-serving assessments produced by errors in self- or social prediction?" *Journal of Personality and Social Psychology* 79 (6): 861–875.

Eshel, Yohanan, Shaul Kimhi, Hadas Marciano, and Bruria Adini. 2022. "Conspiracy claims and secret intentions as predictors of psychological coping and vaccine uptake during the COVID-19 pandemic." *Journal of Psychiatric Research* 151: 311–318. doi: 10.1016/j.jpsychires.2022.04.042.

Hume, David. 1998. *An Enquiry Concerning the Principles of Morals* (Oxford, Oxford University Press). Original edition, 1777.

Imhoff, Roland, and Pia Lamberty. 2017. "Too special to be duped: Need for uniqueness motivates conspiracy beliefs." *European Journal of Social Psychology* 47: 724–734. doi: 10.1002/ejsp.2265.

Imhoff, Roland, and Pia Lamberty. 2020. "A bioweapon or a hoax? The link between distinct conspiracy beliefs about the coronavirus disease (COVID-19) outbreak and pandemic behavior." *Social Psychological and Personality Science* 11 (8): 1110–1118. doi: 10.1177/1948550620934692.

Ioannidis, John P.A., Sally Cripps, and Martin A. Tanner. 2022. "Forecasting for COVID-19 has failed." *International Journal of Forecasting* 38 (2): 423–438. doi: 10.1016/j.ijforecast.2020.08.004.

Jaśko, Katarzyna, Aneta Czernatowicz-Kukuczk, Małgorzata Kossowska, and Anna Z. Czarna. 2015. "Individual differences in response to uncertainty and decision making: The role of behavioral inhibition system and need for closure." *Motivation and Emotion* 39 (4): 541–552. doi: 10.1007/s11031-015-9478-x.

Jefferson, Anneli. 2017. "Born to be biased? Unrealistic optimism and error management theory." *Philosophical Psychology* 30(8): 1159–1175. doi: 10.1080/09515089.2017.1370085.

Jefferson, Anneli, Lisa Bortolotti, and Bojana Kuzmanovic. 2017. "What is unrealistic optimism?" *Consciousness and Cognition* 50: 3–11. doi: 10.1016/j.concog.2016.10.005.

Kruglanski, A. W. (1989). *Lay epistemics and human knowledge: Cognitive and motivational bases*. New York, NY: Plenum Press.

Kruglanski, Arie W., Katarzyna Jasko, and Karl Friston. 2020. "All thinking is 'wishful' thinking." *Trends in Cognitive Science* 24 (6): 413–424.

Kuper-Smith, Benjamin J., Lisa M. Doppelhofer, Yulia Oganian, Gabriela Rosenblau, and Christoph W. Korn. 2021. "Risk perception and optimism during the early stages of the COVID-19 pandemic." *Royal Society Open Science* 8 (11): 210904. doi: 10.1098/rsos.210904.

Kuzmanovic, Bojana, Anneli Jefferson, and Kai Vogeley. 2015. "Self-specific optimism bias in belief updating is associated with high trait optimism." *Journal of Behavioral Decision Making* 28 (3): 281–293. doi: 10.1002/bdm.1849.

Kuzmanovic, Bojana, Anneli Jefferson, and Kai Vogeley. 2016. "The role of the neural reward circuitry in self-referential optimistic belief updates." *Neuroimage* 133 (2016): 151–162. doi: 10.1016/j.neuroimage.2016.02.014.

Kuzmanovic, Bojana, and Lionel Rigoux. 2017. "Valence-dependent belief updating: Computational validation." *Frontiers in Psychology* 8. doi: 10.3389/fpsyg.2017.01087.

Lantian, Anthony, Dominique Muller, Cécile Nurra, and Karen M. Douglas. 2017. "'I know things that they don't know'. The role of need for uniqueness in belief in conspiracy theory." *Social Psychology* 48 (3): 160–173.

Larson, James R., R. Scott Tindale, and Young-Jae Yoon. 2020. "Advice taking by groups: The effects of consensus seeking and member opinion differences." *Group Processes & Intergroup Relations* 23(7):921–942.doi:10.1177/1368430219871349.

Levy, Neil. 2019 "Is conspiracy theorising irrational?" *Social Epistemology Review and Reply Collective* 8 (10): 65–76. Available at: https://wp.me/p1Bfg0-4wW (accessed November 2022).

Mangan, Dan. 2020. "Trump dismissed coronavirus pandemic worry in January—now claims he long warned about it." *CNBC*, March 17 (2020). Available at: https://www.cnbc.com/2020/03/17/trump-dissed-coronavirus-pandemic-worry-now-claims-he-warned-about-it.html. (accessed November 2022).

Murphy-Hollies, Kathleen, and Lisa Bortolotti, L. 2021. "Stories as evidence." *Memory, Mind & Media* 1: E3. doi:10.1017/mem.2021.5.

Photopoulos, Julianna. 2021. "A scientist's opinion: Interview with Professor Arie Kruglanski about our need for cognitive closure during COVID-19." *European Science Media Hub*, April 14 (2021). Available at: https://sciencemediahub.eu/2021/04/14/a-scientists-opinion-interview-with-professor-arie-kruglanski-about-our-need-for-cognitive-closure-during-covid-19/.

Pica, Gennaro, Maxim Milyavsky, Antonio Pierro, and Arie W. Kruglanski. 2021. "The epistemic bases of changes of opinion and choices: The joint effects of the need for cognitive closure, ascribed epistemic authority and quality of advice." *European Journal of Social Psychology* 51 (4–5): 690–702.

Pivovar, Allana, Elder Semprebon, Nichole Perdoncini, Amanda Corelhano, and Cassius Torres-Pereira. 2022. "The effects of the cognitive bias of unrealistic optimism in the adoption of preventive measures against COVID-19 in dentistry." *Revista Brasileira de Medicina do Trabalho* 20 (1): 105–112.

Ratcliff, Chelsea L., and Rebekah Wicke. 2022. "How the public evaluates media representations of uncertain science: An integrated explanatory framework." *Public Understanding of Science*. doi: 10.1177/09636625221122960.

Rice, Orlaith. 2022. "Explaining Swedish exceptionalism in its pandemic response." *The Loop*, March 14 (2022). Available at: https://theloop.ecpr.eu/explaining-swedish-exceptionalism-in-its-pandemic-response/ (accessed November 2022).

Rottweiler, Bettina, and Paul Gill. 2022. "Individual differences in personality moderate the effects of perceived group deprivation on violent extremism: Evidence from a united kingdom nationally representative survey." *Frontiers in Psychology* 13: 790770. doi: 10.3389/fpsyg.2022.790770.

Sachdeva, Ruchika. 2022. "Pandemic, perceived risk, and cognitive dissonance as antecedents to need for cognitive closure," *International Journal of Service Science, Management, Engineering, and Technology (IJSSMET)* 13 (1): 1–20. doi: 10.4018/IJSSMET.298676.

Salgado, Sinué, and Dorthe Berntsen. 2021. "'It won't happen to us': Unrealistic optimism affects COVID-19 risk assessments and attitudes regarding protective behaviour." *Journal of Applied Research in Memory and Cognition* 10 (3): 368–380. doi: 10.1016/j.jarmac.2021.07.006.

Schulz-Hardt, Stefan, Marc Jochims, and Dieter Frey. 2002. "Productive conflict in group decision making: Genuine and contrived dissent as strategies to counteract biased information seeking." *Organizational Behavior and Human Decision Processes* 88 (2): 563–586. doi: 10.1016/S0749-5978(02)00001-8.

Shackel, Nicholas. 2022. "Uncertainty phobia and epistemic forbearance in a pandemic." *Royal Institute of Philosophy Supplement* 92: 271–291. doi: 10.1017/S1358246122000248.

Sharot, Tali, Christoph W. Korn, and Raymond J. Dolan. 2011. "How unrealistic optimism Is maintained in the face of reality." *Nature Neuroscience* 14 (11):1475–1479. Available at: http://www.nature.com/neuro/journal/v14/n11/abs/nn.2949.html#supplementary-information.

Shepperd, James A., William M. P. Klein, Erika A. Waters, and Neil D. Weinstein. 2013. "Taking stock of unrealistic optimism." *Perspectives on Psychological Science* 8 (4): 395–411. doi: 10.1177/1745691613485247.

Shepperd, James A., Erika A. Waters, Neil D. Weinstein, and William M. P. Klein. 2015. "A primer on unrealistic optimism." *Current Directions in Psychological Science* 24 (3): 232–237. doi: 10.1177/0963721414568341.

Shukla, Shanu, Sushanta Kumar Mishra, and Himanshu Rai. 2021. "Optimistic bias, risky behavior, and social norms among Indian college students during COVID-19." *Personality and Individual Differences* 183: 111076. doi: 10.1016/j.paid.2021.111076.

Snyder, C. R., and Howard L. Fromkin. 1977. "Abnormality as a positive characteristic: The development and validation of a scale measuring need for uniqueness." *Journal of Abnormal Psychology* 86 (5): 518–527. doi: 10.1037/0021-843X.86.5.518.

Stewart, Conor. 2022. "Cumulative number of coronavirus deaths in the Nordics 2022." *Statista*, (2022). Available at: https://www.statista.com/statistics/1113834/cumulative-coronavirus-deaths-in-the-nordics/ (accessed November 2022).

Tilner, Alina, Birga Schumpe, and Hans-Peter Erb. 2022. "The need for uniqueness – a motor for social change." Routledge. doi: 10.4324/9780367198459-REPRW108-1.

Walker, Peter. 2020. "Boris Johnson: UK can turn tide of coronavirus in 12 weeks." *The Guardian*, March 19 (2020). https://www.theguardian.com/world/2020/mar/19/boris-johnson-uk-can-turn-tide-of-coronavirus-in-12-weeks.

Wang, Xiuxin, and Du Xiufang 2018. "Why does advice discounting occur? The combined roles of confidence and trust." *Frontiers in Psychology* 9: 2381. doi: 10.3389/fpsyg.2018.02381.

White, Holly A. Mar. 2022. "Need for cognitive closure predicts stress and anxiety of college students during COVID-19 pandemic." *Personality and Individual Differences* 187: 111393. doi: 10.1016/j.paid.2021.111393.

Yaniv, Ilan, and Eli Kleinberger (2000). "Advice taking in decision making: Egocentric discounting and reputation formation." *Organizational Behavior and Human Decision Processes* 83 (2): 260–281. doi: 10.1006/obhd.2000.2909.

3 Feeling lonely

Toward a phenomenological account of loneliness during the COVID-19 pandemic

Flavio Williges

3.1 Introduction

The COVID-19 pandemic was accompanied by a series of emotional responses. Studies carried out in the early stages of the pandemic showed that not only health professionals but also ordinary people, with a lower risk of being infected by the virus, experienced intense forms of fear, anxiety, and depression (Montemurro 2020; Ornell et al. 2020). In subsequent stages, the isolation of the infected, social distancing measures, and the lockdown aroused feelings of discomfort, irritability, worry, sadness, loneliness, grief, and nostalgia (Brooks et al. 2020; Goularte et al. 2021). For most people, this intense and oscillating emotional activity, along with cognitive and behavioral changes such as distraction and lack of focus, converted the emotional experience of the pandemic into something negative. Although our emotional experience has been mainly negative, I contend that such feelings also have a positive outcome that has mostly gone unnoticed so far. I develop this positive significance through a phenomenological analysis of loneliness, an emotion that has been prevalent throughout the pandemic.

Loneliness is often described in the health sciences as a negative feeling arising from the perceived discrepancy between a person's desired and achieved social relations (Bekhet et al. 2008; Dahlberg 2021). It is also defined as an emotional state in which individuals experience a feeling of isolation, detachment, and lack of social support and belongingness (Lampraki et al. 2022). Among philosophers of emotions, on the other hand, loneliness is characterized as an emotion that reacts to the absence of "distinctive kinds of social connection" (Roberts and Krueger 2021, 191). A person feels lonely when he or she values but does not achieve social goods such as "companionship, moral support, physical contact and affection, sympathy, trust, romance, friendship, and the opportunity to act and interact – and so to flourish – as a social agent" (Roberts and Krueger 2021, 191). Thus, feeling lonely means to feel bad for the absence of certain kinds of social involvements and for not experiencing a sense of belonging. If loneliness is an undesirable and painful emotional state in

DOI: 10.4324/9781003310129-4

the sense described, then what positivity could we learn from the painful feelings of loneliness?

The main purpose of this chapter is to argue that feeling lonely in response to the disruptive reality of the pandemic helps us understand the subjective importance of social relations and integration with the world around us. We feel lonely when trapped in our homes, bewildered by empty streets, or cannot reach a friend or a loved one; this feeling reveals things that are important for our happiness and well-being. Therefore, feeling alone is a way of knowing how much one cares about others, misses others and feels lost without them, and how significant and valuable the connection to the world around us is. Also, it offers an opportunity to redirect priorities and even promote more radical changes in one's life.

I do not think, however, that this general point is valid or could be sustained as an indiscriminate truth for every form of loneliness or for every individual.[1] The pandemic experience did not have a standard form. It has been argued that different kinds of people showed complex, diverse experiences during the pandemic, "ranging from dreadful to wonderful" ones (Carel and Kidd 2020; Guruge et al. 2021). Studies show that many individuals experienced loneliness during the pandemic as a form of chronic loneliness, i.e., a severe and incapacitating feeling (Antonelli-Salgado et al. 2021; Banerjee and Rai 2020; Sugaya et al. 2022), while others experienced a rather transient form (Luchetti et al. 2020; Killam 2020; McGinty et al. 2020; Lampraki et al. 2022). I contend that only transient or slightly painful feelings of loneliness might elicit the awareness of the importance and personal value of certain joyful experiences – the ones that were temporarily out of reach during the pandemic.

In order to make my point clearer and more compelling, I begin by describing some general aspects of loneliness during the pandemic based on empirical studies. Then I present a typical analysis of the structure of loneliness in three different but related dimensions: ontological, affective, and cognitive.

Ontologically, I will construct pandemic loneliness not just as an internal feeling but as an embodied emotion with a pervasive affective structure close to the notion of existential feelings introduced by Matthew Ratcliffe (2005, 2008). One way of putting this is to say, as Joel Krueger writes in relation to Dewey's philosophy of emotions, that emotions are not

> comprised of states or processes physically located within the individual subject, and specifically within the subject's brain. Instead, […] emotions are made up of both internal (neural and physiological activity, phenomenal properties and cognitive judgments) *and* external processes, (expressive behavior, ongoing "transactions" with the surrounding environment.
>
> (Krueger 2014, 140)

From this perspective, pandemic loneliness can be conceived as a practical, dynamic, and all-encompassing embodied form of response to the absence of social goods and other significant changes introduced in our surroundings by the pandemic outbreak.

Affectively, loneliness during the pandemic will be characterized by a subjective painful state connected with the perception of social isolation and the experience of not belonging. Such an affective dimension should not be understood merely as a psychological state, but also as a bodily feeling that offers evaluative information about our lives and the world we live in. As a bodily feeling, loneliness had some complex cognitive effects too.

Cognitively, I begin with the insightful analysis of Roberts and Kruger and contend that loneliness is an *emotion of absence* that involves a pro-attitude of approval of the importance of social goods (Roberts and Krueger 2021). Roberts and Krueger's account emphasizes the absence of certain social goods – that is, goods especially connected with social relationships and conviviality. The main difference I introduce regarding the authors' characterization is the emphasis on the special role that the lack of sense of belonging to physical spaces has had in pandemic loneliness.

Considering all these together, I claim that feelings of loneliness are crucial to getting a deep understanding of the things that we have missed during the pandemic and by that acknowledging structures of value and importance in our experience.

My focus will be on developing a phenomenological account of loneliness during the pandemic. But since any account in this area must respond not only to the structure of one's own experience but also to the empirical findings systematized about loneliness in the disciplines of psychiatry and psychology, I also draw on those disciplines as a way of enriching the complexity of loneliness during the pandemic. Since the phenomenological view needs to be connected to a plausible developmental account of existential feelings and bodily feelings, I also draw on pertinent material about the nature of bodily feelings in the phenomenological tradition.

The chapter is divided into six sections. In Section 3.2, I present a general account of loneliness, contrasting chronic and milder forms. In Section 3.3, I characterize the nature of loneliness as being similar to existential feelings – that is, as a pervasive emotion that structures our practical and theoretical activities. In Section 3.4, I provide a detailed analysis of the embodied nature of loneliness. Then, in Section 3.5, I look more directly at the positive role of the emotional experience of loneliness and indicate how the affective and structural features discussed in the previous sections reinforce a characterization of loneliness as an essential part of the way we can better understand our dependence to others and the exchanges we made during the pandemic. Finally, the conclusion, Section 3.6, restates the main topics developed in the chapter and points out the contributions of my account for an analysis of the pandemic as a transformative experience. I also highlight a few limitations of this discussion and present some aspects for further investigation in this research agenda.

3.2 Loneliness during the COVID-19 pandemic

Feelings of loneliness have at least two aspects: level and symptoms. Regarding the level, loneliness is usually either transient or chronic. When an individual's feelings of loneliness vary over time, loneliness is usually referred to as "transient." When it is constant, it is referred to as "chronic" loneliness. Pandemic loneliness encompassed those two different forms of loneliness. Transient loneliness usually has milder symptoms. As an illustration, consider the case presented by psychiatrists John Cacioppo and William Patrick about a lonely middle-aged woman called Kate Bishop. Kate is described as a friendly, small-town girl who grew up in a lively community where she had an active social life but felt tied down. This changed when she moved to a larger city to work and experienced a new routine in which she lacked close connections and social interactions.

> After six months of this very different routine, she realized that she was not sleeping well. In fact, her whole body seemed to be off. If a cold or flu bug was anywhere in her vicinity, she would catch it. When she wasn't traveling or working long hours, or taking yoga classes to try to deal with the back and neck pain from traveling and working those long hours, she spent a great deal of time in front of the TV; eating ice cream straight from the carton. Six months into her new, independent life, Katie Bishop was even beginning to wonder if she would ever be socially acceptable outside the little town that had made her feel so trapped.
>
> (Cacioppo and Patrick 2008, 4–5)

As we can glimpse from the passage, Katie Bishop was feeling a kind of chronic or pathological loneliness. There is no doubt that many have experienced Bishop's depressing mental and physical states during the pandemic (Antonelli-Salgado et al. 2021). Chronic loneliness is a very concerning condition in modern societies, and the pandemic certainly intensified and increased the rate of such an incapacitating condition (Banerjee and Rai 2020). As Cacioppo and Patrick explain, this form of loneliness represents a risk to physical and mental health since it is a painful and even terrifying emotion that can generate "a persistent and self-sustained cycle of negative thoughts, sensations and behaviors" (Cacioppo and Patrick 2008, 7).

However, during the pandemic, not everyone experienced persistent feelings of emptiness and disconnection, self-destructive behavior, or states of paralysis. People started to feel lonely as a reaction to ordinary changes, along with the lack of involvement with friends and family and other forms of social connection. Most people did not feel loneliness in the sense of a mental illness, but rather as a slightly disruptive way of feeling themselves and the world around them, especially in virtue of the absence of social activities or vivid engagement with the world and others. In this kind of case, loneliness is a reaction to the physical impossibility of reaching others and interacting socially with them. Transient feelings of loneliness are not as deep as chronic loneliness, a form of loneliness characterized by an inner experience of social disconnectedness (Roberts and Krueger 2021; Zhong et al. 2017).

Empirical research carried out during the pandemic confirms this assumption: feelings of loneliness ranged from *severe forms* of disconnection (Banerjee and Rai 2020), which included some forms of depression and suicidal ideation (Antonelli-Salgado et al. 2021), to relatively *transient and milder* forms (Folk et al. 2020; Killam 2020; Luchetti et al. 2020) characterized by a distressing and emotionally manageable subjective need for social interaction and contact. Additionally, there may be some relevant differences in the prevalence of loneliness in the general population, with higher levels among older adults and single individuals than among young people and families with children (Lampraki et al. 2022).

In light of this evidence, loneliness during the COVID-19 pandemic may be regarded as having a varying nature for different persons. Some felt a more constant loneliness while others showed more transient forms. Physical and mental health studies also reveal multiple outcomes, ranging from milder to more severe ones. Unless otherwise stated, I will henceforth refer to *loneliness* or *pandemic loneliness* as meaning that bundle of physical and psychological effects. In the next sections, I will offer a detailed description of the structure of this emotion as comprising three components: ontological, affective, and cognitive. It should be noted, however, that these dimensions are being conceptually distinguished for instructive purposes only; they are, in fact, intertwined.

3.3 The ontological structure of pandemic loneliness

The ontological dimension of the affective domain deals with the nature of different kinds of affective states such as emotions, moods, feelings, and emotional dispositions. Despite having been historically marginal, embodied theories of emotions have gained increasing importance in research on emotion in the last decade. In my analysis, I follow a phenomenological approach and maintain that loneliness can be taken as a background and bodily emotion of a particular kind, akin to moods, atmospheres, or existential feelings (Ratcliffe 2005; Trigg 2020). *Feeling lonely* is not restricted in this sense to an "internal feeling" but as having the potential to affect how we notice and deal with our surroundings.

One useful way of highlighting this approach is to consider Matthew Ratcliffe's original analysis of existential feelings.

Ratcliffe described existential feelings as a particular affective state that can be conceived as "ways of finding oneself in the world" that permeate and reveal the totality (internal and external; body and mind) of our experience as being in a certain way (Ratcliffe 2008). Taken this way, affective states make up a background for every "encounter" with the world, both theoretically and practically. As he puts it, as a way of finding oneself in the world, existential feelings do not simply "consist in an experience of being an entity that occupies a spatial and temporal location, alongside a host of other entities." Instead,

> [w]ays of finding oneself in a world are presupposed spaces of experiential possibility, which shape the various ways in which things can be experienced. For example, if one's sense of the world is tainted by a "feeling of unreality", this will affect how all objects of perception appear. They are distant, removed, not quite "there".
>
> (Ratcliffe 2005, 47)

Following Ratcliffe, I would like to maintain that feelings of loneliness during the pandemic have the characteristic of being all-encompassing world orientations that make certain situations or even our presence in the world feel different from pre-pandemic times. Part of this can be formulated by saying that if one's sense of the world is tainted by a feeling of loneliness, this feeling or emotion will affect how one experiences daily places such as buildings, streets, routes, and parks; it will create a sense of belonging to a "new reality," a reality where absence and lack of involvement dominate our experience of our surroundings and of others. Loneliness appears here as a way of being present in the world. That is, loneliness could be conceived as a background emotion that structures our world as something a bit distant and cold, an emotion that makes salient the absence of social goods (Roberts and Krueger 2021). The need to remain inside our homes and to stop traveling, eating in restaurants, or sitting in cafes significantly affected our emotional experience of ourselves and the world around us. Some of those emotional changes yielded joyful experiences and offered new forms of signifying our lives (Carel and Kidd 2020), but others seemed to have the loneliness effect that I have stressed.

Some conceptual specifications are important to clarify my tentative analysis of loneliness using the terminology created to describe existential feelings. Emotions are usually conceptualized as specific attitudes we hold toward objects or events, while existential feelings do not seem intentional because they never target specific objects. In other words, emotions are directed toward specific objects, events, or situations; on the other hand, existential feelings "embrace the world as a whole."

As one might expect, however, things in the affective domain are not always so sharply distinguishable. Although emotions may differ from existential feelings in virtue of being intentionally directed at specific objects, those differences can blur in certain cases. Michael Stocker says, for example, that an emotion can be conceived as "diffuse, pervasive, and lasting, forming our background, as well as the tone, color, affective taste, sensation of activities, relationships and experiences" (Stocker 2004, 137). Ratcliffe (2005, 48) also acknowledges this possibility in connection with certain forms of grief.

3.4 The bodily affective structure of loneliness

The affective analysis in the phenomenological tradition considers that emotions are bodily phenomena that cannot be reduced to internal hedonic qualities situated "in the mind." The body should not be taken in this case as a set or place of sensations, but rather as an intentional structure usually explained by the phenomenological tradition through the difference between the words *Korper* and *Leib*. In German, *Leib* refers "to the lived, feeling and expressive body, whereas the term *Körper* refers to the body as it appears when examined like any other extended object" (Colombetti and Ratcliffe 2012, 146). Conceived as *Leib*, references to the body are not to organs or to the whole body as an objectified entity but as an "intentional object of awareness" (Colombetti and Ratcliffe 2012, 146). As an "intentional object of awareness," feelings experienced in the body offer us an intentional awareness of the world (Slaby 2008). In the case of loneliness, such intentional content cannot be reduced to a visceral desire for connection. Bodily feelings of loneliness are not a craving for the food and drink that alleviate unpleasant sensations, something that is sometimes referred to as an "internal hunger" (Cacioppo and Patrick 2008). Although the idea of an "internal hunger" captures something important about the bodily experience of loneliness, it does not capture the precise nature of the complex bodily feelings of loneliness that were felt during the pandemic. Loneliness during the pandemic entailed not only pangs in our stomachs or some form of physical desire for satisfaction, but something more elusive such as a lack of subtle forms of warmth that accompany social interactions, like intimacy and coziness. In other words, it is crucial that we acknowledge that the "what-it-is-like" quality of feeling lonely cannot be reduced to kinesthetic sensations or muscular feedback that characterizes each emotion (Deonna and Teroni 2012). What is overlooked in the isolated references to hedonic qualities and bodily sensations of loneliness is a very complex set of emotional resonances in our bodies. Such resonances react to what is not present or is missing in the current environment (Roberts and Krueger 2021). In other words, bodily feelings of loneliness have an intentional content because our bodies are affected by absence. I will further explore this intentional aspect of the feeling in Section 3.5.

A promising strategy for capturing the bodily feelings of loneliness during the pandemic concerns the relationship of our bodies with material objects such as household items (family photographs, clothes, furniture) and personal objects that became salient in emotional experiences linked to loneliness. Historian Fay Alberti notes that "alongside verbal narratives and gestures, material objects are the means through which we structure our physical and mental worlds and communicate our emotional experiences to others and ourselves" (Alberti 2019, 180). Given that physical or personal objects are an important form of affirming our own identity and bonds with others, things such as the absence of someone important can be restored by material objects in the environment to which we belong. As Alberti puts it, "Because material objects tell stories about who we are, and where we are in the world, they become especially important when other aspects of ourselves and our identities are destroyed and distant" (Alberti 2019, 180). From this perspective, we can say that the presence of objects of a loved one who has passed away is relevant for capturing an embodied sense of loneliness.[2] We can easily recognize this embodied experience of loneliness connected with objects during the pandemic because many of us turned to objects such as photographs, clothes, books, and other personal items, or to places our loved ones used to attend to create an emotional atmosphere of presence. These objects have the function of reminding the lonely person of happy memories and providing a sense of comfort through the revival of connections with certain people and places. In some cases, these objects may even be the only connection that someone has to their former pre-pandemic life (think, for example, of older individuals who could not visit their offspring or a physician who could not get back home to see their family because of the threat of contagion).

A new bodily experience of familiar objects was part of loneliness. Certain objects have the function of recreating a sense of proximity to everyday things. Our bodily experience of loneliness amid objects and places also occurred in another form. It appears as a form of displacement or detachment from the familiar world. It was not only familiar objects that acquired an emerging reference to absence. Absence seems to be also a constant structure of the places and surrounding context of our daily activities. Let us consider this point in more detail.

Consider our bodily nature and the physical endurance of emptiness or physical absence around us during the pandemic. Bodily affective engagement with reality during the pandemic was not only centered on the contemplation or manipulation of certain objects that reminded us of or moved us by signs of pre-pandemic times, such as a grandchild's toys, workwear, and personal belongings of those whom we were forced to be far from. Feelings of loneliness can also be articulated through the bodily resonances of emptiness "from all sides," "from above," "underneath," and "everywhere."[3] Thus, one way of putting it is to say that loneliness was characterized by bodily feelings of *persistence of the spatial emptiness.* Spatial emptiness can be conceived as a literal bodily feeling since it happened to people left alone at COVID-19 intensive care units or, less literally, as an experience of embracing emptiness and silence at home and in the street during the pandemic. I will consider in more detail this second option.

"Physical" apprehension of emptiness gave rise to a quite clear embodied understanding of displacement, emphasizing the feeling of an isolated "self," marked by distance and separation. The appeal to the self, however, must be well understood. It is not merely an intellectual or objective perception of separation, like a cognitive sense of being isolated or far from others as it happens when we notice that we are physically incapable of reaching others – as an adolescent that is barred from going to a party with some much-loved friends.[4] Spatial emptiness could be described as a part of a large scenario where the anxiety provoked by the uncertainty about the ending of the pandemic, the fear of being contaminated, the forced separation of others significant results in a deep feeling of loneliness and not belonging to the world. One useful way to clarify this is to reflect on our experience of walking on sidewalks of empty streets of big cities during *lockdowns,* as can be seen in the pictures in Figures 3.1 and 3.2.[5]

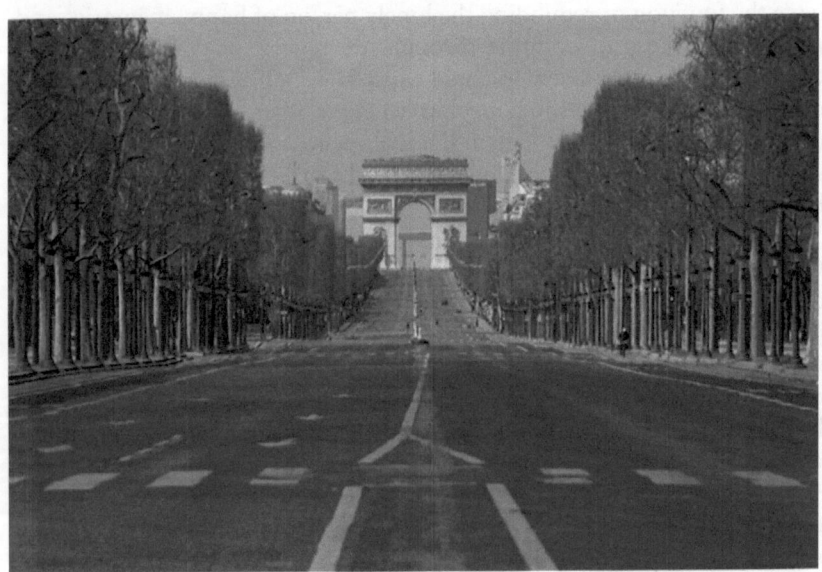

Figure 3.1 Champs Elysées Avenue empty because of COVID-19 containment measures.

(Photo by COM & O, iStock, March 22, 2020).

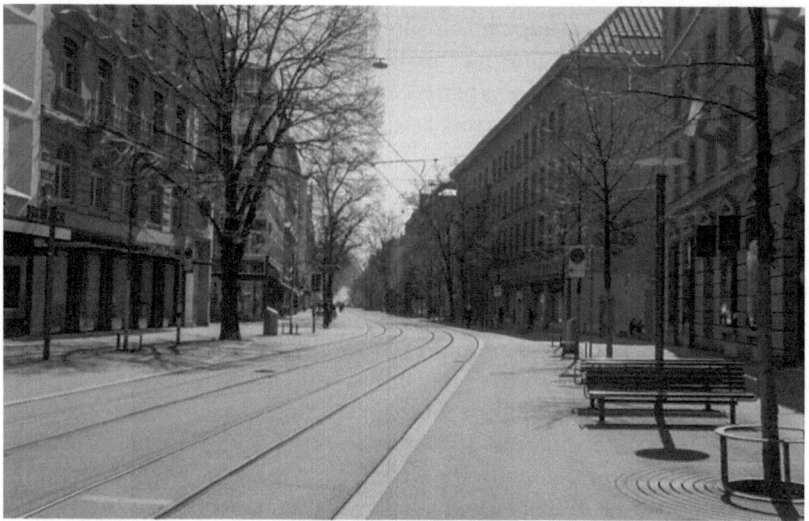

Figure 3.2 Empty streets. Zurich during the coronavirus crisis on a Thursday afternoon.

(Photo by racconbtc, iStock, April 2, 2020).

Although the pictures represent space in an objective way regarding the idea of social isolation, they clearly remind us that feeling lonely is also an effect of being in certain places or getting into a certain atmosphere that open spaces bring to light. Compare this experience of emptiness with the regular practice of walking down the street to go shopping. Usually, the latter experience is accompanied by sounds, people, and some form of environmental excitement. During the pandemic, much of the focus of this practice was transferred to the perception of the absence of other people and the presence of emptiness, which in turn made the surroundings acquire a salience or "reality" usually not perceived. The empty alleys of a grocery store, the silence in shops and streets, and the nature of presentness of all objects and details around us illustrate the vivid, intense aesthetic absence of the ordinary buzz that gives sense to our common world. The absence of people, the lack of sound, and the emptiness created an eerie feeling that is part of the embodied experience of loneliness. A street with large buildings with little or no vegetation may create a feeling of smallness and aloneness, particularly when associated with quietness, making one feel isolated and alone.

The salience of the emptiness – illustrated by the pandemic photographs – shows that loneliness is partially made up of our embodied reaction to absences felt in ordinary places. Experiences of emptiness, smallness, and aloneness that people might experience in open spaces or large buildings deprived of the presence of other people hold some lyricism that constitutes a complex set of psychophysical sensations that flood our experience, shaping our interaction with reality as something lonely. Another way of putting this is to think of it as a form of *withdrawal* from the world, an experience of separation, mainly because of the vividness that "empty" spaces assume, underscoring the absence of a shared reality.

In sum, what we can take from the affective salience of emptiness caused by the pandemic is that the loneliness felt during its most restrictive stages was something painful and contained some degree of affective suffering. At the same time, such feelings did not necessarily hinder other cognitive functions like the ability to recognize the importance of living in a world that is purposeful and existentially appealing, especially for those who had a milder form of loneliness. Mild forms of loneliness, even painful ones, carry this kind of intentional content and invite cognitive processes such as evaluating and even reconsidering the role of social relations and engagement with the world. Now it is time to see how these feelings worked to produce some positive consequences.

3.5 The cognitive dimension of loneliness

In the previous sections, I described pandemic loneliness as a pervasive bodily emotional state that makes us feel the absence of social goods and a disconnection from the world. Implicit in this characterization is the idea that such forms of affection can have a positive effect on the acknowledgment of one's own values and identity. A first step in assessing this is looking into how loneliness is a bodily feeling "directed to the world" (Slaby 2008). This directiveness relates to a certain attraction to absence. Roberts and Krueger (2021, 186) have elegantly argued that loneliness is an emotion that reacts to absence. Loneliness makes absence salient. It calls attention to what is missing or lacking in our regular, daily landscape. In this sense, bodily feelings of loneliness can act as sources of salience; they trigger "alert states," which call our attention to regular activities that one is no longer able to carry out, as well as to objects and events that are significant to the kind of person one is. Loneliness can be seen in this aspect as a *sensitivity of absence*. It is not primarily a type of intellectual perception of absence, but an embodied one that is at the same time affective and cognitive. It directs our attention to aspects of reality that are no longer available: being with loved ones, those who passed away, the things we would like to have.

I take Roberts and Krueger's insightful work on loneliness as a reference for explaining the cognitive input of loneliness. They emphasize the social dimension of loneliness and how it impacts personal identities, insofar as social goods depend on other people. What they mean by "social goods" are things such as "company, moral support, physical contact and affection, sympathy, trust, romance, friendship, and the opportunity to act and interact – and so to flourish – as a social agent" (Roberts and Krueger 2021, 191). Central to this analysis is the idea that the emotional response of feeling lonely reveals the need for meaningful human relationships, a kind of relationship that consists of "being intellectually and emotionally supported by others; receiving reassurance, validation, and love; and being able to express and cultivate those aspects of one's identity that have an essentially social form" (Roberts and Krueger 2021, 191). I take their description as saying that loneliness has a social dimension that tracks the absence of some sort of goods that we consider of fundamental importance to our identity and sense of belonging to the world. However, I will extend their work by stressing loneliness as a way of also recognizing the *lack of belonging to the spaces* we inhabit as much as our dependence on others.

The concept of *belonging* is broad enough to encompass physical spaces. As Allen formulates it, belonging can be defined as a subjective feeling that "one is an integral part of their surrounding systems, including family, friends, school, work environment, communities, cultural groups, and physical places" (Allen et al. 2021, 88). Distancing measures and social isolation left people alienated from their familiar spaces, both socially and personally. Family gatherings, sports venues and practices (e.g., bowling, domino clubs), clubs, academic meetings, and classes became disconnected from our daily experience. All of that can trigger the feeling that people's goal-directedness toward places acquires a distant nature: one does not see space as something that the body belongs to but as a set of objects or entities devoid of personal meaning, interests, and goals. Ordinary places are no longer significant to our activities and personal relations; rather, they become just a nexus of physical points in space without any substantial meaning. This meaning deprivation undermines the subjective feeling of belonging to social and dynamic reality. The surroundings are suddenly converted into geographical structures that make us feel destitute of significant, valuable attachments. The COVID-19 pandemic accelerated such a sense of social disconnection. My suggestion here is that an important part of the loneliness is related to how we integrate our bodies into social space and meaningful activities (Allen et al. 2021, 91). In this way, loneliness is an emotion that reacts to absence, not only to the absence of social goods, as Roberts and Krueger have argued but also to the way we feel ourselves and our existence as being separated or distant from the world we live in. As a sensitivity, loneliness brings to light or reveals one's dependence on others, but also to meaningful integration with "physical" spaces. Loneliness has a cognitive impact in this case because it makes clear what we value most. The type of content revealed is from the domain of importance and care related to sociability, integration, and belonging to the world. It is because my friends and family *matter* to me and I *care* about them that I feel alone and disconnected due to their absence. It is also because I *am concerned* with my purposes and commitments in significant places that my body apprehends the surrounding empty spaces as something quiet, devoid of meaning, and slightly painful. Thus, loneliness offers evaluative knowledge about ourselves and our environment as places that are *meaningful to us*, in the sense that they express our *social identity and existential needs*. Such knowledge tells us the kind of people we are, the commitments we have, and the things that matter to us, especially our dependence on or vulnerability to others and a significant social world, taken here as a space where we can fight for our dreams and ideals of happiness.

Drawing attention to the cognitive and moral role of loneliness during the pandemic does not mean that awareness of it is not present in less tragic times. Prior to the pandemic, we could certainly notice the value of friendship, extended family life, and even experiences of social interaction at work or in leisure activities in ordinary places. We could also notice how engaging with the world is definitional of our sense of being in it. However, after the onset of the pandemic, a novel sense of the importance of others and social contact has arisen. Influenced by feelings of detachment, emptiness, and loneliness, it was possible to recognize that something crucial was at stake. Pandemic loneliness has made transparent the significance or importance of things that were usually not at the forefront. In the end, it has shown that the absence of certain social goods and forms of coexistence is costly to us.

Taken together, all these different aspects make it clear that loneliness during the pandemic has been an experience of bodily disconnection from places, persons, and what comes with them. The experience of being in the world was suddenly converted into circulating through "cold" spaces without warmth or meaning.

3.6 Conclusion

The aim of this chapter has been to examine the emotion of loneliness and, in light of this, to explain how such a painful emotion can have some positive outcomes. I have undertaken the first task by arguing that loneliness during the pandemic should be conceived as a pervasive emotion essentially felt throughout the body. Also, as something capable of giving us a perception of the absence of certain social goods and nonbelonging to familiar places in pre-pandemic times. My account offers a richer understanding of loneliness during the pandemic in that it highlights how our embodied experience of loneliness is a reaction to absence, emptiness, aloneness, and detachment.

It is important to take into account a few shortcomings of my point by considering the relationship between loneliness and other emotions. To be sure, the work of unveiling valuable dimensions of our lives and our sense of belonging does not turn on loneliness alone. Emotions always appear in clusters, one leading to another (Price 2015). Loneliness could appear with feelings of fear, anxiety, sadness, grief, among others. Admittedly, those emotions cooperate to create the "atmosphere" that I linked to loneliness. It can also be said that all of them participate in directing our attention to the centrality of other people and social contact for a purposeful life.

Another shortcoming concerns the scope of my debate on loneliness. I do not claim that the painful emotional experience of loneliness is something good. Many forms of negative emotional experiences intensified by the pandemic constitute forms of suffering. Notwithstanding that, I do claim that emotional experiences of loneliness have significant instrumental value. Such value can be assessed by the way loneliness sensitizes us to our vulnerability to others and belonging to the world in order to flourish.

To close my contribution to this volume, I would like to indicate how my account might contribute to a characterization of the pandemic as a transformative experience (Carel and Kidd 2020). Transformative experiences are life-changing experiences, ones that radically transform who we are. A very influential line of discussion on transformative experience comes from Laurie Paul's work (2014). She defines transformative experience as a kind of experience that affects an individual in two deeply related ways: personally and epistemically. As she wrote, transformative experience "needs to transform our *personality*, values and goals and it also needs to give us *new knowledge*, a knowledge that we would not otherwise obtain" (Paul 2014, 10–16). In other words, a transformative experience is one that radically changes the people who go through it in a way that one "is no longer the same person as before," and the qualities of the process of changing cannot be properly anticipated or imagined by individuals except after they have been through the changes themselves. Havi Carel and Ian Kidd (2020) propose an analysis of the COVID-19 pandemic as a transformative experience. The account of loneliness presented here can be useful to articulate the *epistemic* transformation that is part of the pandemic in the way they have argued. Epistemically, transformative experiences are constituted by new attitudes or qualitative changes in the way we consider some relevant items of our experience. New ways of understanding or new ways of entertaining certain content involve emotional changes. That is, although we might have had a qualitative understanding of what it means to have a certain experience of our dependence on others before the pandemic, we can only fully understand what this means by living through the processes and feeling the emotions it triggered. Emotions like pandemic loneliness have a substantial role in creating this phenomenal or qualitative knowledge. Such knowledge is distinct from the phenomenal experience of simple *qualia*, raw emotions, or unarticulated affective contents. It is characterized by a unique phenomenology that includes felt qualities of suffering and discomfort. It's that discomfort associated with loneliness that makes an absence salient.

In sum, loneliness contributes to understanding the pandemic as a transformative experience because it reveals the need for connection and warmth that accompanies conviviality, in a particular and much deeper way than any propositional apprehension or inferences based on previous experiences or even certain qualitative pre-pandemic consciousness of the importance of social relations. In other words, the pandemic loneliness makes absence salient, and the salience taught us to understand things in a new way, with new connections.

Acknowledgments

For encouragement and helpful comments on earlier versions of this chapter I would like to thank Robson Reis, Leonardo de Mello Ribeiro, Marta Nunes, Flademir Williges, and especially Felipe Nogueira de Carvalho. Many thanks also to Evandro Barbosa for his suggestions and for inviting me to discuss the paper in the Symposium on Pandemic Relations at the University of Pelotas, Brazil, in 2020. For revision and stylistic suggestions, I am grateful to Luiz Coletto.

Notes

1 An important qualification for my argument here has to do with personality differences regarding goods associated with social life. Loneliness is a negative emotion brought about by the perception of a lacking in some social goods that come from socializing, being with others, and giving them and receiving their support (Roberts and Krueger 2021). People with introverted personalities tend not to value interpersonal relationships as much as extroverts, and are thus less susceptible to feeling unpleasantness or unhappiness when deprived of companionship. So it would seem that the thesis advanced here does not hold to the same degree for introverts. Yet, given that loneliness turns on the subjective valuing of social goods, the thesis may still hold for universally, albeit in varying degrees. The acknowledgment of the significance of others for ourselves and of our own vulnerabilities and dependency on others is subjectively felt by everyone, including introverts. I thank an anonymous reviewer of this chapter for having called my attention to this point.

2 Familiar objects appear here as part of an extended experience in the material culture, like the potential of music for bringing about integrative contexts of emotional awareness (Krueger and Szanto 2016).

3 The expression "physical endurance" was used by Etty Hillesum, a young Jewish woman who was imprisoned in the Westerbork ghetto in Holland and later sent to Auschwitz, to describe the affective impact of her therapist and lover. In the intimacy of her diary, she wrote, "He talked and I listened, all surrender, and now and then he put his hand very tenderly on my face. And that's how I went home, with the most conflicting feelings, rebellious ones because I thought he was mean, and tender ones, overflowing with human kindness and warmth. And all the while I was overwhelmed by erotic fantasies brought on by the guileful movements of his hands. For a few days I could do nothing but think of him. Though you couldn't really call it thinking, it was more like a sort of *physical endurance* test he was subjecting me to.

His great supple body threatened me from all sides, it was on top of me, under me, everywhere, it threatened to crush me, I was quite unable to work and thought in horror, my God, what have I let myself in for" (Etty Hillesum, *A Life Interrupted: The Diaries, 1941–1943 and Letters from Westerbork*. New York: Henry Holt and Company, 1966).

4 Many thanks are owed to Felipe Nogueira de Carvalho for discussion here.

5 This spatial sense of loneliness was explored in the material of an advertising campaign by the Finnish Helsinki Missio entity. The campaign consisted of showing busy spots in Helsinki, such as a square then empty because of the pandemic, accompanied by the message, "For some people, this is how the world has always felt. Show the lonely they are not alone" (*Scandinavian Way. Finns use quarantine to support loners*. Scandinavian Way, accessed on April 20, 2020, https://scandinavianway.com.br/finlandia-campanha-solidao-pandemia-coronavirus/). The second photo is from Wuhan, China, in mid-2022 (see Bloomberg, Wuhan Locks Down 1 Million Residents in Echo of Pandemic's Start. July 26, 2022, https://www.bloomberg.com/news/articles/2022-07-27/wuhan-locks-down-1-million-residents-in-echo-of-pandemic-s-start).

References

Alberti, Fay Bound. 2019. *A Biography of Loneliness: The History of an Emotion*. (Oxford: Oxford University Press)

Allen, Kelly-Ann, Kern, Margaret L., Rozek, Christopher S., McInerney, Dennis M., and Slavich, George M. 2021. "Belonging: A review of conceptual issues, an integrative framework, and directions for future research." *Australasian Journal of Psychology*, 73(1): 87–102. DOI 10.1080/00049530.2021.1883409

Antonelli-Salgado, Thyago, Monteiro, Gabriela Massaro Carneiro, Marcon, Grasiela, Roza, Thiago Henrique, Zimerman, Aline, Hoffmann, Maurício Scopel, Cao, Bo, Hauck, Simone, Brunoni, André Russowsky, and Passos, Ives Cavalcante. 2021. "Loneliness, but not social distancing, is associated with the incidence of suicidal ideation during the COVID-19 outbreak: A longitudinal study." *Journal of Affective Disorders*, 290(1): 52–60. DOI: 10.1016/j.jad.2021.04.044

Banerjee, Debanjan, and Rai, Mayank. 2020. "Social isolation in COVID-19: The impact of loneliness." *International Journal of Social Psychiatry*, 66(6): 525–527. DOI: 10.1177/0020764020922269

Bekhet, A.K., Zauszniewski, J.A., and Nakhla, W.E. 2008. "Loneliness: A concept analysis." *Nursing Forum*, 43: 207–213. DOI: 10.1111/j.1744-6198.2008.00114.x

Brooks, Samantha K., Webster, Rebecca K., Smith, Louise E., Woodland, Lisa, Wessely, Simon, Greenberg, Neil, and Rubin, Gideon James. 2020. "The psychological impact of quarantine and how to reduce it: Rapid review of the evidence." *The Lancet*, 395(10227): 912–920. DOI: 10.1016/S0140-6736(20)30460-8.

Cacioppo, John T., and Patrick, William. 2008. *Loneliness: Human Nature and the Need for Social Connection*. (New York: W.W Norton & Company).

Carel, Havi, and Kidd, Ian James. 2020. "Pandemic transformative experience: Havi Carel and Ian James Kidd explain how COVID-19 is changing us." *The Philosophers' Magazine*, 90: 24–31. DOI: 10.5840/tpm20209059

Colombetti, G., and Ratcliffe, M. 2012. "Bodily feeling in depersonalization: A phenomenological account." *Emotion Review*, 4(2): 145–150. DOI: 10.1177/1754073911430131

Dahlberg, Lena. 2021. "Loneliness during the COVID-19 pandemic." *Aging & Mental Health*, 25(7): 1161–1164. DOI: 10.1080/13607863.2021.1875195

Deonna, Julien, and Teroni, Fabrice. 2012. *Emotions: A Philosophical Introduction*. (Oxford: Oxford University Press).

Folk, Dunigan, Okabe-Miyamoto, Karynna, Dunn, Elizabeth, and Lyubomirsky, Sonja. 2020. "Did social connection decline during the first wave of COVID-19? The role of extraversion." *Collabra: Psychology*, 6: 1–13. DOI: 10.1525/collabra.365

Goularte, Jeferson Ferraz, Serafim, Silvia Dubou, Colombo, Rafael, Hogg, Bridget, Caldieraro, Marco Antonio, and Rosa, Adriane Ribeiro. 2021. "COVID-19 and mental health in Brazil: Psychiatric symptoms in the general population." *Journal of Psychiatric Research*, 132: 32–37. DOI 10.1016/j.jpsychires.2020.09.021

Guruge, Sepali, Lamaj, Paula, Lee, Charlotte, Ronquillo, Charlene Esteban, Sidani, Souraya, Leung, Ernest, Ssawe, Andrew, Altenberg, Jason, Amanzai, Hasina, and Morrison, Lynn. 2021. "COVID-19 restrictions: Experiences of immigrant parents in Toronto." *AIMS Public Health* 8(1): 172–185. DOI: 10.3934/publichealth.2021013

Krueger, Joel. 2014. "Dewey's rejection of the emotion/expression distinction." In *Neuroscience, Neurophilosophy and Pragmatism. New Directions in Philosophy and Cognitive Science*, edited by Tȳbor Solymosi, John R. Shook. (London: Palgrave Macmillan).

Krueger, Joel, and Szanto, Thomas. 2016. "Extended emotions." *Philosophy Compass*, 11(12): 863–878. DOI:10.1111/phc3.12390

Killam, Kasley. 2020. "In the midst of the pandemic, loneliness has leveled out." *Scientific American*. August 18. https://www.scientificamerican.com/article/in-the-midst-of-the-pandemic-loneliness-has-leveled-out

Lampraki, Charikleia, Hoffman, Adar, Roquet, Angélique, and Daniela, Jopp. 2022. "Loneliness during COVID-19: Development and influencing factors." *PLoS One* 30: 1–20. DOI: 10.1371/journal.pone.0265900

Luchetti, Martina, Lee, Ji Hyun, Aschwanden, Amanda Sesker, Strickhouser, Jason E., Terraciano, Antonio, and Sutin, Angelina. 2020. "The trajectory of loneliness in response to COVID-19." *American Psychologist*, 75(7): 897–908. DOI: 10.1037/amp0000690

Montemurro, Nicola. 2020. "The emotional impact of COVID-19: From medical staff to common people." *Brain, Behavior, and Immunity*, 87: 232–235. DOI: 10.1016/j.bbi.2020.03.032

Ornell, Felipe, Schuch, Jaqueline B. Sordi, Anne O, and Kessler, Felix Henrique. 2020. "Pandemic fear and COVID-19: Mental health burden and strategies." *Brazilian Journal of Psychiatry* 42(3): 222–235. DOI: 10.1590/1516-4446-2020-0008

Paul, Laurie.2014. *Transformative Experience*. (Oxford: Oxford University Press).

Price, Carolyn. 2015. *Emotion*. (London: Polity Press).

Ratcliffe, M. 2005. "The feeling of being." *Journal of Consciousness Studies*, 12(8–10): 43–60.

Ratcliffe, M. 2008. *Feelings of Being. Phenomenology, Psychiatry and the Sense of Reality*. (Oxford: Oxford University Press).

Roberts, Tom, and Krueger, Joel. 2021. "Loneliness and the emotional experience of absence." *The Southern Journal of Philosophy*, 59(2): 1–20.

Slaby, Jan. 2008. "Affective intentionality and the feeling body." *Phenomenology and the Cognitive Sciences*, 7(4): 429–444. DOI: 10.1007/s11097-007-9083-x

Stocker, Michael. 2004. "Some considerations about intellectual desires and emotions." In *Thinking about Feeling. Contemporary Philosophers on Emotions*, edited by Robert C. Solomon. (Oxford: Oxford University Press). pp. 135–151.

Sugaya, Nagisa, Tetsuya, Yamamoto, Suzuki, Naho, and Chigusa, Uchiumi. 2022. "The transition of social isolation and related psychological factors in 2 mild lockdown periods during the COVID-19 pandemic in japan: longitudinal survey study." *JMIR Public Health and Surveillance*, 8(3): e32694. DOI: 10.2196/32694

Trigg, Dylon. 2020. "The role of atmosphere in shared emotion." *Emotion, Space and Society*, 35, 2020. DOI: 10.1016/j.emospa.2020.100658.

Zhong, Bao-Liang, Chen, Shu-Lin, Tu, Xin, and Conwell, Yeates. 2017. "Loneliness and cognitive function in older adults: findings from the Chinese longitudinal healthy longevity survey." *Journals of Gerontology B Psychological Sciences and Social Sciences*, 72(1): 120–128. DOI: 10.1093/geronb/gbw037

4 From fear to anger

An investigation of the relationship between negative emotions and populism in the context of COVID-19

Matheus de Mesquita Silveira

4.1 Introduction

Since Ancient Greece, the study of rhetoric in philosophy has been drawn to emotions. *Pathē tēs psychēs* – the affections of the soul, or, simply, emotions – were one of the focuses of Greek investigations into the ability of rhetoricians to manipulate the emotional states of their audience. The relevance of these analyses in ancient times derived from the acuity given to the study of particular types of emotions. After all, some ancient intuitions concerning anger, pity, shame, or envy are echoed by contemporary investigations on the subject in various areas of science. Although the investigation carried out in this chapter is not based on an exegesis of classical authors, the philosophical relevance of the study of emotions as they pertain to adherence to political discourse remains. The present chapter focuses on the manipulation of fear and anger by populist rhetoric in the wake of the COVID-19 pandemic.

Infectious diseases have been present since time immemorial, but the contemporary world provides a particularly fertile ground for the spread of pathogens. Ferguson et al. (2020) use HIV, Ebola, Zika, and H1N1 as examples. The authors stress that globalized life facilitates the emergence of pandemics, which bring in their wake major political and social consequences that impact the biopsychic structure of individuals. Since the World Health Organization (WHO) recognized COVID-19 as a pandemic, misinformation and disinformation about the virus have driven insecurity, fear, and disbelief on a global scale. Malta, Rimoin, and Strathdee (2020) note that insufficient control measures and the absence of an adequate psychological response tend to aggravate the emotional overload present in a pandemic world. As a result, growing uncertainties have direct consequences on the mental health of individuals, which impact their reading of reality and decision-making in the public sphere.

The question is whether there is a corollary effect of fear and anger concomitant with the pandemic of COVID-19. Luo et al. (2021) reviewed 44 articles addressing the presence of fear during the pandemic, with a sample size of 52,462. A combined average of 18.57 was found for

DOI: 10.4324/9781003310129-5

fearful dispositions related to COVID-19, slightly higher in women (20.67) than in men (18.21). However, the results presented by meta-regression analysis indicate no significant association between such emotion and the age of the participants. The intergenerational average points to the homogeneity of fear among generational groups, which grew up in very different social and cultural contexts (especially concerning technology, health care, and medicine). The research concludes that the average fear related to COVID-19 was high worldwide, pointing to the need to pay attention to the effects of the pandemic on the emotional structure and mental health of individuals.

Concerning anger, Smith et al. (2021) found that 56.1% of survey participants reported having arguments, feeling angry, or having a fight with someone because of the COVID-19 pandemic. The research associated factors such as age and the possibility of experiencing financial insecurity due to COVID-19 as relevant to confrontations between individuals and groups. Another relevant factor is that a greater dependence on social media as a source of information about COVID-19 is associated with anger, given that such associations remained significant even when controlled for sociodemographic characteristics. Allington et al. (2020) state that misinformation and conspiracy theories about COVID-19 spread rapidly through social media and were associated with decreased adherence to government guidelines. Although endorsement of a face-covering conspiracy theory was not associated with anger in the study by Smith et al. (2021), this behavior was strongly associated with interpersonal confrontation. In this scenario, the disinformation and conspiracy theories typical of the far-right populist discourses of the 21st century may have contributed to the increase in tension between individuals and groups.

The context of social anxiety combined with chronic fear is posed by Jost et al. (2003) as influential for the advancement of political conservatism. The point is that the maintenance of prevailing social signs influences one's perception of the reduction of uncertainty, regardless of whether it is real or imaginary. Mudde (2007) adds to this position by arguing that anxiety is not directly related to political extremism but does provide a fertile ground for ideological aspects contingent on this political spectrum, such as authoritarianism and fascism. In this sense, an important resource for understanding the growth of these forms of populism in the context of COVID-19 is direct investigation of the emotional dispositions that underlie these political attitudes.

Druckman and McDermott (2008) developed an approach focusing on the effect of emotions on social dispositions and high-risk behaviors, but without considering the influence of dispositional differences and social contexts. Therefore, in order to address this issue, an integrated approach is needed to systematically assess the way in which variations in fear and anger are relevant factors in the political proclivities of individuals. Adding this element can provide a better understanding of differential susceptibility to various environmental contingencies – notably, the role that the contemporary context has played in this process. In this sense, the present chapter will focus on the impact that fear and anger have on social behavior inherent to the populist advance of extremist bias within the COVID-19 scenario worldwide.

4.2 Pandemic stressors and the psychobiological bases of fear

Fear is a natural reaction to potentially lethal threats. Indeed, McEwen (2007) argues that this emotion is an adaptive response to infectious diseases, consisting of an expected protective reaction. Morens, Folkers, and Fauci (2008, 717) emphasize that "emerging infections remain among the principal challenges to human survival." Regarding viral pandemics, Towers et al. (2020) document the presence of fear and stress throughout the history of various outbreaks. This is true with COVID-19, where the presence of stressors that intensify fear and anger is empirically verifiable, and their manifestation is underwritten by real-world data.

The viral agent of COVID-19 is undetectable by the senses, and symptoms become manifest only days after infection. The consequences are similar to those described by Cheung (2015) in relation to Ebola. The author states that the submicroscopic properties of the virus generate stress due to uncertainty regarding the risk of exposure to contamination, intensifying fear. After onset of the initial symptoms, the development of COVID-19 is debilitating and deeply distressing. Krishnamoorthy et al. (2020) report that, as patients struggle with physically stressful symptoms, they become aware of the possibility of dying alone. Isolation also affects the relatives of those infected, constituting a stressor that intensifies fear-related responses in all those involved.

> The most important subgroup, i.e., the victims of the infection, face the fear of dying from the disease, isolation from family, losing their job, facing discrimination and getting stigmatized by the society. All these problems have in turn increased the fear of social isolation, loneliness, fear of getting the disease and dying, staying away from family, anxiety, depression, stress, insomnia, sleep disturbances and psychological distress.
>
> (Krishnamoorthy et al. 2020, 1)

Quarantine is also a stressful experience on a psychological and social level. Brooks et al. (2020) describe loss of freedom, financial insecurity, separation from friends and family, social stigma, and uncertainty about exposure to illness as emotional stressors in this scenario. This context is regarded by Arwady et al. (2015) as recurrent in pandemic periods. According to the author, public health measures to curb the spread of the virus, such as social distancing and banning gatherings, have a dual effect:

(i) they intensify fear reactions prompted by the social context of the catastrophe and (ii) incite anger and unrest in response to loss of freedom. In this scenario, it is plausible to address that fear increases the emotional stress of confinement, while anger elicits an aggressive disposition, increasing the risk of contamination by persons breaking quarantine.

Steimer (2002) points out that fear is an acute stress response, not only felt but physiologically detectable. In other words, it is an adaptation that focuses the individual's attention on potentially dangerous situations – a behavioral reaction to environmental changes. In pandemic settings, Farmer (2001) notes that fear is intensified when traditional referents for the control of viral disease collapse or are invalidated. In this scenario, the emotional response acquires renewed motivational strength to drive defensive behavior or escape, both physical and mental. While physical escape involves withdrawing one's body from the space of the threat, mental escape can entail a denial of danger itself.

> The main function of fear and anxiety is to act as a signal of danger, threat, or motivational conflict, and to trigger appropriate adaptive responses. [...] Ethologists define fear as a motivational state aroused by specific stimuli that give rise to defensive behavior or escape.
>
> (Steimer 2002, 233)

Accordingly, fear-associated behavioral patterns were categorized by Bracha (2004) as fight-or-flight responses. The author argues that such inclinations can trigger an exponential domino effect of aggressive actions in the social and political domain. Regarding pandemics, Shultz et al. (2016a) define that fear can be triggered by a threat regarding a potentially traumatic event, regardless of whether the danger is real or imagined.[1] As a motivating force, this emotion can spread gregariously and be highly contagious. Like a virus, fear spreads among groups that share similar anxieties or concerns and is fed back by the perception that individuals have of the same behaviors in one another.

> These fear-related behaviors can be an individual or collective response to a perceived threat or to an actual exposure to a potentially traumatizing event. These behaviors are rarely founded on clear reasoning or accurate perception of risks, yet they can shape events powerfully and coalesce into the collective actions of families, social groups, and entire neighborhoods.
>
> (Shultz et al. 2016a, 304–305)

Kendler et al. (2008) emphasize that individuals are differentially predisposed to react fearfully in response to unusual circumstances, which leads to a difference in sensitivity to threat perception. Thus, it is plausible to consider that psychobiological systems exhibit plasticity in the fear reaction as a response to external groups, and that this differentiation may even be able to influence ideological belonging. On the one hand, certain circumstances favor cooperation with strangers and the exploration of new interactions, despite the risk of exposure to possible confrontations. Otherwise, alternative conditions would benefit less cooperation, with greater fear and mistrust being fundamental to survival. Considering that these variations are adaptive, and these behavioral traits are psychobiological constitutional among social mammals, it is plausible to consider that they still exert some influence on contemporary decision-making.

Regarding COVID-19, it is still quite difficult to quantify prosocial actions within the spectrum of interpersonal relationships that have effectively mitigated fear by preserving personal safety. Beyond breaks in quarantine, some people are still maintaining social distance and mitigating the spread of the virus. However, it became clear in the first years of the pandemic that fear-related behaviors created highly negative consequences, from increased risk of contamination to an explosion of aggressiveness, compounded by the populism of extremist discourses aimed at the segregation of social groups. To understand this relationship, one must arguably investigate how emotions influence social perception.

4.3 The influence of fear and anger on social perception

The multidisciplinary perspective proposed in this chapter seeks to investigate the relationships between emotional dispositions and sociopolitical behavior both from the standpoint of cultural and social contexts, as well as through an understanding of the psychobiological foundations that constitute emotions. For instance, Kosfeld et al. (2005) found that oxytocin modulates trust behaviors, and this process regulates anxiety and influences the formation of social bonds. Stenner (2005), in turn, found that the perception of social threat potentiates authoritarianism, while Canetti-Nisim et al. (2009) found that the perception of danger influences political attitudes toward minorities. Based on experimental research on emotions, Halperin, Canetti-Nisim, and Hirsch-Hoefler (2009) found that adherence to hate speech is influenced by fear. It is noteworthy that the methodological plurality of these different positions helps to explain how fear conditions the perception of external groups and social behaviors related to the unknown.

Emotional states can be distinguished by their valence dimension, in which emotions of the same spectrum tend to correlate. For example, negative emotional experiences such as anger and fear can co-occur in specific contexts. Marcus, Neuman, and MacKuen's (2000) theory of political emotions is circumscribed within this theoretical framework. The authors understand the emotional dimension as structured within an elbow room between enthusiasm and anxiety, respectively associated with dispositional psychobiological threat-monitoring systems.

When one regards fear as a natural response to threats, it becomes plausible to place uncertainty regarding the presence of danger in the COVID-19 context as a strong behavioral trigger in the search for situational control. Rico, Guinjoan, and Anduiza (2017) believe that the perception that a given context is the result of uncontrollable circumstances implies that the individual lacks a clear intuition of how the threat can be avoided. The sense of uncertainty that governs fear states generally translates into increased vigilance, information seeking, and systematic judgment processing. However, the effort to avoid damage and reduce uncertainties does not imply greater judiciousness regarding one's sources of information and does not prevent aversive emotions from influencing judgments.

Background and social context can make individuals, even when endowed with the same psychobiological structure, react differently to identical stimuli. Therefore, there are differences regarding the antecedents and consequences of different emotions within the same valence field. MacKuen et al. (2010) integrate aversion behavior into their theory of political emotions, which encompasses negative reactions such as anger, disgust, contempt, and hatred. The authors stress that individuals move across familiar environments based on established habits. Within this sphere, when faced with groups, causes, discourses, or symbols that deconstruct this familiarity, some of the aforementioned emotions can be expected to be elicited.

> Aversion – which includes feelings of anger, disgust, contempt, and hatred – signals the need to confront an adversary. When familiar aversive stimuli are encountered, people rely on previously learned routines to manage these situations, just as they do for familiar rewarding circumstances. They often simply ignore uncomfortable information or, alternatively, bolster their own views by seeking conforming information.
>
> (Mackuen et al. 2010, 441)

Small, Lerner, and Fischhoff (2006) point out that emotions are intrinsic to moral judgments in a way that is consistent with the central paradigm of emotion appraisal theories. For example, angry reactions can be triggered by a failure of expectation toward those believed to be able to cope with a given situation. In the political field, it is plausible to consider that anger arises as a response to a perceived threat to the social structure to which one is accustomed. Likewise, it can be triggered by deliberate or negligent behavior by others, particularly if they are in leadership positions. Isbell and Lair (2013), in turn, highlight that emotional states regulate and constitute judgments both within and beyond the specific circumstances that elicit them. The authors state that negative emotions intensify the perception of the illegitimacy and injustice of an action or event, being substantive to the composition of the perception of degradation of the integrity of those who perceive it as such.

The argument up to this point is that emotions not only arise in response to specific situations but also influence the perception and consequent interpretation of events – even those that are, apparently, not directly related. Individuals who are afraid are predisposed to perceive social contexts as more unpredictable and determined by circumstances beyond their control. The response to this scenario is an increase in aggression. Once imbued with anger, they are more likely to blame others and judge actions that harm them as unfair. In a scenario such as COVID-19, it is plausible to consider that emotions are influencing the social and political perceptions of individuals. To move further on this question, the next step will be to understand the psychobiological bases that connect fear and anger to political preferences.

4.3.1 Connecting fear and anger to political preferences

The review of the political, psychological, and biological literature presented earlier suggests that individuals with high levels of fear are more prone to aggressive behavior. Antony et al. (2005) note that one's level of chronic fear reflects one's threshold for comfort with the lack of familiarity with others, be they institutions, social groups, or particular individuals. The authors believe one of the social consequences of this behavioral disposition is the emergence of substantial underlying biases against political and social out-groups. This is exactly the type of fear that is present during pandemics, like COVID-19. It is noted that this emotional state potentiates political stances of aversion toward immigrants or ethnic minorities, intensifying one's interpretation of these groups as threats to a particular vision of social order. This phobic aversion is manifested by adherence to punitive policies directed against out-groups for the sake of community protection, notably through exclusionary guidelines such as segregation or support for anti-immigration laws.

The previous argument represents only one layer in explaining the influence of chronic fear on social and political behavior. Schreiber et al. (2012) suggest that political preferences are linked to negative emotions and one's sense of threat. Santos, Meyer-Lindenberg, and Deruelle (2010) propose that influences of this nature inform the stereotyping of external groups and are constitutive of social fear. This reflects the position of Hatemi and McDermott (2012), who suggest adherence to political ideologies is influenced by the human psychobiological constitution.

> Most of the correlation between social fear and immigration attitudes was due to a common genetic factor. This suggests that genes do not directly affect specific attitudes, but rather genetic propensity influences the disposition and operation of an emotive condition, which then manifests toward many targets, including strangers and out-groups, when elicited.
>
> (Hatemi and McDermott 2012, 529)

Hatemi et al. (2011) present suggestive evidence that N-methyl-D-aspartate, glutamate, serotonin, dopamine, and G protein-coupled receptors are implicated in political preferences on the liberalism–conservatism axis. These receptors are associated with cognitive-behavioral performance, both with respect to modulation of aggression, anxiety, impulsivity, fear conditioning, and social behavior, as well as with prosocial cooperation and learning. This point is relevant, as it shows that the argument does not involve biological reductionism concerning political preferences, but rather that psychobiological systems influence the perception of culturally informed contexts. In other words, genetic influence is one of the foundations of social experience, but it is not the only one, and cultural constructs matter, as individuals learn who the out-group is through social reinforcement.

Here the argument goes in the direction of a close relation, through psychobiological systems, between political attitudes toward out-groups and the chronic fear characteristic of pandemics. The findings of Hatemi et al. (2013) suggest that social fear derives in part from psychobiological systems, through which variation in response to threats can arise in a population. The point is that the way in which fear is triggered and remains present in an individual is influenced by their natural structure, while the target group to which related emotions are directed will be constituted by the sociocultural construct of which they are part. The social disposition of fear is grounded on psychobiological systems whose role it is to regulate the level of anxiety and sensitivity to the perception of external threats, which are dysfunctionally potentiated in contexts such as COVID-19. In turn, cultural elements and personal experiences will determine who or what will be identified as an out-group.

> These dispositions might then influence individual differences in such areas as discomfort around novel situations and people, expressed as either social phobic-fear or political attitudes, depending on the domain. In this way, social fear provides a measure of the anxiety individuals experience toward unfamiliar others, and this fear and negative attitudes toward political out-groups covary because they share a common genetic origin.
>
> (Hatemi et al. 2013, 283)

The link between chronic fear and prejudice toward out-groups is expressed in different ways in non-pandemic contexts. These attitudes are usually institutionalized and manifest themselves in an observable manner in ordinary political stances, e.g., toward immigration and segregation. In contexts such as COVID-19, the constant presence of a fear stimulus and the emergence of a large-scale phobia are constituted, at least in part, by psychobiological systems. The hypothesis is that a pandemic of fear would potentiate existing dispositions and make individuals more susceptible to emotional manipulation by populist rhetoric, which can intensify manifestations against specific groups identified as out-groups.

4.4 Populism and its relationship to fear and anger

One can reach something of a consensus definition of populism by considering a core set of basic characteristics. Mudde (2004) defines this political practice as a *subtle ideology* that aims to divide society into relatively homogeneous, antagonistic groups. The author classifies these groups as *the corrupt elite* and *the pure people*. In the context of COVID-19, populist governments, guided by extremist ideologies, made ample use of speeches in which they pitted *honest and hardworking folks* (the pure people) against health organizations (the corrupt elite), presenting them as being in opposition to the alleged general will of the people – supported by *upstanding citizen* rhetoric.

> I define populism as an ideology that considers society to be ultimately separated into two homogeneous and antagonistic groups, "the pure people" versus "the corrupt elite", and which argues that politics should be an expression of the *volonté générale* (general will) of the people.
>
> (Mudde 2004, 543)

COVID-19 has heightened aversion against any restrictions on *citizens' rights* based on the absolute primacy of an alleged sovereignty of the people. These practices are exemplified in official speeches which encouraged disobedience to practices such as social distancing or mask-wearing. Stanley (2008) reinforces this point by conceiving populism as composed of four central elements: (i) a division between homogeneous groups, (ii) praise for the pure people and defamation of the corrupt elite, (iii) an antagonistic relationship between the groups classified as the people and the elite, and (iv) the rhetoric of popular sovereignty. This creates a Manichaean political struggle of the *common sense of the pure people* against the *malign power of the selfish elite*.

The aforementioned rhetoric is effective in directing anger by enhancing the specific functions attributed to this emotion. Its relationship with fear is somewhat more complex, since fear can motivate one to escape from confrontation, which presents a problem for notably warlike ideological structures. In this case, empowering the population through rhetoric that offers it an enemy it can beat is a characteristic strategy of extremist ideologies. Of course, not every individual will react in the same way to identical stimuli; after all, not everyone is equally beset by the anxiety and fear caused by COVID-19. It again bears stressing that there are individual differences in emotional dispositions, and this influences the way individuals adhere to such practices.

Hatemi et al. (2013) point out that, although there is a standard genetic disposition that influences social fear and attitudes toward segregation, there is no relationship between a specific gene, one's disposition of fear, and political preferences that is reducible to a purely biological level. The authors state that there are divergent dispositions of aversion to strange individuals, but prolonged exposure to the unknown makes it familiar and no longer unknown. This strengthens the argument that the definition of *unknown* may change over time, with culture and personal experience being relevant factors. The dispositional nature of biologically informed negative emotions will hardly be fixed; it is plastic and can be modulated by different personal and collective contexts. Thus, both the chronic fear that underlies social phobia and cultural constructs play an important role in attitudes toward out-groups.

> If one or both parents have high levels of self-report phobic-fears, there is a significant, but modest correlation with more conservative offspring attitudes and a lesser but significant correlation with out-group attitudes. These findings provide some hint that the causal path operates through fear and not through attitudes; yet education of the parents has an important role in mediating fear of out-groups. In addition, the findings also hint at the potential for passive gene-environment covariation, where the parents create a specific home environment influenced by their own genetic characteristics, which may be competing (e.g., education vs. fear).
>
> (Hatemi et al. 2013, 287)

Panizza (2005) states that populist uprisings occur as a result of frustration with the political system's unresponsiveness to popular demands. Vasilopoulou, Halikiopoulou, and Exadaktylos (2014) add that the ascription of responsibility is present in populist politics, highlighting in particular the *blame transfer* rhetoric. In turn, Hameleers, Bos, and de Vreese (2017, 871) state that "populism is inherently about attributing blame to others while absolving the people of responsibility." Responsibility is assigned to someone else, characterized as a unified bloc as opposed to the *pure people*, by building the image of an external agent that prevents the in-group from achieving its goals. The authors conclude that negative emotions find fertile ground in populism due to the causal apprehension in which an *outsider* is responsible for the problems faced by individuals.

Aversion to leadership in crisis contexts was associated by Steenbergen and Ellis (2006) with the belief that the threat is controllable, inclining individuals to blame institutions for the situation in which they find themselves. In turn, Rico, Guinjoan, and Anduiza (2017) state that attributing blame is key to the emergence of aggressive behaviors. This lends plausibility to the idea that causal relationships play a relevant role in the emotional apprehension of the actions of authorities in times of crisis. In the context of the COVID-19 pandemic, feeling angry about protective measures relates to a certainty on the part of individuals regarding the capacity of institutions to control the virus – responsibility for which is assigned in advance by populist rhetoric to an out-group (i.e., the WHO and the scientists who are investigating the disease).[2] The argument is that the responsibility ascribed to an out-group and the breach of expectations incites anger and triggers negative judgments of negligence (if the threat is perceived as real) or deceit (if the threat is perceived as false).

> However, the key point that causes anger in politics may be that the agent over whom we nominally have control has not acted in ways that benefit us. Recent research in evolutionary psychology has argued that anger arises when the other party is not placing "sufficient" weight on [our] welfare.
>
> (Steenbergen and Ellis 2006, 689)

Capelos (2013) demonstrated that aggressive emotions are automatic responses to political candidates perceived as *immoral*. In fact, Steenbergen and Ellis (2006) reinforce this point and place moral motivations as the main reason for aversion to US president Bill Clinton after his extramarital affair with Monica Lewinsky. Rico, Guinjoan, and Anduiza (2017) point out that sociopolitical scenarios in which anger results from the perception of injustice, real or imagined, are based on the frustration of a reward perceived by specific groups as legitimately theirs. In this sense, aggressive emotions stem from the perception of those responsible as being in control of the situation and able to take a different course of action than the one chosen.

As noted earlier, populist rhetoric aims to address fear by introducing a palpable threat to the *pure people*. The response of extremist ideologies to assuage this emotion is not to acknowledge the other but to reinforce usually degrading stereotypes. It should be noted that the state of chronic stress caused by COVID-19 intensifies the search for content that helps individuals understand and face new threats – whether they are true or not.[3] This discourse does not aim to eliminate fear as a whole, but rather to reinforce the drive to *fight* for the empowerment of specific groups and the consequent directing of aggression toward out-groups. As a result, *escape* behavior is eliminated through warlike and Manichaean rhetorical elements. Thus, regardless of whether fear or anger is more or less present, individuals have their ordinary political apprehension shaped by these emotions.

4.4.1 Populist rhetoric and information mediated by fear and anger

Moral appraisals motivated by anger are central to the populist belief system. Hawkins (2010, 8) views this phenomenon as "a way of interpreting the moral basis or legitimacy of a political system." Indeed, moralism permeates the rhetoric of populism, in which the vices of the *corrupt elite* are placed in contrast to the virtues of the *pure people*, with the relationship between the two defined by antagonism. Whether as a discourse or as a worldview, the author emphasizes that populism grows among politicians and citizens when there is a perception of widespread violations of culturally rooted social signs and norms.

> [A] populist worldview, or a Manichaean outlook that identify as Good with a unified will of the people and Evil with a conspiring minority, and they convey this set of ideas with a characteristic language – a discourse – full of bellicose, moralizing rhetoric emphasizing the recent subversion of the political system.
>
> (Hawkins 2010, 29)

In the equation between fear and anger, Petersen (2010) points out that the former predisposes to a search for information and what is familiar, while the latter is a response to a perceived violation of rules, in which intentionality is a relevant factor. In the context of COVID-19, access to information in populist governments did not operate through official channels. On the contrary, the intended content reached the *pure people* via their peers, through messages and memes shared on social media. This strategy not only perpetuates the Manichaean dichotomy but serves to assuage fear and transform it into anger directed at the *corrupt elite*, which is blamed for harming the economy, placing the *pure people* in dire straits. Responsibility is shifted from the government to health-care organizations and institutions; fear of the virus is mitigated and turns to anger against those who *conceal the truth* or *are not good enough to contain the threat* – in this case, health officials and scientists.

Albertson and Gadarian (2015) found that individuals tend to trust experts as a way to reduce anxiety in fearful contexts. At first, this inclination is in conflict with both populist Manichaeism and extremist ideologies. However, Hallowell (2005, 57) stresses that "as a specialist in learning disabilities, I have found that the most dangerous disability is not any formally diagnosable condition like dyslexia or ADD. It is fear." That is, fear impairs cognitive processes associated with differentiated learning and understanding. The argument is that, although the fear generated by the presence of a threat such as COVID-19 inclines individuals to a greater search for knowledge, it makes it difficult for them to process and understand information.

The criteria that separate a reliable source from fake news are guided by familiarity with the source of the news. In this scenario, information coming from the in-group is perceived as more reliable than official communications from health organizations. The context of COVID-19 has intensified the efficiency of the spread of populist propaganda through unofficial information channels. In this setting, the fear-driven search for information is manipulated in two ways: (i) threat mitigation by discrediting science and (ii) holding health agencies responsible for adverse situations. The result is a heightened sense of security and increased aggression, targeted at out-groups duly identified by the Manichaean rhetoric of populism.

COVID-19 showed the world as a dangerous place, and this fear still influences individuals' reactions. Although not necessarily directly violent, populism approaches authoritarianism through its policies of segregation. Although whether populism and authoritarianism are personality traits or political ideologies is a matter of debate among social psychologists, Pettigrew (2017) argues that these two perspectives are not in conflict. The author believes inclinations of this type begin as a personality trait that leads to engagement with political extremisms. In this perspective, the motivation lies in the manipulation of fear into anger through hate speech, with Manichaean rhetoric engaging different groups and leading them to consider heads of state such as US former-president Donald Trump and Brazilian president Jair Bolsonaro representative in issues of public health and national sovereignty.[4] After all, they are on the side of the *pure people* against the *corrupt elite*. Much of the support their constituency offers to their policies of segregating out-groups and discrediting health organizations derives from this point.

> Authoritarianism is an intensely studied syndrome the effects of which are surprisingly consistent across the globe. Several traits characterize the syndrome: deference to authority, aggression toward outgroups, a rigidly hierarchical view of the world, and resistance to new experience. Authoritarianism is typically triggered by threat and fear, and authoritarians tend to view the world as a very dangerous and threatening place.
>
> (Pettigrew 2017, 108)

In the context of COVID-19, social anxiety provoked by chronic fear becomes a more influential driver of political leanings. This position is supported by Shultz et al. (2016b), who believe the relationship between this emotion and conservative tendencies is significant in individuals with extreme phobic dispositions. It does not necessarily follow from this that conservatism is phobic or that individuals with social phobia are conservative, but rather that chronic fear increases the likelihood of adhering to this political axis. In turn, Mudde and Kaltwasser (2017) stress that the core ideas of populism are vague enough to encompass different points of view, aggregating different ideologies into a single discourse. Rico, Guinjoan, and Anduiza (2017) add further support for this point by stating that anger inclines individuals to follow superficial stereotypes. Hence, the way in which negative emotions affect information processing is a relevant factor in engaging with populist positions and extremist ideologies.

Many believe that "the people" should take the most important decisions instead of delegating its sovereign power to professional politicians. This notwithstanding, populist attitudes are often latent, i.e., lying dormant or hidden until circumstances are suitable for their development or manifestation.

(Mudde and Kaltwasser 2017, 99)

A review of the conditions that explain the emergence of populism shows that it proliferates through different forms of resentment toward society. Betz (2002, 198) states that "populist rhetoric is designed to tap feelings of resentment and exploit them politically." In the case of popular resentment, the author maintains that negative emotions are the basis of a feeling of frustration, illegitimate harm, identification of an out-group as responsible, and the consequent desire for retaliation. Demertzis (2006, 105), in turn, emphasizes that anger is an "emotional opposition to unequal and unjust situations." Therefore, it is plausible to consider fear and anger as core elements of the feeling of resentment inherent to characterizations of a populist outbreak.

Although no estimation of the regular effects of emotions on political behavior can be demonstrated with experimental data alone, the empirical relevance of the studies presented herein underpins some broader causal claims. In particular, it highlights the argument that populist rhetoric fueled negative emotions directed at WHO guidelines and the scientists responsible for the fight against COVID-19. Moffitt (2015) points out that the populist emphasis on the use of *moral terms* contributes to amplifying anger, turning it into hate. Therefore, the way in which the rhetoric of populism conveyed information regarding the core events of the contemporary context places emphasis on the *injustice to the pure people* and the *responsibility of the corrupt elite* in fighting the pandemic.

Mudde and Kaltwasser (2017) point to a reciprocal relationship between negative emotions and populism, which results in a supply-and-demand effect. In other words, individuals with chronic fear process information with greater difficulty, as they are more receptive to Manichaean reductions, providing fertile ground for populist rhetoric to incite anger and turn it into hatred. Regardless of the causal direction, while fear exerts an indirect influence, anger is directly involved with adherence to ideological extremisms. In this respect, there is no reason to differentiate populism on the right-left axis, as both can manipulate these emotions toward appraisals of injustice and social culpability.[5]

Anger is a catalyst in activating latent segregationist inclinations, which are already widespread in society. After all, the breadth of populist discourse allows it to be adopted by voters of different political orientations. Because it is a simplistic ideology lacking any pragmatic content, it can operate as a host of ideological extremisms, which can develop on either side of the right-left axis. The simple answers offered by populism are seductive in times of uncertainty, and the contemporary context is a fertile ground for its proliferation. In conclusion, in addition to COVID-19, there is a pandemic of fear and its consequent manipulation by populist rhetoric, which turns it into anger, directing this emotion so as to feed it back into political attitudes guided by hatred.

4.5 Conclusion

The present chapter used a multidisciplinary approach to conduct an empirically informed investigation into how the emotions of fear and anger influenced sociopolitical attitudes in the setting of COVID-19. The data presented herein suggest a relationship between the stressful context caused by the risk of virus spread and the existence of a state of chronic fear, which proved to be fertile ground for the development (or intensification of relevant phobias), increasing social stigma and discrimination directed at out-groups. Based on an investigation of negative emotions associated with the lack of familiarity and uncertainty typical of a pandemic context, an exploratory argument was made as to how adherence to populism and segregation policies, influenced by traits of social phobia, was intensified during the pandemic.

Fear proved to be particularly relevant to the populist advance during COVID-19 in an indirect manner, which can be understood in two main aspects. First, as a protective factor, essential for the survival of the species. In this case, the fear of threats such as infectious disease is widespread, yet understandable, as it serves a function (to reduce the risk of contamination). Second, as a risk factor, i.e., a situation in which fear can spread contagiously within a population. In other words, this is an emotion that creates, propagates, and amplifies itself in a feedback loop.

The impact of fear on populism was manifested indirectly both in the pandemic and in previous contexts. Indeed, this emotion seems to affect individuals in different ways and its initial emotional affect is not necessarily uniform. Conversely, fear dispositions tend to differ among the population, which is inclined to react differentially to the unknown – explained, in part, by plastic variation of psychobiological systems as a behavioral drive. These effects are conditioned throughout the lives of individuals by their personal experiences within the culture they inhabit, shaping attachment patterns and triggering social fear of out-groups through psychobiological systems.

The plasticity of psychobiological systems is influenced by sociocultural factors and individual experiences, forming the *biopsychosocial* character of contemporary social behaviors. In this sense, many political leanings are influenced by evolutionary adaptations apart from the contemporary context. After all, fear is an adaptive reaction to unfamiliar situations, avoiding potentially dangerous encounters and offering enhanced protection from the unknown. These behavioral traits are still present and may be redirected by cultural triggers that influence the covariation of negative emotions and aggressive attitudes toward out-groups. Fear and anger are avenues through which segregationist actions can emerge – and a significant way in which psychobiological systems have influenced judgments regarding out-groups in the context of COVID-19.

Regarding the way individuals process information and apprehend social contexts, emotions of the same valence can have different behavioral consequences. The findings presented herein show that populist attitudes are asynchronously motivated and influenced by the emotions of fear and anger. While fear drives a search for information, it simultaneously hinders the cognitive processing thereof; it is also associated with anxiety toward the unknown. Anger, in turn, incites confrontation and demands for punishment, and is easily placed in the populist rhetoric of the *pure people* against the *corrupt elite*s. It thus provides a direct vector to engage individuals in aggressive behavior against out-groups through hate speech.

The different theoretical approaches converge in maintaining that the manipulation of negative emotions is an important factor in adherence to segregated ideologies. Chronic fear is systematically related to *being afraid of the unknown*, hindering the processing of information even as it inclines individuals to search for information. This makes individuals more susceptible to the segregated, simplistic explanations typical of populist rhetoric. Likewise, populist Manichaeism has behavioral implications in the social sphere by directly linking evaluative inclinations driven by aggressive emotions toward specific groups. In the context of COVID-19, anger transformed by hate speech served as a springboard for populism to grow from extremist ideological biases.

Considering that the definition of what is *unknown* is contextual and changes over time, prejudices against specific groups cannot be biologically rooted in psychobiological systems inherent to emotional responses such as fear and anger. In contemporary society, aversions to out-groups are expressed by segregationist attitudes such as opposition to migration or, in the case of COVID-19, to ethnic groups superficially and wrongfully identified with the disease. The point is that this behavior tends to manifest itself in different ways in the future, but will still be motivated by negative emotions. Fear and anger are not harmful in and of themselves; on the contrary, they played an important role in the survival of the species and are still relevant in the contemporary world. Suggesting that prejudices are inevitable or, fallaciously, *genetic* is to deny that the content of *chronic social fears* is substantiated by hate speech, supported by populist rhetoric. In other words, although emotions are biologically constituted, angry attitudes are triggered by specific circumstances relating to cultural constructs and political ideologies.

In conclusion, a broad scenario can be outlined for the rise of populism in the post-COVID-19 crisis. Considering that chronic fear underlies pandemic contexts, it tends to remain present and self-propagate even after the initial threat of the virus has been neutralized. Populist campaigns based on the manipulation of negative emotions will find individuals receptive to a typically Manichean rhetoric regarding contemporary sociopolitical conditions. Given the cognitive and behavioral consequences of fear (i.e., a greater search for information while being less able to process it), there is fertile ground for fear to turn into anger. This process tends to make individuals politically active and willing to support segregationist policies toward out-groups. The chronic influence of these emotions decreases the likelihood of a careful examination of populist discourses, resulting in greater difficulty in fighting post-truth policies (such as fake news propagated through social media). Thus, the greater emotional predisposition to populism raises the need for affirmative emotional policies that respond to both the threat of the virus and the *pandemic of fear* that underlies the contemporary context.

Notes

1 Shultz et al. (2016b) note that, during the 2013–2016 Ebola outbreak, social behaviors were modified by fear in several key points: (i) fear and stress interfered with cognitive processing; (ii) personal assessment of risk was hampered by lack of information – individuals' risk assessments were poor even with good information; (iii) individual actions were strongly influenced by the actions of other individuals, leading to mass *herd* behavior; and (iv) fear-driven actions escalated, compounded by a collapse of cultural references regarding systems of governance and public order. The authors add that this state of fear persists and tends to influence assessments of future risk even after the apparent containment of the threat.

2 For example, on his official Twitter account, the then-president of Brazil, Jair Bolsonaro, wrote that "the WHO, after my demonstration, takes a stand against mandatory vaccination. So now they start to get it right" (October 22, 2020a. Tweet), and later writes, "good night everyone. Mandatory vaccine here only on fire" (October 24, 2020b. Tweet).

3 Bento et al. (2020) shows that searches for *coronavirus* increased 36% after the first case announcement but decreased to baseline in a couple of weeks. However, the research was conducted relatively early in the pandemic, and the authors state that more-elaborate policy responses were not yet part of the public discourse. Kim et al. (2020) examined the implications of exposure to misinformation about COVID-19 using a RISP model. The results showed that misinformation exposure reduced information insufficiency, which increased heuristic processing, leading to a less systematic apprehension of information. Li and Zheng (2022) also applied the RISP model to examine factors contributing to online information seeking about COVID-19. The study found that the high threat appraisal caused by the pandemic triggered fear and anxiety, which motivated the responders to search for related information on the internet.

4 Rico and Anduiza (2019) noted that populist ideas are widespread in European democracies. Pettigrew (2017) reports a similar phenomenon in the

United States. The author describes five factors that influence the uncritical acceptance of Donald Trump by his supporters: (i) authoritarianism, (ii) social dominance orientation (i.e., social familiarity with dominant groups), (iii) prejudice, (iv) intergroup contact (i.e., a low level of contact with outgroups), and (v) relative deprivation, compounded by the feeling that *others* are more advantaged than their own community.

5 Hoggett, Wilkinson, and Beedell (2013) consider that resentment is related to greater adherence to the radical right-wing populism and to policies contrary to social welfare. Likewise, Oliver and Rahn (2016) associate anger with Trump's electoral victory. Rico, Guinjoan, and Anduiza (2017), in turn, report that, although their research is restricted to the left-wing populist advance in Spain with the growth of *Podemos*, the primacy of anger is consistent with different expressions of populism on the right-left axis.

References

Albertson, B.; Gadarian, S. K. 2015. *Anxious Politics: Democratic Citizenship in a Threatening World*. New York: Cambridge University Press.

Allington, D.; Duffy, B.; Wessely, S.; Dhavan, N.; Rubin, J. 2020. "Health-protective behaviour, social media usage and conspiracy belief during the COVID-19 public health emergency." *Psychological Medicine*, 1–7. doi: 10.1017/S003329172000224X

Antony, M. M.; Rowa, K.; Liss, A.; Swallow, S. R.; Swinson, R. P. 2005. "Social comparison processes in social phobia." *Behavior Therapy*, 36(1): 65–75.

Arwady, M. A.; Bawo, L.; Hunter, J. C.; Massaquoi, M.; Matanock, A. M.; Dahn, B.; Ayscue, P.; Nyenswah, T. G.; Forrester, J. D.; Hensley, L.; Monroe, B.; Schoepp, R. J.; Chen, T.; Schaecher, K. E.; George, T.; Rouse, T.; Schafer, I. J.; Pillai, S. K.; De Cock, K. M. 2015. "Evolution of Ebola virus disease from exotic infection to global health priority, Liberia, mid-2014." *Emerging Infectious Diseases*, 21(4): 578–584.

Bento, A. I.; Nguyen, T.; Wing, C.; Lozano-Rojas, F.; Ahn, Y. Y.; Simon, K. 2020. "Evidence from internet search data shows information-seeking responses to news of local COVID-19 cases. Proceedings National." *Academy of Science USA*, 117: 11220–11222.

Betz, H. G. 2002. "Conditions favouring the success and failure of radical right-wing populist parties in contemporary democracies." In Yves Mény and Yves Surel (Eds.), *Democracies and the Populist Challenge*, 197–213. New York: Palgrave.

Bolsonaro, J. M. (@jairbolsonaro). "the WHO (…)" Oct 22, 2020a, 15h23. [Tweet]. Available at: https://bit.ly/3rwEt2R. Access in: October 31, 2022.

Bolsonaro, J. M. (@jairbolsonaro). "Good night everyone (…)." Oct 24, 2020b, 19h36. [Tweet]. Available at: https://bit.ly/39oXldK. Access in: October 31, 2022.

Bracha, H. S. 2004. "Freeze, flight, fight, fright, faint: Adaptationist perspectives on the acute stress response spectrum." *CNS Spectrums*, 9(9): 679–685.

Brooks, S. K.; Webster, R. K.; Smith, L. E.; Woodland, L.; Wessely, S.; Greenberg, N.; Rubin, G. J. 2020. "The psychological impact of quarantine and how to reduce it: Rapid review of the evidence." *The Lancet*, 395: 912–920. doi:10.1016/s0140-6736(20)30460-8

Canetti-Nisim, D.; Halperin, E.; Sharvit, K.; Hobfoll, S. E. 2009. "A new stress-based model of political extremism." *Journal of Conflict Resolution*, 53(3): 363–389.

Capelos, T. 2013. "Understanding anxiety and aversion: The origins and consequences of affectivity in political campaigns." In *Emotions in Politics*, 39–59. Basingstoke: Palgrave Macmillan.

Cheung, E.Y. 2015. "An outbreak of fear, rumours and stigma: Psychosocial support for the Ebola virus disease outbreak in West Africa." *Intervention*, 13(1): 70–76.

Demertzis, N. 2006. "Emotions and populism." In *Emotion, Politics and Society*, 103–122. London: Palgrave Macmillan.

Druckman, J.; McDermott, R. 2008. "Emotion and the framing of risky choice." *Political Behavior*, 30(3): 297–321.

Farmer, P. 2001. *Infections and Inequalities: The Modern Plagues.* Berkeley: University of California Press.

Ferguson, N. M.; Laydon, D.; Nedjati-Gilani, G.; Imai, N.; Ainslie, K.; Baguelin, M.; Bhatia, S.; Boonyasiri, A.; Cucunubá, Z.; Cuomo-Dannenburg, G.; Dighe, A.; Dorigatti, I.; Fu, H.; Gaythorpe, K.; Green, W.; Hamlet, A.; Hinsley, W.; Okell, L. C.; Elsland, S.; Thompson, H.; Verity, R.; Volz, E.; Wang, H.; Wang, Y.; Walker, P. G. T.; Walters, C.; Winskill, P.; Whittaker, C.; Donnelly, C. A.; Riley, S.; Ghani, A. C. 2020. "Report 9: Impact of non-pharmaceutical interventions (npis) to reduce Covid-19 mortality and healthcare demand." *Imperial College London.* doi: https://doi.org/10.25561/77482

Hallowell, E. M. 2005. "Overloaded circuits: Why smart people underperform." *Harvard Business Review*, 83(1): 54–62.

Halperin, E.; Canetti-Nisim, D.; Hirsch-Hoefler, S. 2009. "The central role of group-based hatred as an emotional antecedent of political intolerance: Evidence from Israel." *Political Psychology*, 30(1): 93–123.

Hameleers, M.; Bos, L.; de Vreese, C. H. 2017. "'They did it' the effects of emotionalized blame attribution in populist communication." *Communication Research*, 44(6): 870–900.

Hatemi, P. K.; Gillespie, N. A.; Eaves, L. J.; Maher, B. S.; Webb, B. T.; Heath, A. C.; Medland, S. E.; Smyth, D. C.; Beeby, H. N.; Gordon, S. D.; Montgomery, G. W.; Zhu, G.; Byrne, E. M.; Martin, N. G. 2011. "A genome-wide analysis of liberal and conservative political attitudes." *The Journal of Politics*, 73: 271–285.

Hatemi, P. K.; McDermott. R. 2012. "The genetics of politics: Discovery, challenges, and progress." *Trends in Genetics*, 28(10): 525–533.

Hatemi, P. K.; McDermott, R.; Eaves, L. J.; Kendler, K. S.; Neale, M. C. 2013. "Fear as a disposition and an emotional state: A genetic and environmental approach to out-group political preferences." *American Journal of Political Science*, 57(2): 279–293. doi: 10.1111/ajps.1

Hoggett, P.; Wilkinson, H.; Beedell, P. 2013. "Fairness and the politics of resentment." *Journal of Social Policy*, 42(3): 567–585.

Isbell, L. M.; Lair, E. C. 2013. "Moods, emotions, and evaluations as information." In *The Oxford Handbook of Social Cognition*, 435–462. Oxford: Oxford University Press.

Jost, J. T.; Glaser, J.; Kruglanski, A. W.; Sulloway, F. J. 2003. "Political conservatism as motivated social cognition." *Psychological Bulletin*, 129(3): 339–375.

Kendler, K. S.; Gardner, C. O.; Annas, P.; Lichtenstein, P. 2008. "The development of fears from early adolescence to young adulthood: A multivariate study." *Psychological Medicine*, 38(12): 1759–1769.

Kim, H. K.; Ahn, J.; Atkinson, L.; Kahlor, L. A. 2020. "Effects of Covid-19 misinformation on information seeking, avoidance, and processing: A multicountry comparative study." *Science Communication*, 42(5): 586–615. doi: 10.1177/1075547020959670

Kosfeld, M.; Heinrichs, M.; Zak, P. J.; Fischbacher, U.; Fehr, E. 2005. "Oxytocin increases trust in humans." *Nature*, 435(7042): 673–676.

Krishnamoorthy, Y.; Nagarajan, R.; Saya, G. K.; Menon, V. 2020. "Prevalence of psychological morbidities among general population, healthcare workers and Covid-19 patients amidst the Covid-19 pandemic: a systematic review and meta-analysis." *Psychiatry Research*, 113382. doi: 10.1016/j.psychres.2020.113382

Li, J.; Zheng, H. 2022. "Online information seeking and disease prevention intent during covid-19 outbreak." *Journalism and Mass Communication Quarterly*, 99(1): 69–88. doi: 10.1177/1077699020961518

Luo, F.; Gheshlagh, R. G.; Dalvand, S.; Saedmoucheshi, S; Li, Q. 2021. "Systematic review and meta-analysis of fear of Covid-19." *Frontiers in Psychology*, 12: 661078. doi: 10.3389/fpsyg.2021.661078

MacKuen, M.; Wolak, J.; Keele, L.; Marcus, G. E. 2010. "Civic engagements: Resolute partisanship or reflective deliberation." *American Journal of Political Science*, 54(2): 440–458.

Malta, M.; Rimoin, A. W.; Strathdee, S. A. 2020. "The coronavirus 2019-epidemic: Is hindsight 20/20." *E-Clinical Medicine* 20: 100289. doi: 10.1016/j.eclinm.2020.100289

Marcus, G. E.; Neuman, W. R.; MacKuen, M. 2000. *Affective Intelligence and Political Judgment*. Chicago: University of Chicago Press.

McEwen, B. S. 2007. "Physiology and neurobiology of stress and adaptation: Central role of the brain." *Physiology Review*, 87: 873–904. doi: 10.1152/physrev.00041.2006

Moffitt, B. 2015. "How to perform crisis: A model for understanding the key role of crisis in contemporary populism." *Government and Opposition*, 50(2): 189–217.

Morens, D. M.; Folkers, G. K.; Fauci, A. S. 2008. "Emerging infections: A perpetual challenge." *The Lancet Infectious Diseases*, 8: 710–719.

Mudde, C. 2004. "The populist zeitgeist." *Government and Opposition*, 39(4): 542–563.

Mudde, C. 2007. *Populist Radical Right Parties in Europe*. Cambridge: Cambridge University Press.

Mudde, C.; Kaltwasser, C. R. 2017. *Populism: A Very Short Introduction*. Oxford: Oxford University Press.

Oliver, J. E.; Rahn, W. M. 2016. "Rise of the trumpenvolk: Populism in the 2016 election." *The Annals of the American Academy of Political and Social Science*, 667(1): 189–206.

Panizza, F. 2005. "Introduction: Populism and the mirror of democracy." In *Populism and the Mirror of Democracy*, 1–31. London: Verso.

Petersen, M. B. 2010. Distinct emotions, distinct domains: Anger, anxiety and perceptions of intentionality. *Journal of Politics*, 72(2): 357–365.

Pettigrew, T. F. 2017. "Social psychological perspectives on Trump supporters." *Journal of Social and Political Psychology*, 1(5): 107–116. doi: 10.5964/jspp.v5i1.750

Rico, G.; Anduiza, E. 2019. "Economic correlates of populist attitudes: An analysis of nine European countries in the aftermath of the great recession." *Acta Politic*, 54: 371–397. doi: 10.1057/s41269-017-0068-7

Rico, G.; Guinjoan, M.; Anduiza, E. 2017. "The emotional underpinnings of populism: How anger and fear affect populist attitudes." *Swiss Political Science Review*, 23(4): 444–461.

Santos, A.; Meyer-Lindenberg, A.; Deruelle, C. 2010. "Absence of racial, but not gender, stereo-typing in Williams syndrome children." *Current Biology*, 20(7): 307–308.

Schreiber, D. M.; Simmons, A. N.; Dawes, C. T.; Flagan, T.; Fowler, J. H.; Paulus, M. P. 2012. "Red brain, blue brain: Evaluative processes differ in democrats and republicans." *PLoS One*, 8(2): e52970. doi: 10.1371/journal.pone.0052970

Shultz, J. M.; Althouse, B. M.; Baingana, F.; Cooper, J. L.; Espinola, M.; Greene, M. C.; Espinel, Z.; McCoy, C. B.; Mazurik, L.; Rechkemmer, A. 2016a. Fear factor: The unseen perils of the Ebola outbreak. *Bulletin of the Atomic Scientists*, 72(5): 304–310. doi:10.1080/00963402.2016.1216515

Shultz, J. M.; Cooper, J. L.; Baingana, F.; Oquendo, M. A.; Espinel, Z.; Althouse, B. M.; Marcelin, L. H.; Towers, S.; Espinola, M.; McCoy, C. B.; Mazurik, L.; Wainberg, M. L.; Neria, Y.; Rechkemmer, A. 2016b. "The role of fear-related behaviors in the 2013–2016 west Africa Ebola virus disease outbreak." *Current Psychiatry Reports*, 18: 104. doi: 10.1007/s11920-016-0741-y

Small, D. A.; Lerner, J. S.; Fischhoff, B. 2006. "Emotion priming and attributions for terrorism: Americans' reactions in a national field experiment." *Political Psychology*, 27(2): 289–298.

Smith, L. E.; Duffy, B.; Moxham-Hall, V.; Strang, L.; Wessely, S.; Rubin, G. J. 2021. "Anger and confrontation during COVID-19 pandemic: A national cross-sectional survey in the UK." *Journal of the Royal Society of Medicine*, 114(2): 77–90. doi: 10.1177/0141076820962068

Stanley, B. 2008. "The thin ideology of populism." *Journal of Political Ideologies*, 13(1): 95–110.

Steenbergen, M. R.; Ellis, C. 2006. "Fear and loathing in American elections: Context, traits, and negative candidate affect." In *Feeling Politics: Emotion in Political Information Processing*, 109–133. New York: Palgrave Macmillan.

Steimer, T. 2002. "The biology of fear and anxiety-related behaviors." *Dialogues in Clinical Neuroscience*, 4(3): 231–249.

Stenner, K. 2005. *The Authoritarian Dynamic: Cambridge Studies in Public Opinion and Political Psychology*. New York: Cambridge University Press.

Towers, S.; Afzal, S.; Bernal, G.; Bliss, N.; Brown, S.; Espinoza, B.; Jackson, J.; Judson-Garcia, J.; Khan, M.; Lin, M.; Mamada, M.; Moreno, V. M.; Nazari, F.; Okuneye, K.; Ross, M. L.; Rodriguez, C.; Medlock, J.; Ebert, D.; Castillo-Chavez C. 2020. "Mass media and the contagion of fear: The case of Ebola in America." *PLoS One*, 10(6): e0129179. doi: 10.1371/journal.pone.0129179

Vasilopoulou, S.; Halikiopoulou. D; Exadaktylos, T. 2014. Greece in crisis: Austerity, populism and the politics of blame. *Journal of Common Market Studies*, 52(2): 388–402.

5   "Nobody makes it alone"

Toward a relational view of resilience

Martina Orlandi

5.1 Introduction

The COVID-19 pandemic and the unprecedented challenges it has presented have led to a striking increase in calls to be "resilient." To give a few examples, Canada's prime minister Justin Trudeau praised Canadian's resilience during the pandemic,[1] universities released guidelines for "how to build resilience,"[2] newspapers routinely ran stories of entrepreneurs reinventing their businesses after closing down. A quick Google search on "resilience" and "COVID" yields more than 300,000 results.

Resilience, commonly conceived as the capacity to overcome setbacks, has traditionally enjoyed a positive reputation. Psychological studies have linked resilience to traits like successful regulation of negative emotions, human growth, and subjective well-being (cf. Sisto et al. 2019; Chen et al. 2018; Kong et al. 2018). Philosophical research, on the other hand, has emphasized that, among the advantages of a gritty attitude, "the inertia in the agent's expectations of success will help to protect her against temporary dips in confidence that might otherwise lead her to quit" (Paul and Morton 2019, 196).[3]

But the COVID-19 pandemic has also exposed the limits of resilience, especially when calls for it target individuals who are marginalized. In 2021, writer and film director Zandashé Brown tweeted,

> I dream of never being called resilient again in my life. I'm exhausted by strength. I want support. I want softness. I want ease. I want to be amongst kin. Not patted on the back for how well I take a hit. Or for how many.[4]

Brown's insight captures how calls for resilience often place an emotional burden on *individuals* to find ways to persist through difficult circumstances when what is most needed is instead government support and structural change. My chapter builds on the lived experience of women and minorities like Brown and proposes that we rethink resilience in favor of a new view that contributes to well-being and takes into consideration systemic inequality.

DOI: 10.4324/9781003310129-6

The chapter has two aims. The first aim is to show that the reason why calls for resilience are inadequate is that we have an *individualistic* notion of resilience. I do this in Sections 5.2 and 5.3 where I argue that this individualistic notion is flawed in two ways: (i) at best, it fails to insulate from burnout, and at worst, it can contribute to it by generating psychological harm because it can be experienced as cognitively burdensome, and (ii) it fails to attend to systemic injustices because it discounts how structural oppression can undercut success in overcoming setbacks. In light of this, the second aim of the chapter is to propose a recharacterization of resilience as a *relational* notion that takes into account structural support as well as conditions of oppression and marginalization. I do this in Sections 5.4 and 5.5 where I develop this relational notion of resilience drawing from feminist work on relational views of autonomy and propose a new notion that structurally mirrors causally relational views of autonomy (Sherwin and Stockdale 2017; Mackenzie and Stoljar 2000; Downie and Llewellyn 2012). According to this latter notion of resilience, oppression, lack of material conditions, or lack of structural support can all be external elements that impact its exercise. A relational notion then turns calls for resilience into something that fosters well-being and takes into consideration structural oppression.

Reconceptualizing resilience is both timely and important for not only theoretical but also practical reasons. Theoretically, an analysis of the drawbacks of the individualistic notion of resilience can deepen our understanding of the notion and how it intersects with psychological and sociopolitical frameworks. In this sense, an examination of resilience can contribute to filling in a crucial gap. But an analysis of resilience is also important for practical reasons: understanding the limits of an individualistic notion of resilience, particularly during precarious times (like the COVID-19 pandemic), urges us to reckon even more with the impact that systemic inequality has on people's lives. A relational account of resilience exposes problems with current practices of calling for resilience in response to crises and offers a framework that is better positioned to inform public responses to such crises in ways that benefit individuals and social groups.

5.2 How the individualistic notion of resilience can foster ill-being

Resilience has traditionally been regarded in positive terms, and this reputation has been further reinforced by empirical evidence that shows its advantageous aspects. Chen et al., for example, argue that resilience is comprised of multiple factors that involve strength in facing setbacks, tenacity in overcoming them, and optimism in believing one will succeed (Chen et al. 2018, 1). As such, resilience, and the optimism component specifically, has been linked to the successful regulation of negative emotions whose neural response is inhibited by positive thinking (Chen et al. 2018, 3). Several other studies show that resilience is also associated with "enhance[d] subjective well-being" (Kong et al. 2018, 755). Defined as a multidimensional concept, it has been suggested that hopeful thinking present in resilience plays an important "mediator role" between resilience and subjective well-being, which then leads to "more positive evaluations about cognitive and affective dimensions of life" (Satici 2016, 72).[5]

Focusing on resilience in children, Mandleco and Peery have suggested that resilience is tied to a "higher degree of self-control" and "competence" when facing "frustrations," "threats," difficult family situations, and "dislocation" (Mandleco and Peery 2000, 99–103). Maintaining a positive outlook, a crucial component in resilience, has also been positively related to better health (Smith 2006, 228), as well as mindfulness, positive affect, and self-esteem (Bajaj and Pande 2015, 64; Liu et al. 2014).

Although there is no universally received definition (Mandleco and Peery 2000), resilience is often understood as a successful adaptation that involves recovering from hardships by employing emotional and cognitive resources aimed at restoring an optimistic drive to persevere. It is precisely this dynamic that has led researchers to identify the drawbacks of resilience.

In what follows, I draw on empirical evidence to suggest that resilience, particularly if characterized as individual strength of will, can in some circumstances contribute to individuals' ill-being because it can be experienced as cognitively and emotionally burdensome.

This suggestion, however, will not be uncontroversial. The reason why is that even during a challenging time like the COVID-19 pandemic, in which we have seen worryingly high rates of burnout, a large number of studies conducted with health-care workers suggests a negative correlation between resilience and burnout.[6] For example, a cross-sectional study conducted on a sample of 196 health-care workers (including nurses and doctors) in Portugal in June 2021 found that "during a pandemic situation, higher levels of resilience associated both with lower levels of emotional exhaustion and depersonalization" and that the employment of resilience as "personal resources" successfully decreased "negative consequences of job strain, such as burnout" (Ferreira and Gomes 2021, 1, 2). Another study conducted in July 2020 on 377 midwives and nurses in Turkey found that a high level of psychological resilience acted as a "protective" factor against burnout and depression. Yörük and Güler further argue that "[t]here was a negative, weak, and significant correlation between depression and all subdimensions of resilience" (Yörük and Güler 2021, 393). In an integrative review of the literature on health-care workers' resilience, Baskin and Bartlett emphasize there is an "inverse relationship between resilience and burnout" with nurses experiencing burnout also experiencing low resilience scores (Baskin and Bartlett 2021, 2338).

In what follows, I do not intend to argue against these studies. But in light of such relevant evidence that shows how resilience can contribute to preventing burnout, I think a couple of reflections are worthwhile.

First, as some researchers themselves point out, the COVID-19 pandemic is still ongoing, and this means that the long-term effects of resilience on burnout as a result of the pandemic are still unknown. These preliminary studies then, although helpful, have limitations. Baskin and Bartlett are among those who urge caution in their integrative review, remarking that the COVID-19 pandemic, far from being over, might have surprising effects (ibid., 2338).

Among these surprising effects, I suggest that resilience fatigue might be a reasonable one to expect. Since the notion of resilience, individualistically conceived, involves the employment of resources to overcome challenges and setbacks, it is not unreasonable to hypothesize that such resources, which presumably require psychological and physical energy, might deplete over time. Treglown et al., for example, argue that resilience is a dynamic process where the individual interacts with the environment by negotiating and managing resources in response to a stressor. In light of this, resilience can influence the number of resources employed and thus the likelihood of burnout development – whereby burnout means "an internal and emotional response to external stressors that consume, exceed, and deplete our personal and social resources" (Treglown et al. 2016, 3).

Particularly in circumstances where individuals struggle to count on external support, relying exclusively on one's own personal resources can reveal its limits. This has been the case for a consistent portion of health-care workers who, in spite of high resilience scores, still experienced significant levels of burnout. A *New York Times* COVID-19 briefing from January 2022 reported that around one in five health-care workers has left their job since the beginning of the pandemic.[7] The Canadian Medical Association has reported that more than half of physicians experienced rates of burnout, a rate that is almost double pre-pandemic levels.[8] In Ontario alone, the COVID-19 advisory has reported that "[i]n spring 2020, the prevalence of severe burnout was 30%–40%. By spring 2021, rates >60% were found in Canadian physicians, nurses, and other health-care professionals."[9]

Burnout is not a new problem is health-care settings. A large study conducted on 5445 US physicians between 2017 and 2018, for example, found that 29% of physicians with the highest possible resilience score still experienced burnout, thus showing that "burnout rates were substantial even among the most resilient physicians" (West et al. 2020, 1). West et al. appropriately suggest that successful ways of reducing burnout should focus on addressing "system issues" in the clinical care environment (2020, 1). Interestingly, this suggestion seems in harmony with other studies conducted in Italy during the first wave of the COVID-19 pandemic. Catania et al. (2021), for example, highlight how lack of personal protective equipment (PPE) and staff issues played an important role in negatively affecting health-care workers' well-being (notice how lack of PPE and organizational challenges are *system* issues as West et al. and not lack of individual resources). Catania et al. 2021 also report that increased resilience during the COVID-19 pandemic was aided by a sense of community and teamwork – which, again, are not individual resources. One of the health professionals, for example, said, "We are growing as a team: we feel like an army that is fighting against a common enemy" (Catania et al. 2020, 409).

The harmful effects of the individualistic notion of resilience are particularly evident for people who experience marginalization. Brody et al. 2016, for example, found that an individualistic "unrelenting determination to succeed" that involves "high aspirations, unwavering persistence, investment in education, and avoidance of activities that sidetrack success" can have detrimental effects on the health of people who are marginalized, such as increased production of "stress hormones (like cortisol, adrenaline and noradrenaline)" and "substantial risks of developing diabetes or hypertension" (Brody et al. 2016, 1; Miller, Chen, Brody 2014, 2).

The story of Misbah Noor, a former elementary school teacher from Pakistan who immigrated to Canada in 2015 with her family, might be a fitting example. Noor recalls her struggles when she first settled in the country: the challenge of finding a job that provided her family a living wage, the disorientation of dealing with bureaucracy in another language, the discomfort of seeing her husband, previously a bank manager at a well-known bank in Pakistan, only to find jobs as a carpet installer. Over the years, Noor's family eventually overcame these setbacks and built a happy life for herself and her family, but this resilience came with a cost that Noor herself acknowledges. Noor writes,

> [T]he stress of the past seven years had lasting effects. After going through so much, I still feel tired and anxious over everyday problems. I feel like my memory was affected by chronic stress, and my husband now has high blood pressure, cholesterol and diabetes. We believe this is also connected. This is the price we paid to get to the place where we are now.
>
> (Noor 2022)

These deleterious aspects of resilience are also in harmony with psychological research conducted in different but complementary fields. With respect to empathy, for example, Paul Bloom has famously argued that feeling what others feel by, say, picking up their suffering or anxiety, can be exhausting and eventually lead to refraining from helping others in order to preserve mental resources (Paul 2016). With respect to self-control, Roy Baumeister has suggested that the energy required to exercise self-control can, similarly to a muscle, deplete over time (Baumeister et al. 2007, 351). In a well-known study, Baumeister shows that participants who successfully resisted eating chocolate and cookies failed to exercise self-control in subsequent tasks compared to those who gave into the temptation of indulging in the chocolate (Baumeister et al. 2007, 352).[10]

That resilience can be perceived as cognitively draining is also evident if this one is characterized in terms of willpower (Paul and Morton 2019, 176). Characterizing resilience in this way inevitably portrays individuals who *give up* as weak-willed. But this is questionable. As Jennifer Morton and Sarah Paul suggest, for example, resilience (what Morton and Paul call "grit", I am using the two terms interchangeably here) possesses an epistemic dimension that willpower cannot account for. On their view, quitting does not simply amount to giving up on one's goal, but it involves a loss of confidence that trying again will yield success. In this sense, abandoning a goal is caused not by moments of weakness which are often transitory, but by a "stable change in view about the relative value of the goal or activity" (ibid., 177). If giving up is not a weakness, then this highlights even more sharply the limitations of characterizing resilience as strength of will.

Taken as a whole, the empirical evidence presented in this section is at least indicative of the fact that resilience does not insulate against burnout. And this is particularly relevant for the purposes of my argument in the following way. An important lesson we should take from the COVID-19 pandemic is that a collective, relational notion of resilience – as involving a range of material, social, and psychological networks of support – is better equipped at fostering well-being in the long-term, as compared to an individualistic notion that conceives resilience as a function of personal resources.

5.3 How the individual notion of resilience discounts structural injustices

In the previous section, I have drawn on empirical evidence to suggest that resilience can cause ill-being by being experienced as mentally taxing and burdensome, particularly when calls for resilience target people who experience marginalization. In this section, I turn to a sociopolitical framework to suggest that calls for resilience, in addition to causing psychological harm, also discount the role that structural and systemic prejudices play with respect to vulnerable minorities. They do so by unduly shifting the responsibility of addressing structural issues onto individuals who are marginalized when the burden should instead be on institutions to resolve systemic problems. The claim I am making draws on the experience and voices of marginalized people themselves, particularly when tragic events happen, and in the research done to examine the sociopolitical consequences of individualized resilience.

Goodkind, Brinkman, and Elliott, for example, argue that talk of individual resilience "expends resources developing resilience among those considered "at risk" (even if they have yet to experience adverse life events or trauma) rather than addressing macro-level causes of oppression" (Goodkind et al. 2020, 319). This leads to "ignor[ing] power and context" and thus "encouraging people to be individually resilient is a way they are blamed for their own oppression and societal inequality" (Goodkind et al. 2020, 319).

Daniel Markovits has recently advanced a similar claim with respect to meritocracy (Markovits 2019). Speaking of university settings, Markovits claims that society's emphasis on merit as a key to success fails to take into consideration "patterns of inequality" that function as gatekeepers of American elite schools and effectively prevent access to a large portion of students who fall outside of the 1%. These patterns, Markovits emphasizes, are not the result of individual failings, but rather they are the results of accumulated structural inequalities and thus cannot be overcome through individual merit, as exceptional as the latter can be. Markovits says,

> Meritocracy's promise of equality – the theory that anyone can succeed simply by excelling, because meritocratic universities admit students based on academic achievement and employers hire workers based on skill – proves false in practice. The emphasis on excellence, whatever its motivation in principle, in fact produces admissions competitions and labor markets in which people from modest and even middle-class backgrounds cannot succeed. Exceptional cases always exist, but in general, children from poor or even middle-class households simply cannot compete in the battle for places at elite universities with rich children who have imbibed massive, sustained, planned, and practiced investment from birth or even in the womb. Workers with ordinary training, in turn, cannot compete with the immensely skilled and enormously industrious workers produced by the elite training.
>
> (Markovits 2019, 71–72)

Drawing on Markovits' claim, resilience seems to act in similar ways and brings about similarly pernicious effects. Characterizing success as a function of persistence entails attributing failure in large part to a lack of perseverance. This approach, in turn, transfers the responsibility of any achievement onto the single individual, entailing that success would have occurred if only one had just "tried one more time." But when confronted with structural prejudice, marginalized people cannot be expected (nor is it fair to expect them) to employ their individual resources to cut through systemic injustices and inequality. The latter are by definition structural; thus they require structural (not individualistic) intervention. Again, as Markovits remarks, exceptional cases of individual success exist, but these are not enough to legitimize an individualistic solution to systemic issues. In this sense, resilience is not sufficient to insulate from failure when systemic injustices are at play.

Jennifer Morton and Sarah Paul further argue that grit is not a capacity isolated from its context, but is indeed "ecologically constrained" (Paul and Morton 2019, 179). When it comes to "contexts of poverty or severe discrimination," Morton and Paul suggest that "[p]ublic policies and educational programs aimed at promoting the development of grit without an eye to the effect of context may [...] risk doing more harm than good" (Paul and Morton 2019, 179). This is not to suggest that those who experience "severe material and emotional scarcity" should quit but simply that they should be alert to the "evidence that pure effort will not be enough" (ibid., 202).

Conceiving success in individual terms is problematic because it also shifts the responsibility of success onto the individual's resources. In doing so, not only might we be distracted from how systemic injustices often impact minorities' trajectory in life, but it may also hinder social justice. Elizabeth Harrison argues that an "overemphasis on the ability of those at the sharp end of economic downturn to 'bounce back'" may come at "the cost of understanding the nature of structural factors," "it depoliticizes and shifts responsibility for dealing with crisis away from those in power" (Harrison 2013, 99).

With respect to marginalized youth, Dorothy Bottrell argues that an individualized focus on resilience "loses young people's legitimate critique and social protest based in their collective experiences of institutions and communities and their recognition of configurations of power in the interrelations of identifiable social groups" (Bottrell 2009, 333). This, Bottrell suggests, undermines social change because it "look[s] to the resilient individual, self-inventing for prosperity and success, with no regard for the adverse conditions that stack the odds against success for the disadvantaged and marginalized" (Bottrell 2009, 334). An individualistic notion of resilience, in this sense, "may shift the emphasis from positive adaptation despite adversity to positive adaptation *to* adversity" (Bottrell 2009, 334).

This claim is at odds with ordinary discourse that often touts resilience (similarly to how it touts individual merit) as an equalizer for success. But the glorification of resilience as a path to self-realization reinforces a narrative that is doubly false: on the one hand, it unfairly urges marginalized people to exclusively rely on their own resources – regardless of conditions of oppression – when they should instead benefit from structural support (and it unduly characterizes minorities' struggles as self-inflicted because they are "not resilient enough"). On the other hand, it also portrays individuals' success as self-made through resilience, discounting that successful individuals may often enjoy the advantage of a variety of factors, among which race, gender, and wealth.

This false narrative is particularly evident when tragic events occur, and it is exemplified by the many who have encouraged resilience during the COVID-19 pandemic. But outsourcing social change to individual resilience is not a pandemic-specific phenomenon. In 2005, after Hurricane Katrina hit New Orleans, its citizens were repeatedly told to be resilient. However, Anne Gisleson, a survivor, points out that encouragement to be resilient "puts the onus on the person to fix the things that should be a civic priority," thereby "tak[ing] the power structures off the hook" (Attenberg 2020). Studies conducted during the COVID-19 pandemic to assess the mental well-being of health-care workers found that

> [t]he risk of depression was significantly higher in midwives, those who were under 35, those who worked 49 h or more per week, those who stated their health status as bad or moderate, and those who evaluated their economic status as low or middle.
>
> (Yörük and Güler 2021, 393)

5.4 Toward a relational view of resilience

So far, I have argued that the COVID-19 pandemic has helped reveal that the individualistic notion of resilience is flawed in two ways: (a) it can generate psychological harm because it is experienced as cognitively burdensome, and (b) it fails to attend to systemic injustices because it discounts how structural oppression can undercut vulnerable minorities' success in overcoming setbacks. In light of these limits, in this section, I suggest that we abandon the individualistic notion of resilience in favor of a new one. I argue that we should think of resilience in *relational* terms; that is, we should characterize the notion of resilience as one that takes into account structural support as well as conditions of oppression and marginalization.

The notion of relational resilience I will propose has some points in common with the notion of "collective resilience" that Goodkind et al. (2020) propose. In a study aimed at advancing an alternative characterization of individualistic resilience, Goodkind et al. advance the idea of collective resilience as one that "promote[s] social support, connection, and collective action" and that can be developed through an "empowerment process" with the "potential to create structural and systemic change via the development of critical consciousness and collective action" (Goodkind et al. 2020, 319).

However, while Goodkind et al. developed a notion tailored to psychology and social work, in what follows, I advance a philosophical notion of relational resilience that is situated and inspired by feminist work on relational views of autonomy (Sherwin and Stockdale 2017; Mackenzie and Stoljar 2000; Downie and Llewellyn 2012). In what follows, I propose a relational notion of resilience that can be impacted by social and historical contexts of oppression and marginalization in a similar way as autonomy can be impacted by oppression.

The individualistic notion of autonomy was historically conceptualized as a capacity to self-govern and a state of self-sufficiency (Stoljar 2018). However, feminist authors have convincingly shown the inadequacy of this individualistic conception of autonomy and, instead, have advanced a notion of autonomy that is a function of social relationships and conditions of oppression. In what follows, I briefly summarize three main theories of relational autonomy (procedural or substantive, and causal or constitutive) in order to lay the ground for sketching my notion of relational resilience.[11]

Procedural theories of autonomy generally claim that conditions of oppression can (but do not necessarily) undermine autonomy, provided that the individual maintains the ability to engage in a process of critical reflection on their choices and preferences and revise them in virtue of whether they accept them or not. Gerald Dworkin, for example, argues that autonomy involves "the capacity of a person critically to reflect upon, and then attempt to accept or change, his or her preferences, desires, values, and ideals," where such a change is a direct result of critical reflection (Dworkin 1988, 48). Dworkin emphasizes that this ability to self-reflect must not be viewed in overly intellectualistic terms but that anyone "with a minimal education, may without being aware of it be conducting [their] life in ways which indicate that [they] ha[ve] shaped and molded [their] life according to reflective procedures" (ibid., 17). Self-reflection on one's conduct is exemplified, Dworkin argues, by "what [the individual] tries to change in his life, what [the individual] criticizes about others, the satisfaction he manifests (or fails to) in his work, family, and community" (ibid., 17).

Identifying (or not identifying) with the motivations that shape one's choices and preferences is then a necessary but not sufficient condition for being autonomous because autonomy requires, in addition to an evaluative element, also a second-order capacity to change one's first-order preferences in light of self-reflection (Dworkin 1988, 20). It is through the exercise of this capacity that "persons define their nature, give meaning and coherence to their lives, and take responsibility for the kind of person they are" (ibid., 20).

According to this view, autonomy is a "contentless notion" (ibid., 110) in the sense that "there is no specific content to the decisions an autonomous person takes" (Dworkin, 108). Dworkin argues that "[s]omeone who wishes to be the kind of person who does whatever the doctor orders is as autonomous as the person who wants to evaluate those orders for himself" (ibid., 108–109). In this sense, the theory leaves room for "the possibility of a patient granting complete authority to a doctor" and still counting as autonomous (ibid., 109). Along similar lines, Marylin

Friedman also holds a content-neutral conception of autonomy (Friedman 2003, 3) and argues that "a person is autonomous so long as the manner in which she reaches and makes her choices" occurs "in the right way or it coheres appropriately with her perspective as a whole" (ibid., 19). Friedman claims that

> [s]omeone can autonomously give up her own future autonomy, for example, by entering a religious order requiring unconditional obedience to church authority. She will become nonautonomous in her behavior after making and adhering to that sort of choice, but this does not mean that she was nonautonomous when first making the choice.
>
> (Ibid., 19)

The only way in which one fails to be procedurally independent according to Dworkin is when second-order reflections, "the choice of the kind of person one wants to become" are "influenced by other persons or circumstances in such a fashion that we do not view those evaluations as being the person's own" (ibid., 18). This can happen for example when someone gets hypnotized, manipulated, coercively persuaded, or subliminally influenced (ibid., 18). But if a person's capacity to self-reflect has not been manipulated, coerced, and so forth, and if the person meets the requisite identification, then they are, in Dworkin's view, autonomous.

A worry that has been advanced by proponents of strong *substantive* theories of autonomy is that a contentless notion of autonomy, such as the one defended by procedural theories, fails to capture cases where an individual may technically meet the criteria for self-reflection but come to make decisions or choices whose result does not appear to be autonomous (Charles 2010, Stoljar 2000). For this reason, substantive theorists argue that the content of the self-reflection process plays a decisive role regarding attributions of autonomy. Sonya Charles, for example, argues that certain decisions that derive from "false beliefs that rely on subordinating reasoning and perpetuate oppression should not count as autonomous" (Charles 2010, 413). Among these decisions are "decisions that reflect a certain devaluation of self (or lack of self-worth)" (ibid., 413). Charles is careful to specify that it is not decisions that spark from false beliefs that alter the verdict on autonomy, but a subset of these decisions: those that result from false beliefs that are a form of "internalized oppression" because they rely on "subordinating reasoning *and* perpetuate oppressive systems" (ibid., 416).

To clarify, Charles discusses Thomas Hill's case of *The Deferential Wife*, who agrees with claims of gender equality, and yet believes and derives happiness from the conviction that the role of a woman is to serve her family. She tends to adopt her husband's preferences without developing her own, and when she does, she conceives of them as less worthy. While procedural theorists would likely consider *The Deferential Wife* autonomous because there is no evident coercion or manipulation, Charles argues that the case of *The Deferential Wife* should not be considered autonomous because *The Deferential Wife*'s choices and decisions stem precisely from those false beliefs that are a result of internalized oppression and, particularly, "oppressive norms of femininity" (ibid., 419).

On a weaker version of the substantive conception of autonomy, Paul Benson proposes a view that "incorporates normative content" without imposing normative constraints on "the types of actions agents might autonomously perform or the content of the motives or values that lead them to act" (Benson 2005, 125). The normative content that Benson has in mind involves "agents' attitudes toward their own authority to speak and answer for their decisions" (ibid., 125). In this sense, Benson's view sits in between strong substantive theories of autonomy and contentless views. One of the advantages of such a moderate substantive view is that the account "is well suited for feminist efforts to analyze possibilities for women's autonomy within oppressive social arrangements" (ibid., 125). In particular, Benson's view makes room for cases where women may autonomously "criticize and resist misogynist conventions even if they have internalized some aspects of traditional femininity that are hostile to their interests" provided that they have "a sense of their authority as reasoning, potentially answerable agents" (ibid., 137).

Benson motivates the account by pointing out that socialization and oppressive practices are pervasive and that acknowledging this fact should lead us to accept that "autonomous agency is compatible with making some seriously mistaken or unwarranted normative judgments, embracing some harmful values, or maintaining some attitudes that are inimical to agents' own interests" (ibid., 131). Failure to accept this, Benson continues, results in a "fairly radical skepticism" about autonomy that is implied by strong substantive theories of autonomy, and that, according to him, is too costly. According to Benson, it is possible to "recognize prospects for autonomous action within the scope of false or harmful norms without having to erase impairments of autonomy from the catalog of injuries that oppressive practices perpetuate" (ibid., 131).

Autonomy is a capacity that is not developed in isolation, it can be influenced and shaped, positively or negatively, by external factors like social relationships and sociohistorical conditions of oppression. The lack of sociohistorical conditions of oppression and the presence of social relationships can for example foster the development of autonomy, while the presence of sociohistorical conditions of oppression and the lack of social relationships can hinder its development.[12] The distinction between procedural and substantive views further reveals two different approaches to how external elements like conditions of oppression can influence the capacity to be autonomous. Procedural theorists generally conceive of external elements having a *causal* influence on autonomy, without necessarily hindering it. In this sense, conditions of oppression can hinder, say, the capacity for self-reflection, albeit not necessarily. Annette Baier, for example, suggests that factors like social relationships can influence a person's autonomy because persons are "essentially successors" whose personality should not be conceived of as having developed in isolation, but rather it is their "relations to others and in their response to their own recognized genesis" (Baier 1985, 85). The causal relation then lies in how earlier and later phases of a person's life are connected with the former "causally influenc[ing]" the latter (Baier 1985, 85). Baier points out that

> [t]he fact that a person has a life history, and that a people collectively have a history, depends upon the humbler fact that each person has a childhood in which a cultural heritage is transmitted, ready for adolescent rejection and adult discriminating selection and contribution. Persons come after and before other persons.
>
> (Ibid.)

In contrast to the theories previously described, others suggest that some external elements necessarily hinder autonomy. These *substantive* theorists generally "see interpersonal and social factors as conceptually necessary for autonomy" instead of "contributory factors" (Christman 2004, 149).

Marina Oshana, for example, argues that "[p]ersons cannot be autonomous unless the satisfaction of certain social conditions is guaranteed" (Oshana 2006, 94). Oshana suggests that we distinguish between the "capacity for autonomy" and the "condition of being autonomous" (ibid., 20). Accordingly, autonomy is in part "*constituted* by social relations that are extrinsic to facts about the psychological states of the individual" (Oshana 2006, 20, italics mine).

In arguing this, Oshana's argument diverges from procedural and causal theories because it argues that "the state of being autonomous is primarily a function of the external situation a person finds himself in rather than being predominately a function of a person's psychological state or practical skills" (ibid., 6). Oshana employs several examples, like the voluntary slave and the subservient homemaker Harriet, to emphasize that a lack of "authoritative control" over "the management of their choices, actions, and goals" makes the authority in question "vulnerable to interference" where this vulnerability is due to "social status and relations to others," and it is not sufficient for autonomy (ibid., 75).

5.5 Resilience as causally relational

I have briefly summarized the three main approaches to autonomy in order to lay the groundwork for the theory of resilience that I advance in this section. In what follows, I propose that we do for the notion of resilience what feminist philosophers have done for the notion of autonomy. That is, I suggest that we endorse a new characterization of the notion of resilience that is *relational*, that fosters well-being, and that takes into account structural injustice. Given that the literature on resilience is not particularly large and that, to my knowledge, there is currently no systematic view of relational resilience, in what follows, my aim is not to propose a detailed account of relational resilience, but rather to outline some features of this new characterization that I hope will spark a future conversation about how and why we should rethink resilience.

With respect to relational autonomy, John Christman writes that relational views "emphasize the role that background social dynamics and power structures play in the enjoyment and development of autonomy" (Christman 2004, 143). I suggest that a relational view of resilience should be motivated by a similar approach. In particular, the view of relational resilience that I suggest should replace the current individualistic notion is one that is *causally* relational and that takes into account how external factors such as social relationships, support networks, as well as sociohistorical conditions, can foster or undermine the capacity of being resilient.

Relational theorists argue that autonomy is not a capacity that is developed in isolation, but one that recognizes that we are "socially embedded" (ibid., 144). Similarly, for the capacity to be resilient, the resources that individuals must employ to overcome setbacks are not accrued in isolation, but they are socially embedded as well. Being able to successfully "bounce back" involves both psychological and material resources, both of which can be crucially influenced by sociohistorical conditions, oppression, and social relationships. Material resources are often employed by those who are privileged, and the wealthy can rely on support networks while also being free from most conditions of oppression. Instead, people who are oppressed lack the same resources and social supports for structural and systemic reasons.[13]

When it comes to catastrophic events, such as the COVID-19 pandemic, material considerations intersect with considerations of fairness because encouragements to be resilient that target marginalized individuals discount that what is indeed needed is structural support (and not individual strength) to solve social and collective issues. A lack of material means can in turn impact the psychological resources needed to overcome challenges because a lack of material and social support can generate a psychological state of isolation and deplete the mental resources that would be employed to be resilient. (Recall the earlier case of Misbah Noor, who explains how the struggles of settling in Canada had negative physical and emotional effects.)

With that said, I am not suggesting that conditions of oppression *necessarily* undermine resilience (they *can*), nor that people that experience oppression cannot have the capacity of being resilient. The reason why I claim this is because I do not rule out that individuals who are marginalized or oppressed can be resilient. Rather, my aim is to introduce a view of resilience that takes into consideration social factors as playing a more central role in the capacity of being resilient compared to the individualistic notion of resilience. If this is correct, a notion that is sensitive to how external elements can impact resilience goes beyond the limitations of the individualistic characterization. A *causally relational* view is one that resists embracing the doubly false narrative of failed resilience that shifts responsibility to individuals regardless of sociohistorical conditions of oppression and unjustly praises success stories without taking into consideration privileged support networks. In resisting this narrative, a causally relational notion of resilience puts the responsibility where it is due by placing accountability on structures rather than individual strength.

I have said that sociohistorical conditions of oppression can undermine the capacity to be resilient, albeit not as necessarily. I now want to further suggest that there is an element that is necessarily impacted by a causally relational view of resilience, and it is *calls* for being resilient. What I mean by this is that if we sincerely rethink resilience and we embrace a causally relational notion of resilience, then we are committed to say that when it comes to individuals who have a history of oppression and marginalization, this history of oppression and marginalization *invalidates* individual *calls* for being resilient. Let me explain.

A view of resilience that incorporates awareness that conditions of oppression can undermine the capacity of being resilient renders individual encouragements to be resilient ethically dubious, particularly when directed at individuals who have a history of oppression and marginalization. Calls for resilience are inappropriate in this case because in discounting the role that structural injustices can play in undermining the capacity of being resilient, they also discount that what is instead needed is structural support. Structural and systemic injustices that are at the heart of conditions of oppression and marginalization must be counteracted with structural solutions. Thus, the examples I have cited at the beginning of this chapter of politicians' and universities' encouragements to be resilient during the COVID-19 pandemic are not appropriate under a causally relational characterization of resilience for the same reason why it would not be appropriate to encourage a person who is financially precarious to "pull themselves up by their own bootstraps."

Sensitivity and consideration for sociohistorical conditions of oppression make it the case that individual calls for being resilient that target marginalized people run into moral failure. Again, this does not entail that individuals who are oppressed or marginalized cannot be resilient, but it does mean that when it comes to setbacks, the burden to be resilient should not be shifted onto them. It is society at large that should instead provide structural support. To cite again the words of Zandashé Brown that I quoted at the outset:

I dream of never being called resilient again in my life. I'm exhausted by strength. I want support. I want softness. I want ease. I want to be amongst kin. Not patted on the back for how well I take a hit. Or for how many.

It becomes clear that awareness of the mental toll that individualized resilience can cause (especially in long stretches of time like the years that involved the COVID-19 pandemic) makes calls for resilience ethically questionable because they can lead to negative consequences.

In conclusion, my view of relational resilience is positioned as a hybrid that has shares similarities with both procedural and substantive views. Structurally, it is in harmony with causally procedural views of autonomy insofar as it acknowledges that the presence or lack of sociohistorical conditions of oppression and social relationships *can* impact the capacity of being resilient, but not necessarily. But it is in harmony with substantive views of autonomy because it claims that conditions of oppression *necessarily* invalidate calls for being resilient.

5.6 Conclusion

The aim of this chapter has been twofold: to examine the limits of an individualistic notion of resilience and, in light of this, to lay the groundwork for a new notion of resilience that is fundamentally relational.

With respect to the first aim, I have argued that an individualistic notion of resilience can cause psychological harm, particularly when calls for resilience target individuals with a history of oppression. Because this notion of resilience involves individuals relying exclusively on their own resources and energy, calls to persevere can be experienced as burdensome and eventually lead to burnout and mental exhaustion.

But conceiving resilience in individual terms also has sociopolitical consequences because it discounts the role that structural inequality plays for oppressed individuals when it comes to overcoming setbacks. People who experience marginalization cannot and should not be expected to rely on individual resources when calls for resilience are employed as a solution to structural problems. This limitation has been even more evident during the COVID-19 pandemic when encouragements to be resilient should have been rightly replaced by more economic, social, psychological, and health support on behalf of government institutions. For similar reasons, we should expect these limitations again when we face future crises. An individualistic notion of resilience then paints a narrative that is doubly false: it shifts the responsibility of solving structural issues onto individuals unduly blaming those experiencing oppression for failing to individually overcome setbacks; and it fairly praises those who succeed while discounting hidden privileges.

In light of the limits of the individualistic notion of resilience, in the second half of the chapter, I suggested that we rethink resilience and move toward a characterization that is causally relational. I have framed this new view of resilience within the feminist literature on relational autonomy and have argued that a causally relational notion of resilience takes into account how external elements such as historical conditions of oppression and structural inequality can impact the resources needed to be resilient. It does so by suggesting that conditions of oppression can, although not necessarily, undermine the capacity of being resilient.

Acknowledgments

Many thanks to the audience at the Pacific American Philosophical Association Committee on the Status of Women in Academia and particularly to Kathryn Norlock, Suze Berkhout, Catherine Clune-Taylor, and Kathryn Norlock. I am especially grateful to Sarah Stroud, Sarah Paul and Constantine Sandis for helpful feedback on earlier drafts of this chapter, an anonymous referee, and Katie Stockdale and Nicole Fice for written comments.

Notes

1 As reported here: https://toronto.citynews.ca/2021/07/01/trudeaus-canada-day-message-2021/
2 See here: https://developingchild.harvard.edu/resources/how-to-help-families-and-staff-build-resilience-during-the-covid-19-outbreak/
3 See also Calhoun (2018) and Calhoun (2009) for more on this.
4 See here: https://twitter.com/zandashe/status/1394805726825099279
5 On the relationship between hope and resilience see also Stockdale (2021a, Ch. 5).
6 There is no universally received definition of burnout, but the phenomenon is commonly characterized by a cluster of symptoms involving "a state of mental exhaustion, depersonalization, and a decreased sense of personal accomplishment" (Lacy and Chan 2018, 311).
7 As reported here: https://www.nytimes.com/2022/01/14/briefing/coronavirus-briefing-a-pandemic-burnout-crisis.html?searchResultPosition=2
8 As reported here: https://globalnews.ca/news/8889103/covid-burnout-destroyed-health-workers/
9 As reported here: https://covid19-sciencetable.ca/sciencebrief/burnout-in-hospital-based-healthcare-workers-during-covid-19/
10 It is important to note that Baumeister's theory has been recently questioned. See Hagger et al. (2016) for more on this. However, I believe that the theory's conceptual import is still worth discussing.
11 I borrow this set up from Stoljar (2018). The literature on autonomy is vast and complex. I want to stress here that I do not intend to provide an exhaustive, in-depth review of the theories nor to defend a particular one. My aim is more modest than that, and it is simply to give the reader a conceptual map of those features of the main theories of autonomy that are salient for my characterization of relational resilience.

12 The idea that external factors can impact the capacity to be resilient is already present in some psychological literature. Mandleco and Peery, for example, list a series of external factors that can affect resilience (Mandleco and Peery 2000, 101). Some are more individualistic such as adults and peers, but others like health-care and social service agencies are structural. What I am suggesting here is that there is more work to be done to stress this causal connection between systems and resilience.
13 A question that I do not explore here, but that is worth asking, is whether the presence (and influence) of external factors can affect attribution of praise with respect to the individual capacity of being resilient. I think that, to a certain extent as well as depending on the degree of influence that these factors have, the answer should be "yes." I am grateful to an anonymous referee for pressing me on this.

References

Attenberg, J. 2020. "Is resilience overrated?" *The New York Times*.
Baier, A., 1985, *Postures of the Mind. Essays on Mind and Morals*, Minneapolis: University of Minnesota Press.
Bajaj, B., Pande, N. 2015. "Mediating role of resilience in the impact of mindfulness on life satisfaction and affect as indices of subjective well-being." *Personality and Individual Differences*, 93, 63–67.
Baskin, R. G., Bartlett, R. 2021. "Healthcare worker resilience during the COVID-19 pandemic: An integrative review." *Journal of Nursing Management*, 29(8), 2329–2342.
Baumeister, Roy F., Vohs, Kathleen D., Tice, Dianne M. 2007. "The strength model of self-control." *Current Directions in Psychological Science*, 16, 351–355.
Benson, P. 2005. "Feminist intuitions and the normative substance of autonomy," in James Stacey Taylor (ed.), *Personal Anatomy*, Cambridge: Cambridge University Press, pp. 124–142.
Bottrell, D. 2009. "Understanding 'marginal' perspectives: Towards a social theory of resilience."*QualitativeSocialWork*,8(3),321–339.doi:10.1177/1473325009337840.
Brody, GH, Yu, T., Miller, GE, Chen, E. 2016. "Resilience in adolescence, health, and psychosocial outcomes." *Pediatrics*, 138(6), e20161042.
Calhoun, C. 2009. "What good is commitment?" *Ethics*, 119(4), 613–641.
Calhoun, C. 2018. *Doing Valuable Time: The Present, the Future, and Meaningful Living*, New York: OUP.
Catania, G., Zanini, M., Hayter, M., Timmins, F., Dasso, N., Ottonello, G., Aleo, G., Sasso, L., Bagnasco, A. 2021. "Lessons from Italian front-line nurses' experiences during the COVID-19 pandemic: A qualitative descriptive study." *Journal of Nursing Management*, 29(3), 404–411.
Charles, S. 2010, "How should feminist autonomy theorists respond to the problem of internalized oppression?" *Social Theory and Practice*, 36(3), 409–428.
Chen, D., Wu, J., Yao, Z. et al. 2018. "Negative association between resilience and event-related potentials evoked by negative emotion." *Scientific Reports*, 8, 7149.
Christman, J. 2004. "Relational autonomy, liberal individualism, and the social constitution of selves." *Philosophical Studies*, 117, 143–164.
Downie, J., Llewellyn, J., 2012. *Being Relational: Reflections on Relational Theory and Health Law*. Vancouver, CA: UBC Press.

Dworkin, G. 1988. *The Theory and Practice of Autonomy.* Cambridge: Cambridge University Press.

Ferreira, Pedro, Gomes, Sofia. 2021. "The role of resilience in reducing burnout: A study with healthcare workers during the COVID-19 pandemic." *Social Sciences, 10*(9), 317.

Friedman, M., 1997, "Autonomy and social relationships: Rethinking the feminist critique," in D.T. Meyers (ed.), *Feminists Rethink the Self*, Boulder, CO: Westview, pp. 40–61.

Friedman, M., 2003, *Autonomy, Gender, Politics.* New York: Oxford University Press.

Goodkind, S, Brinkman, B. G., Elliott, K. 2020. "Redefining resilience and reframing resistance: Empowerment programming with black girls to address societal inequities." *Behavioral Medicine, 46*(3–4), 317–329. doi: 10.1080/08964289.2020.1748864

Hagger, Martin S., Nikos, L. D. Chatzisarantis, et al. 2016. "A multilab preregistered replication of the ego-depletion effect." *Perspectives on Psychological Science, 11*, 546–573.

Harrison, E. 2013. "Bouncing back: Recession, resilience and everyday lives." *Critical Social Policy, 33*(1), 97–113.

Kong, F., Ma, X., You, X., Xiang, Y. 2018. "The resilient brain: Psychological resilience mediates the effect of amplitude of low-frequency fluctuations in orbitofrontal cortex on subjective well- being in young healthy adults." *Social Cognitive and Affective Neuroscience, 13*(7), 755–763.

Lacy, B. E., Chan, J. L. 2018. "Physician burnout: The hidden health care crisis." *Clinical Gastroenterology and Hepatology, 16*(3), 311–317.

Liu, Y., Wang, Z., Zhou, C., Li, T. 2014. "Affect and self-esteem as mediators between trait resilience and psychological adjustment." *Personality and Individual Differences, 66*, 92–97.

Mackenzie, C., N. Stoljar (eds.). 2000. *Relational Autonomy: Feminist Perspectives on Autonomy, Agency and the Social Self.* New York: Oxford University Press.

Mandleco B. L., Peery J. C. 2000. "An organizational framework for conceptualizing resilience in children." *Journal of Child and Adolescent Psychiatric Nursing, 13*(3), 99.

Markovits, D. 2019. *The Meritocracy Trap: How America's Foundational Myth Feeds Inequality, Dismantles the Middle Class, and Devours the Elite.* Penguin Books.

Miller, G. E., Chen, E., Brody, G. H. 2014. "Can upward mobility cost you your health?" *The New York Times – The Great Divide.*

Noor, M. 2022. "Moving to Canada was harder than I thought. I'm not sure I'd do it again." CBC.

Oshana, M. 2006. *Personal Autonomy in Society.* Aldershot: Ashgate Publishing.

Paul, Garrett Michael. 2016, "Questioning tales of 'ordinary magic': 'Resilience' and neo liberal reasoning." *The British Journal of Social Work, 46*(7), 1909–1925. doi: 10.1093/bjsw/bcv017

Paul, S., Morton, J. 2019. "Grit." *Ethics, 129*(2), 175–203.

Satici, S. A. 2016. "Psychological vulnerability, resilience, and subjective well-being: The mediating role of hope." *Personality and Individual Differences, 102*, 68–73.

Sherwin, S., Stockdale, K. 2017. "Whither bioethics now? The promise of relational theory." *International Journal of Feminist Approaches to Bioethics, 10*(1), 7–29.

Sisto, A., Vicinanza, F., Campanozzi, L. L., Ricci, G., Tartaglini, D., Tambone, V. 2019. "Towards a transversal definition of psychological resilience: A literature review." *Medicina (Kaunas, Lithuania)*, 55(11), 745.

Smith, T. W. 2006. "Personality as risk and resilience in physical health." *Current Directions in Psychological Science, 15*(5), 227–231.

Stockdale, K. 2021a. *Hope Under Oppression*. New York: Oxford University Press.

Stockdale, K. 2021b. "Hope, solidarity, and justice." *Feminist Philosophy Quarterly, 7*(2).

Stoljar, N. 2000. "Autonomy and the feminist intuition," in Catriona Mackenzie and Natalie Stoljar (eds.), *Relational Autonomy: Feminist Perspectives on Autonomy, Agency, and the Social Self*, New York: Oxford University Press, pp. 94–111.

Stoljar, N. 2018. "Feminist Perspectives on Autonomy," in Edward N. Zalta (ed.), *The Stanford Encyclopedia of Philosophy* (Winter 2018 Edition). https://plato.stanford.edu/archives/win2018/entries/feminism-autonomy/

Treglown, L., Palaiou, K., Zarola, A., Furnham, A. 2016. "The dark side of resilience and burnout: A moderation-mediation model." *PLoS One, 11*(6). https://doi.org/10.1371/journal.pone.0156279

West, Colin P., Dyrbye, Liselotte N., Sinsky, Christine, Trockel, Mickey, Tutty, Michael, Nedelec, Laurence, Carlasare, Lindsey E., Shanafelt, Tait D., 2020. "Resilience and burnout among physicians and the general US working population." *JAMA Network Open, 3*(7), e209385. doi: 10.1001/jamanetworkopen.2020.9385

Yörük, S., Güler, D. 2021. "The relationship between psychological resilience, burnout, stress, and sociodemographic factors with depression in nurses and midwives during the COVID-19 pandemic: A cross-sectional study in Turkey." *Perspectives in Psychiatric Care, 57*(1), 390–398.

Part II
Virtues and traits of character

6 The COVID-19 pandemic and the language of virtues

Denis Coitinho

I

The current COVID-19 pandemic has substantially altered our daily routines. In order to try and save lives, drastic measures have been taken, such as the closure of shops, the banning of large gatherings of people, and the suspension of live classes in schools and universities. This has led to serious economic problems, such as the closure of small businesses, the loss of jobs, and the reduction of salaries. However, in addition to all these changes, it seems that the pandemic has introduced another new factor, which is the obligatory use of the language of virtues. Ever since the onset of COVID-19, people have been encouraged to be constantly virtuous in their daily behavior. By way of illustration, the health services have insisted that the population should use face coverings in public settings, clean their hands with antiseptic gel, and isolate socially from other people when necessary. They have also stressed the importance of forward planning. The media have set up influential solidarity campaigns, which have included encouraging people to show empathy toward those who are most vulnerable to COVID-19, such as older or homeless individuals. Psychologists have emphasized the importance of being permanently aware of the need to be resilient in times of domestic confinement through maintaining self-discipline in order to avoid mental health problems. And although monetary profit is a cornerstone of free market economies like Brazil's and other countries, public opinion has clearly condemned all profiteering during this time of crisis and has censured anyone who tries to excessively raise the prices of essential goods, especially medical items such as surgical gloves and masks, facial screens, and ventilators.

Although this new social demand for virtues is most welcome, three problems can be identified in relation to it, the first of which is practical, the second theoretical, and the third political. The practical problem is that virtue is acquired, both morally and intellectually, through a process of habituation, and this takes time. It is not enough simply to say that one should be wise, supportive, resilient, and just for people's acts to become automatically virtuous. It is necessary to carry out virtuous acts in order to

DOI: 10.4324/9781003310129-8

reach this goal. As Aristotle has taught us, we become just, moderate, and courageous by undertaking acts of justice, moderation, and courage. In *Intelligent Virtue*, Julia Annas gives us the interesting analogy of virtue and practical abilities such as playing the piano, in the sense that virtue can also be learned through exercise and habit. For instance, in order to be loyal, we must learn how to act loyally, which implies observing examples of loyalty before we carry out acts. This is not a theoretical knowledge of what is right or wrong, but a practical knowledge of "knowledge how" rather than "knowledge that." Although we often know that doing a certain thing is wrong, sometimes we go ahead and do it anyway, and this form of *akrasia* is a psychological phenomenon that is quite common in our daily lives.[1]

Let us refer to the virtue of autonomy in order to emphasize the point made earlier more strongly. As an intellectual virtue, it signals a disposition to undertake investigation independently, thus demonstrating the capacity to think for oneself, which implies the courage to use one's own reason without resorting to heteroregulation. Looked at from an educational point of view, student autonomy is considered a desirable quality that may be understood as a personal disposition to investigate and find solutions oneself. But simply saying that students should be autonomous is not sufficient since regular practice is essential for acquiring this virtue. To give an example, the educational system in Finland is well-known for encouraging students from an early age to be protagonists in the process of learning, and this includes establishing personal goals and solving problems. In this project-based approach, transversal competencies are of crucial importance, whereas a content-based educational methodology does not appear to nurture student autonomy.[2]

Over and above the practical problem of not being educated to act virtuously, we are also confronted with a theoretical problem in the political domain. A liberal and democratic state of the type found in many western countries does not demand virtuous behavior from its citizens in order to avoid accusations of paternalism. In contemporary times, the basic idea behind the separation of the public and private spheres of action is to preserve the individual freedom of each citizen. The state should not act as a parental figure who decides how individuals should live their lives, which religion they should practice, or what is morally right or wrong. At most, the state can demand obedience to certain laws relating to public morality – that is, those concerning harmful actions such as murder, robbery, rape, or kidnapping. To illustrate, the Brazilian penal code stipulates the following: "In the case of murder, the penalty shall be a prison sentence of between six and twenty years" (PC, 121). Its limits are established in the field of positive virtues, as it will not encourage solidarity, resilience, loyalty, or courage, nor will it punish agents who do not possess these virtues. Moral demand in the private sphere is thus a feature of community-based political models of justice.

The apparent paradox here is that in extreme situations like war or the COVID-19 pandemic, we must be able to count on the virtuous behavior of the citizens to be successful and win the fight. But how is this possible if the citizens have not been educated to display this type of behavior? We have seen that people will applaud the courage of health professionals in confronting a dangerous virus, yet we do not demand that all citizens show courage collectively. So how can we escape the paradox in such situations?

The third problem concerns the lack of clarity as to what constitutes "justice" and how it may affect our major political, social, and economic institutions. For clarity, is equality a normative standard that should characterize them all? If that is so, can they guarantee access to health care for all citizens in both the public and private sectors, and ensure that those who are infected will be able to find places in ICUs where they can be linked up to ventilators? Even though Brazil has a public health system that supposedly guarantees free access to health care, there is still a marked difference in medical treatment between the public and private sectors. For example, there may be a shortage of beds in the public system and an excess in the private system, and there is currently no mechanism in place that ensures that health care is always available to all citizens.

I believe that one way to solve this problem would be to create a bridge between the public and private spheres. Although it is important to protect individual freedoms and rights by keeping the two sectors separate, it seems inefficient to maintain this separation when the key aim is to guarantee free access to health care for everyone. In my view, it should be possible to establish a connection between rights and virtues, and a good starting point would be to consider Adam Smith's holistic strategy in his theory of moral sentiments. Smith was an important figure in the Scottish Enlightenment who, while defending the distinction between the public and private spheres, he attempted to harmoniously integrate the social and personal domains by bringing together the psychological, moral, political, legal, and economic spheres through an inclusivist concept of virtues as a means of achieving individual and collective happiness. He correctly defended the neutrality of state ethics but accepted that the state should have a prescriptive role in society.

Having said all this, in the rest of this chapter, I shall first try to clarify the importance of the virtues and show how personal character can be a valid form of approach in this context. Following that, I will outline the inclusivist theory of virtues postulated by Adam Smith in *The Theory of Moral Sentiments* (TMS). I shall then defend the concept of justice as an essential public virtue for specifying human rights and duties in the social sphere. Lastly, I will set out some final considerations for resolving the problem of the connection between rights and virtues.

II

The virtues have an important role to play as a normative standard for social behavior, especially in terms of how we should live our lives, and this has been the case throughout human history. In early civilization, the cardinal virtues of prudence, temperance, courage, and justice were considered essential for the well-being of individuals and the welfare of the whole of society. During the Middle Ages, the theological virtues of faith, hope, and charity also became central virtues as the moral standards of all Christians. In more recent times, other epistemic and moral virtues were included as essential parameters for a successful life, such as curiosity, self-reliance, integrity, resilience, solidarity, and humility, despite the great influence of principialistic theories such as Kantism and utilitarianism in our lives. These virtues were not restricted only to western cultures, and in Buddhism, for example, eternity, happiness, self-awareness, and purity were considered essential qualities in the quest for the most perfect state that a human being could hope to aspire to. Confucianism also indicates five virtues as crucial for personal and social happiness, and these are loving one's neighbor, being just, acting in accordance with moral principles, cultivating knowledge and sincerity, and maintaining awareness of godliness. But what do virtues really consist of, and why are they desirable?

Virtues are behavioral traits that cause people to act in a socially desirable way. In other words, a virtue is a permanent feature of individual character that manifests itself in ordinary actions, and it is a good quality for an individual to possess because it may lead to personal happiness or success in society. To give an example, a prudent person is someone who normally acts with common sense and a balanced approach, and who has the capacity to make sensible decisions, and a just person is someone who recognizes the rights of others, both in a distributive and retributive sense, and is not greedy. On the other hand, a moderate person possesses the quality of self-restraint and can control their desires and appetites, similar to a courageous person who can face challenges and confront their own fears.

We consider this kind of behavior to be desirable because we believe that a person who does not possess these qualities will find it difficult to be successful in life. It would be very problematic to live in a society where its citizens displayed a lack of generosity, along with dishonesty, disloyalty, arrogance, and vanity. This shows that we consider certain standards essential to the way we live our lives, and we value greatly people's determination to become better individuals since it is the repetition of good acts which form their personal character.

However, we must now ask ourselves if individual character is indeed a reliable psychological determinant for action. Many would say that it is not since the circumstances of the act, such as the environmental context and the social dynamics, would appear to have a vital influence on human decisions. This stance is known in the relevant literature as "situationism" and is skeptical in relation to the reliability of moral character. By way of illustration, in "Character" (2010, 355–401), Merrit, Doris, and Harman refer to various experiments in the field of social psychology in order to defend the thesis that individual traits of moral character are not robust; i.e., they are not consistent over a wide range of relevant situations. One of the experiments described was carried out by Isen and Levin and revealed that people who came across a ten-cent coin were twice as likely to help someone who had dropped their papers as those who had not come across the coin. Another experiment by Darley and Batson showed that carefree pedestrians were six times more helpful to disabled people than preoccupied pedestrians. Likewise, Mathews and Cannon demonstrated that even surrounding noise can have an influence on human behavior. The results of the experiment noted that people who were exposed to normal conditions of noise were five times more likely to help a disabled person who had dropped some books than those who were distracted by the noise of a lawnmower.[3]

Based on these and other experiments, such as the one by Milgram which attempts to show how agents are influenced by obedience to an external authority, the "situationists" have concluded that the traits of moral character are not consistent, especially when we take into consideration a wide range of relevant situations that appear to influence individual decisions. They also consider that although moral character is stable over time, it should be viewed consistently in a particular situation and that there is no strong correlation between one specific virtue and others. Although I believe that the empirical evidence which seeks to emphasize the limits of moral reasoning is relevant, this does not prove that virtues do not exist or that they cannot serve as motivation for certain acts and that therefore virtuous character is merely an illusion. I maintain that this evidence can only show that in many circumstances we are the victims of external influences that also motivate human acts since virtuous character is not a normative standard that is immune to the forces of the outside world.

Let us now look more closely at Milgram's experiment referred to earlier. Known as the experiment in obedience to authority as created by Stanley Milgram, its aim was to show that people are clearly susceptible to external authority in their deliberations, decision-making, and actions such that moral character is not a reliable variable. The experiment was undertaken at the University of Yale in 1961, and its aim was to prove that people have a tendency to obey uncritically certain rules stipulated by a higher authority. Participants were led to believe that they were involved in an innovative educational experiment in which they would give electric shocks to a particular student in order to make the process of learning easier. The shocks varied between 15 and 450 volts, and each time the student gave a wrong answer the teacher was supposed to increase the level of shock administered. It turned out that only those who were playing the role of teacher were actually being tested, as the students were, in fact, actors who pretended to feel pain. In the same way, those who were responsible for conducting the experiment were either academic staff involved in the research or even actors. Some very impressive data was collected from this experiment: 65% of the "teachers" continued to administer shocks to the maximum limit of 450 volts, while all of them administered shocks of at least 300 volts.[4]

It was therefore proved that 65% of a total of 40 "teachers" aged between 20 and 50 years were strongly influenced by an external authority – i.e., those who were responsible for organizing the experiment. But the experiment also revealed that 35% (14) of the "teachers" stopped increasing the voltage before they reached the permitted maximum level of 450 volts. It should also be remembered that, as the force of the shocks was increased, the "students" pretended to cry out and begged for the experiment to be stopped. And even though the majority of the "teachers" accepted the instruction of their "superiors" to go up to the permitted maximum level of 450 volts, some of them refused to continue, and one of them, referred to as the "teacher of the Old Testament," gave up because of moral and religious reasons. Even though the person in charge of the experiment encouraged the "teachers" by saying things like, "Please continue," "The experiment needs you to continue," "It's absolutely essential that you continue," or "You really have to continue," the "teacher of the Old Testament" was extremely concerned about the welfare and good health of the "student," and insisted that he did, in fact, have a choice and that meant he was going to cease administering the electric shocks (Milgram 1963, 371–378).

This example appears to demonstrate the importance of the agent's virtuous character. This is because the "teacher of the Old Testament" displayed prudence in attaching more importance to the welfare of the "student" rather than to the success of the experiment. This showed his autonomy in acting in a self-determined way, in considering illegitimate the authority of the person in charge of the experiment, in feeling compassion for the "student's" suffering, and in manifesting his own integrity in the sense that his action corresponded to the set of values and principles he considered to be correct, such as the dignity and physical welfare of the "student," thus signaling that he had deliberated carefully about the consequences of the experiment.[5]

Of course, this does not prove that in certain circumstances agents are not influenced by the outside world. However, it appears to show that, in many cases relevant to day-to-day, life moral character is the motivational source of specific actions. It also indicates that, in general, virtues are intrinsically linked with the behavior of the agent, as in the example given earlier of the connection between prudence, autonomy, compassion, and integrity. We should remember that Aristotle considered prudence (the ability to identify the necessary means to ensure a good outcome for a specific action) as an intellectual virtue that is a precondition for all the other important virtues, whether they be moral, such as courage, moderation, justice, and generosity, or epistemic, such as humility, curiosity, and integrity. It is also important to consider the fact that even though certain individuals are influenced by the outside world, it does not mean that they should not be virtuous unless there is some natural impediment to being so. This does not seem to be the case since we can refer to real examples of virtuous people, such as "the teacher of the Old Testament" in Milgram's experiment, as well as other well-known cases, such as those of Socrates, Nelson Mandela, and Sophie Scholl, who acted virtuously even though they were putting their own lives at risk.

Although this is not definitive proof that moral character is indeed reliable, I nevertheless maintain that it is a sufficient one, even for "situationists," of the value of virtues in our daily lives. Perhaps this is because of our strong belief in our capacity for truthfulness and our disposition to become better persons. At the end of the day, without this expectation, it seems that our lives would hardly be worth living.

III

In *The Wealth of Nations* (*WN*), Adam Smith states, "It is not from the benevolence of the butcher, the brewer, or the baker, that we expect our dinner, but from regard to their own interest," and this appears to stem from a somewhat equivocal view within Smithian thought. In *TMS*, Smith begins by claiming that, no matter how self-centered we may be, we also have a natural interest in the happiness and misfortunes of others (Smith 1976, I.i.1.1). Rather than affirming that self-interest and self-love are the only egoistical motivators of agents, Smith believes that, as members of a moral and political community, we have moral sentiments that force us to take into account both the happiness and the misfortunes of others. This implies considering sympathy as the protagonist's capacity to put themselves in the place of another person and to adopt sentiments of resentment and gratitude as essential criteria for the disapproval or approval of an action – i.e., as a criterion of propriety for it, together with an increase in general rules to correct the inconvenience of our transitory emotions – and this conclusion is arrived at through the judgment of the impartial spectator (Smith 1976, I.i.3.4).

In order to know whether a certain action is right or wrong, we need to be able to rely on the approval of an observer who has the imaginative capacity to identify sentiments of gratitude and resentment in others, as these sentiments provide the normative basis for the approval or disapproval of the action in question. Thus, the impartial spectator will be "the person inside the heart" and "the great judge and arbiter" of the suitability of the action (Smith 1976, III.2.32), and they will have the capacity not only to approve the behavior of others but to view themselves both as an individual and as a member of a moral community by means of their sympathy with their peers. This implies that they have the capacity to assess, impartially or at least in reciprocal terms, the behavior and human motivation of others. This means they will represent established social attitudes and are therefore the very voice of society (Smith 1976, I.i.4.6).

It should be emphasized that, in addition to the general characteristics of a moral theory based on sentiments, Smith sets out an ingenious virtue theory in Parts VI and VII of *TMS*. In Part 7, entitled "Of Systems of Moral Philosophy," he examines the limits of the main moral virtue theories and defends the link that exists between the traditional virtues of prudence, benevolence, justice, and self-command for both individual and collective happiness, as well as defending sympathy as the main principle for the approval of human behavior. The limits of these traditional theories, such as the Platonic, the Aristotelian, the Stoical, the Epicurean, and even those of Hutcheson and Hume, can be explained by the partial and imperfect form in which they describe human and social nature. For Smith,

> [f]rom some one or other of those principles which I have been endeavouring to unfold, every system of morality that ever had any reputation in the world has, perhaps, ultimately been derived. As they are all of them, in this respect, founded upon natural principles, they are all of them in some measure in the right. But as many of them are derived from a partial and imperfect view of nature, there are many of them too in some respects in the wrong.
>
> (Smith 1976, VII.i.1)

Having identified the descriptive limitations of the traditional theories, Smith's next step is to observe that there are two central questions that must be dealt with by moral philosophy, that is, the nature of virtue and the principle of the approval of behavior. In the second Section of Part VII in *TMS*, Smith analyses the main answers given to the question concerning the nature of virtue and begins by considering those theories that explain it as the proper controlling and direction of our affections, such as the virtue of propriety, whose main proponents are Plato, Aristotle, and the Stoics (especially Zenon). He then examines Epicurean philosophy, which asserts that virtue is found in prudence; that is, it consists only in the search for our own self-interest and happiness. He ends by analyzing the position of Hutcheson in defending the idea that virtue is found in benevolence or rather that virtue is rooted in the affections that relate to the happiness of others (Smith 1976, VII.II.1–3).

Following his investigation into the range of answers given regarding the nature of virtue, in the third Section of Part VII, Smith examines the answers given concerning the nature of the principle of the approval of agents' behavior. He rejects the self-centered arguments of Hobbes, Mandeville, and Pufendorf who identify self-love as the only principle for the approval of the behavior and motivation of agents. He also rejects Cudworth's rationalist position, which identifies reason as the principle of absolute approval, since he himself asserts that perceptions of right and wrong are rooted in sentiment and are not like an intuition or personal interpretation (which is the position defended by Hutcheson), but rather lie in the virtue of sympathy.

The main point I wish to make here is that Smith's conception of virtues appears to be inclusivist rather than exclusivist, and he does not deny the importance of the virtues of prudence, justice, benevolence, and self-command. The main problem with traditional theories is that they do not admit that we need to possess a range of different virtues in order to achieve personal and social happiness. For instance, in the economic domain, the virtue of prudence is essential in identifying the means which are necessary for subsistence. In the moral domain, the virtue of benevolence is crucial in the sense that it looks to the welfare of others without self-interest. In the judicial and political domain justice, it is seen as an essential virtue in protecting the common good, as well as providing qualities such as probity and leadership. The virtue of self-command can be considered as a metavirtue – that is, as a precondition for all the other virtues and a means of achieving propriety, the most important virtue in being able to control one's own emotions.[6]

For Smith, virtue is a normal trait of character that is revered by members of a community because of its capacity to bring happiness. Thus, it is "excellence, something uncommonly great and beautiful, which rises far above what is vulgar and ordinary" (Smith 1976, I.ii. 1). In a similar vein to Aristotle, the measure of virtue is a mean and neither excess nor deficiency (Smith 1976, I.ii. 1). In line with classical tradition, Smith considers all the virtues to be artificial, including probity, generosity, prudence, and frankness. What is more important is that the virtues are acquired through habit since following the rules, for example, is viewed as satisfactory because it is approved by the impartial observer, and repetition is the best way of forming a virtuous character (Smith 1976, III.2).

But which virtues are necessary for guaranteeing a successful life both for individuals and for society? In Part VI of *TMS*, which was only published in the sixth and final edition of the book in 1790, Smith analyzes the nature of virtue by examining individual character and how it affects the happiness of a particular person, as well as how it affects the happiness of others. He notes that we require prudence in our individual quest for happiness and justice and benevolence in seeking the happiness of others since it is justice that prevents us from doing harm to them and benevolence that impels us to help them. In addition to these virtues, self-command is taken to be the most effective measure, while virtue is more important in the control of emotions (Smith, 1976, VI. concl. 1–2). It seems only right to say that this theory links in a harmonious way with the Aristotelian virtue of prudence and the Christian virtue of benevolence, as well as with the Stoical virtue of self-command. It also includes an important modern conception of justice in the sense that it may be considered a negative virtue or a positive duty since it is based on the recognized rights of the individuals in a particular community.

My final comment on the Smithian distinction between positive and negative virtues is that although virtuous behavior may be desirable and laudable from a personal point of view, only justice is demanded by the public domain. To quote Smith's own words:

> And upon this is founded that remarkable distinction between justice and all the other social virtues, which has of late been particularly insisted upon by an author of very great and original genius, that we feel ourselves to be under a stricter obligation to act according to justice, than agreeably to friendship, charity, or generosity; that the practice of these last mentioned virtues seems to be left in some measure to our own choice, but that, somehow or other, we feel ourselves to be in a peculiar manner tied, bound, and obliged to the observation of justice.
>
> (Smith 1976, II.ii. 1.5)

This appears to imply a liberal conception of justice, in that it stipulates the ethical neutrality of the state since acts of generosity, friendship, or charity are a question of personal choice. Benevolence, for example, is a voluntary and disinterested virtue, and if it is not present, it is not subject to legal censure but simply becomes the object of displeasure. Justice, on the other hand, prevents us from doing harm to others and violating their right to life, property, and reputation, to illustrate. It is because of this that punishment is meted out to those who infringe on the rights of others (Smith 1976, II.ii. 1.9), and it is restricted to acts such as assault, robbery, murder, and rape. But in addition to its being a vitally important liberal achievement, Smith stresses that it acts as a normative force in society and a defense of positive virtues. While society can prescribe rules that prohibit certain offenses and establish corresponding retribution for the perpetrator, a judicious legislator would also take public welfare into account in their judgment (Smith 1976, II.ii.1.8).

I have referred at length to Smith's theory of virtues because it provides the bridge which is so necessary for reconciling the private and public domains. Moreover, his theory considers justice to be the central pillar of the whole social edifice, especially in terms of bridging the empathetic gap, in the sense that sympathy becomes weaker in proportion to the distance between individuals. Fair play is one of the criteria used by Smith, which means that he considers it acceptable to pursue self-interest if you play fairly with others and avoid lies, deception, and fraud in financial dealings, for example (Smith 1976, II.ii.2.2). In *WN*, in addition to recognizing the vital role of the state in resolving social problems, such as the reduction of poverty, access to education, and the construction of roads and communication systems, Smith defends the principle of fair taxation and stipulates that the higher the amount of money received, the higher the rate of tax paid should be (Smith 1976, Vol.2, V.ii.b.3).

IV

Justice is recognized as one of the most important moral virtues and is specifically public in nature. Like all virtues, it is a trait of character that is at the heart of the flourishment of a successful life. Since it is a moral virtue, it can be seen as a multiple trait that links the various emotions of the individual – that is, their choices, values, desires, perceptions, attitudes, interests, expectations, and sensitivities. As McDowell says, virtue requires a reliable sensitivity and implies behaving correctly. For example, generosity implies giving the appropriate attention to the feelings of others as a prerequisite for acting in a certain way (McDowell 1997, 141–147). Bearing this in mind, we can understand justice as a trait of character – that is, as a tendency to act in a just way.

As the tradition emphasizes, the virtue of justice has an intrinsic relationship with other people. It is a trait of character that is nurtured through habit, and it consists in giving other people their due, whether it be in terms of the distribution of goods or punishment for an illegal act. In *Ethica Nicomachea*, Aristotle defines justice as the disposition of the soul to do what is just, as well as to act justly and desire what is just, which implies the perfection of behavior. It is important to point out that a just person cannot be overambitious; that is, they cannot expect more than their just desserts. Justice is therefore often considered to be the principle moral virtue since it is perfect in relation to other individuals and in the relationships which an individual maintains with their community (Aristotle 1999, V, 1129 a 5–1129 b 35).

In this sense, therefore, justice is the moral virtue *par excellence* in relation to other people. This appears to clearly show the public or social character of the virtue of justice, which seems to encapsulate all the other moral virtues, such as generosity, benevolence, clemency, and equity. For instance, equity (*epieikeia*) is the virtue that interprets the law by giving it greater flexibility and determining what is considered just in each situation. It is for this reason that equity is better than legal justice, even though it is not better in an unrestricted context. Equity, therefore, corrects the law when the latter is guilty of omission because of its generality, especially since the law cannot cover all possible situations, which is clearly shown when it is necessary to proclaim a governmental decree. When a determined situation is undefined, the rule that covers it will also be undefined, "as the lead standard is in Lesbian building." Lead adapts itself to the shape of the stone because it is malleable, and in the same way, a governmental decree adapts itself to a particular legal situation (Aristotle 1999, V, 1137 b 29–32).

As I have said, justice, as perceived in the classical tradition, is both a moral quality of the individual and a civic virtue, since it is central to the unity of individual and political existence, bringing about both personal and collective happiness. The capacity of an agent to recognize the relevant features of a particular case to give what is due to others stems from a disposition to achieve justice, but it is also a public virtue that wishes to ensure social stability in the correct way, and this is a point which has often been emphasized by more modern writers. Adam Smith, to give an example, sees justice as a negative virtue in the sense that its application is not linked to the freedom of will of the agent since it can be demanded by force when the violation of legal rules causes resentment among the members of a particular community, which is a fundamental element in all types of punishment. Justice, therefore, considers the harmful tendency of the actions that have brought about this resentment, especially in relation to the empathetic resentment of the impartial spectator. This is why it is considered to be a negative virtue, as it implies a disposition not to cause harm to others and to respect the rights of individuals to life, freedom, and propriety. It is also a social virtue with a specific characteristic: it is obligatory for all citizens, and thus different from such social virtues as generosity, charity, and friendship, which can be chosen freely, while only not acting justly is subject to legal punishment. This conception of justice emphasizes the criterion of impartiality since the acceptable measure of correction will be decided by the impartial observer. In this way, we become just by learning to judge ourselves through the eyes of others, and this implies recognition of the equality of all individuals.[7]

It is important to note that contemporary literature on virtues is more concerned with public rather than personal justice and with the necessary conditions for establishing a just society. In his theory of justice as fairness, John Rawls, by way of illustration, identifies justice as the primary virtue in political, social and economic institutions such as the national constitution, the family, and property. His fundamental idea is that each individual possesses an inviolable morality based on justice, which may not be disrespected even in the case of improved social welfare, thus guaranteeing the freedom and equality of citizens in the face of natural and social arbitrariness. Independently of how the concept of justice may be defined, it is generally that institutions are just when there no arbitrary distinction is made between individuals and when rules determine the equilibrium between conflicting demands. In other words, this means that justice is interpreted as being the same as fairness (Rawls 1999, 3–5).

Although social justice is the principal focus of Rawls' theory, he also expresses an important concern with justice as a virtue in a wider sense. People are characterized by having a sense of justice and a conception of what is good or rather a rational capacity for following a particular life plan. In turn, having a sense of justice means having the natural capacity to know intuitively what is right and wrong, or what is just and unjust. For instance, we know intuitively that it is wrong to punish an innocent person or to obtain a maximum level of personal happiness through the suffering of an innocent person.[8]

In section 9 of *A Theory of Justice*, Rawls compares the sense of justice to the sense of grammaticality we possess in relation to utterances in our mother tongue. He refers to Chomsky's theory of generative grammar, which states that each person has a moral grammar, or rather, the competence of knowing what is right and wrong or just and unjust in everyday situations. However, the performance of the individual is related to many variables, such as whether the public institutions that are responsible for their formation are just, or whether they have a positive disposition toward justice. At any rate, the individual must possess at least a minimal sense of justice that permits them to live together with other people – that is, which allows them to be a citizen who accepts certain obligations and demands certain rights. In other words, the individual must have at least a minimally just character in order to be able to combat feelings such as avarice, envy, cruelty, and insensitivity. This appears to lead us to the confirmation of the criterion of reciprocity, which is identified in the moral senses analyzed. These senses are highly reliable and include the ones that defend the premise that, to illustrate, religious intolerance and racial discrimination are unjust. They are the starting point for the construction of the principles of justice, which are chosen in a situation of symmetry – that is, a situation of clear equality among individuals as moral persons (Rawls 1999, 10–19).

Despite the difficulty of determining exactly what justice consists of, it is my understanding that through the various well-known reflections on this theme, we can identify the relevant normative criteria of equity, impartiality, and reciprocity. The virtue of justice also demands equality and allows us to determine that individual actions are just, both in a distributive and retributive sense, while making it possible to identify injustices, especially in the social practices established by public institutions, in the sense that justice is a normative social standard rather than an individual one.[9]

As noted earlier, a just person can be identified as someone who possesses the virtue of equity (*epieikeia*) – that is, the capacity to recognize the relevant features of a particular case in order to give to others what is due to them as the result of a disposition to see justice done – and this may sometimes mean that the agent gives up their own rights in such cases. A fair decision also tends to determine exactly what is just in each situation, thus correcting the generality of the law. In certain cases, justice seems to demand that a positive law is broken, even though we are morally obliged to obey this law but consider it unjust, as might be the case with Nazism or with the segregationist laws of the United States or South Africa. In these countries, a just individual would have to commit certain acts of disobedience to achieve their desire for justice, and the acts of Martin Luther King Jr. and Nelson Mandela might be good examples through which we would be able to understand better the behavior of a person who possesses the virtue of justice. In turn, impartiality is taken to be the disposition not to cause harm to others, and this leads us to recognize the rights to life, liberty, and property, for instance, as well as the public obligation which stems from this recognition. Here the measurement of justice is given by other people, and therefore it is social, as is the case with the figure of the impartial spectator. Let us imagine a judge who is trying a case of corruption without considering the accused party, but only taking into account the relevant facts of the crime, its materiality, and so on, while duly obeying the law. On the other hand, reciprocity is the normative criterion that prevents any arbitrary distinction from being made between individuals by giving the same weight to their conflicting demands. To illustrate, a just person would not consider it right to punish someone who is innocent or to punish a guilty person too severely merely for reasons of prevention. This is rooted in the disposition to consider all individuals within a situation of symmetry where they each have the same rights and duties, which seems to reveal a natural basis for mutual confidence and affection.[10]

V

Having analyzed the importance of virtues in our lives and exploring in detail Adam Smith's proposal concerning the link between these virtues and the guarantee of happiness, with special attention to the fundamental characteristics of the public virtue of justice, we can now return to our original question and conclude that the problems which arose with the onset of the COVID-19 pandemic may be resolved more efficiently by establishing a bridge between the spheres of personal and public morality. We can do this by linking certain personal moral and epistemic virtues with a range of public virtues, and an example of this is the link between the personal virtues of prudence, benevolence, and self-command, and the public virtue of justice as postulated by Adam Smith's theory.

It is, of course, of fundamental importance to carry out an accurate analysis in order to identify which virtues are currently necessary to reconcile the personal and public domains, since these virtues are the normative standards that have been established over time. For instance, the virtue of courage was central in classical antiquity, especially since wars were a constant feature and well-being was closely associated with victory. In the Middle Ages, the virtue of charity was essential for anyone who aspired to be a good person, whereas in modern times, curiosity became a more relevant virtue since well-being was directly related to scientific discovery. However, nowadays, the list of most relevant virtues seems to be quite different. And, with this in mind, it could be the case that Smith's proposal reveals anachronism.

Therefore, in addition to prudence, self-command, benevolence, and justice, which other virtues are necessary for building the bridge between the private and public spheres, thus guaranteeing personal and collective stability? Autonomy may be important in ensuring that citizens can think for themselves and make independent decisions, thereby increasing personal responsibility. In this connection, integrity seems also relevant since it implies a disposition for acting coherently based on the values and beliefs that are assumed by agents. By the same token, humility seems fundamental in counteracting arrogance and vanity, while tolerance seems crucial for living in a diverse society and is also essential in the field of politics. In addition to these personal virtues, I believe that justice is the most important virtue in the major political, social, and economic institutions of a democratic society, by guaranteeing equal liberty and equality of opportunity and welfare, which in turn ensures equal rights to health care for the protection of all lives, considering that good health is a basic good that should be equitably distributed.

Of course, the solutions proposed in this chapter are only a first draft and are in no way intended to be the final word on the virtues that are fundamental to our social lives. But I believe this is a promising route of investigation that will require public consensus and collective effort so that we may arrive at a better understanding of its many problems and consider how the findings of such an investigation could be applied in practice.

Notes

1 For Julia Annas, virtue can be understood as a stable disposition of the agent's character in order to be seen as a person's tendency to be a certain way. Also, it can be understood as a disposition that is a deep characteristic of the agent, being the virtue the mark of its character. Furthermore, she points out that this disposition, which is active, requires habituation and experience, habituation achieved through education in the family and school and that cannot be seen as a routine due to the need for constant monitoring for personal improvement. See Annas (2011, 1–15).

2 On the success of the Finnish educational model, see the interesting article by Remo Bastos, "The Surprising Success of the Finnish Educational System in Global Scenario of Commodified Education." See Bastos (2017, 802–825).

3 For more details on the experiments carried out and cited by the "situationists," see the chapter by Merrit, Doris, and Harman, "Character" (Merritt, Doris, and Harman 2010, 356–357).

4 For further clarification of the research, its methodology and its results, see the article by Milgram, "Behavioral Study of Obedience" (Milgram 1963, 371–374).

5 Roberts and Wood, in *Intellectual Virtues* (2007), analyze this case, clarifying the character traits manifested in the action: (i) he positioning himself to obtain a maximal relevant information about the "student," doing so with skill and good judgment; (ii) he showed good judgment about conflicting values when deciding for the well-being of the "student"; (iii) he showed epistemic caution about the ostensible authority manifested by the person responsible for the experiment when claiming to know what he was doing and by offering sufficient arguments against that authority; (iv) he demonstrated the virtue of compassion and conscientiousness in the situation; and (v) he demonstrated respect for a moral authority that transcended human authority that could be arbitrary. See Roberts and Wood (2007, 318–319).

6 Robert Shaver correctly observes that Smith's moral theory is attractive in avoiding two familiar caricatures – namely, that of the Aristotelian virtuous agent, who deliberates correctly without making use of universal rules, and that of the Kantian moral agent, who takes as criterion of the action the duties and not its feeling in front of the case. He says that Smith takes the agent's character as the normative source of moral evaluation, but without forgetting the importance of deontic concepts such as duties. See Shaver (2006, 208).

7 Adam Smith says that justice is a negative virtue that forbids us from harming our neighbors. He comments that the person who refrains from violating the rights of others, or the state, or the reputation of his neighbors, would surely have very little positive merit. However, with this abstention, it fulfills all the necessary requirements to be considered a just person, fulfilling her public obligation. See Smith 1976, II.ii.I.2.

8 In the article "The Sense of Justice," Rawls argues that the sense of justice is not only connected with the moral sentiments of resentment, indignation, and guilt but also with the natural attitudes of mutual trust and affection. See Rawls 1963, 281–282.

9 In this regard, it is important to note that the central argument of John Rawls' theory of justice seems to be that, from a social point of view, we can reach a consensus on what counts as having a public moral-political value independently of private beliefs of good, such as political and moral principles of equal liberty (first principle of justice), fair equality of opportunity, and common good's difference principle (second principle of justice), which are socially accepted in contemporary democratic societies. See Rawls (1999, 10–15).

10 On reciprocity in a naturalistic sense, one can think that in cooperative species, such as the human one, there is a clear aversion to inequality since the basis of cooperation seems to be reciprocity. For example, hunting large mammals in the Pleistocene was only possible with human cooperative work, which resulted in a certain understanding of equality among cooperators, as well as a criterion for blaming noncooperators. See Lebar (2018, 6–7). See also Buchanan and Powell (2018, 26–34; 121–123).

References

Annas, Julia. 2011. *Intelligent Virtue*. Oxford: Oxford University Press.

Aristotle. 1999. *Nicomachean Ethics*. Trans. Terence Irwin. 2a. ed. Indianapolis: Hackett.

Bastos, Remo Moreira Brito. 2017. "The surprising success of the Finnish educational system in global scenario of commodified education." *Revista Brasileira de Educação*, Vol. 22, N. 70: 802–825.

Buchanan, Allen., Powell, Russell. 2018. *The Evolution of Moral Progress: A Biocultural Theory*. New York: Oxford University Press.

Lebar, Mark. (Ed.). 2018. *Justice. The Virtues*. New York: Oxford University Press.

McDowell, John. 1997. "Virtue and reason." In Crisp, Roger, Slote, Michael (Eds.). *Virtue Ethics*. New York: Oxford University Press, 141–162.

Merritt, Maria, Doris, John M., Harman, Gilbert. 2010. "Character." In Doris, John M. (Ed.). *The Moral Psychology Handbook*. Oxford: Oxford University Press: 355–401.

Milgram, Stanley. 1963. "Behavioral study of obedience." *Journal of Abnormal and Social Psychology*, Vol. 67, N. 4: 371–378.

Rawls, John. 1963. "The sense of justice." *Philosophical Review*, Vol. 72, N. 3: 281–305.

Rawls, John. 1999. *A Theory of Justice*. Revised Edition. Cambridge, MA: Harvard University Press.

Roberts, Robert C., Wood, W. Jay. 2007. *Intellectual Virtues: An Essay in Regulative Epistemology*. New York: Oxford University Press, 257–285.

Shaver, Robert. 2006. *Virtues, utility, and rules*. In *The Cambridge Companion to Adam Smith*. New York: Cambridge University Press, 89–213.

Smith, Adam. 1976a. *An Inquiry into the Nature and Causes of the Wealth of Nations*. Volumes I and II. Edited by R. H. Campbell and A. S. Skinner, textual editor W. B. Todd. The Glasgow Edition of the Works and Correspondence of Adam Smith, Vol. 2. Oxford: Oxford University Press.

Smith, Adam. 1976b. *The Theory of Moral Sentiments*. Edited by Raphael, D. D. and Macfie, A. L. The Glasgow Edition of the Works and Correspondence of Adam Smith. Oxford: Oxford University Press.

7 An alternative model of ethics for global crises

Confucian relationism

Jana S. Rošker

7.1 Introduction

Drawing on Confucian relational ethics, this chapter explores the connection between the cultural conditionality of Confucian moral philosophies and their possible implications for crisis resolution strategies. The desire to write about this topic arose in me immediately after the onset of the COVID-19 pandemic. As I write these lines, it appears that the pandemic has largely been brought under control. But what we have learned from this experience is that in critical times, our mutual responsibility requires us to act in ways that are often uncomfortable or even painful. In such times, philosophy can show us how to use this crisis as an opportunity to cultivate our sense of togetherness and mutual aid. Moreover, in uncertain times, it can awaken in us an awareness of our individual mortality and moral responsibility. Since every pandemic is a crisis of global proportions, all of humanity must be engaged to find a strategic solution to it. Therefore, knowledge and thoughts from different cultures and times may well prove helpful in such times.

Thus, in such situations, it is especially important to consider ideas and ethical theories from different cultures. Dialogues between different forms of such intellectual legacies are therefore not only advisable but also necessary and the most sensible thing to do. Such exchanges, which could or should take place in the context of the current developments of globalization, are important and valuable not only in terms of solving the current pandemic crisis but also when taking into account other global problems that it is accompanied by and linked to, such as the constant environmental disasters,[1] the ever-widening gap between rich and poor, the resulting migration crises, and so on.

Indeed, solving such problems requires the cooperation and solidarity of the entire world population – something that will only be possible if there can be a mutual understanding between different cultures and civilizations. As a sinologist who is working on Chinese intellectual history, I will focus on the Chinese experience in this context and, in particular, as the title of this chapter suggests, on Confucian philosophy and ethics.

DOI: 10.4324/9781003310129-9

Many people believe that human beings tend to be self-interested and guided by immediate goals. If it is not curbed by appropriate information and hindered by insights into the existential significance of the relationship between the individual and society, this tendency becomes even more apparent in times of crisis. Especially in the modern world, concern about the risks of community contagion seems abstract and less important than the preservation of individual freedoms. If we are to develop other principles and embrace the values of cooperation and solidarity, we must modify and reshape our thinking so that it can proceed from a communal or social rather than an egocentric perspective. Indeed, the COVID-19 pandemic has shown that we need to put our moral theories into action in order to change our individual performances. It is in this context that Confucian relational ethics can certainly offer us useful and valuable alternatives, for, as we shall see, it is based on a different conception of humanity from that which has historically prevailed in Western culture. Within the framework of traditional Confucian ethics, personalities are constituted not by an emphasis on their individual particularities but by their vital embeddedness in a dynamic social network created by their relationships with their fellow human beings. As such, this ethics can provide us with a whole range of valuable foundations for new forms of mutual empathy and solidarity, which are certainly among the most solid foundations for new crisis-solving strategies. Such transculturally conditioned theoretical foundations can help us to create new models of intersubjectivity and new foundations for more human-centered politics, legislation, and decision-making systems.

7.2 Confucianism: Original teachings vs. ideological doctrine

As a sinologist, I cannot forget that the coronavirus, which can cause a lung disease with high contagiousness and mortality, first appeared in China, and thus in the very cultural-linguistic space that is the core of my personal and professional interests, and therefore essential to the fundamental content of my research. However, although the onset of the pandemic can be located in this area, this is not the only reason why it is worthwhile to investigate the connection between China and the entirety of East Asia on the one hand and the COVID-19 pandemic on the other. Initially, as the infection spread on a global scale and assumed pandemic proportions, it quickly became clear that it was the Sinic cultural and linguistic area,[2] rather than the Euro-American regions, that was more effective in stemming the tide of this viral epidemic and partly even eradicating it.

The research on which this chapter is based has clearly shown that in seeking an answer to the question of the reasons for the greater efficiency and effectiveness of Sinic cultural spaces in the initial phases of the pandemic, it is necessary to refute the unfounded claim that this is due to the allegedly autocratic practices of Sinic states, which act 'top-down'[3] and can do so because of the traditional 'obedience' of their people. On the contrary, in the months following the epidemic, it became clear that measures were less effective in Sinic autocratic systems than in those countries of the region that are liberal democracies, such as Taiwan or South Korea. In this chapter, I start from the assumption that the real reasons for this better performance are more likely to be found in Confucian relational ethics, which does not start from the notion of an isolated individual and within which the contextualized human Self and society are placed in a mutually complementary relationship.

What underlies all liberal axiological systems, and what therefore constitutes the crucial moral foundation of today's global modernization, are the European Enlightenment values based on the idea of a free and autonomous individual subject. The recent pandemic has clearly shown that these values in their present form can no longer function as a coherent moral force even for Europe, let alone for all currently globalized and highly differentiated societies. However, the ideas of free and autonomous subjectivity and humanism are among the ideational foundations of modernization and constitute an important part of the European intellectual heritage, which still serves as the basis for numerous legal and ideological paradigms of today's societies.

It is, therefore, necessary to revive, improve and update the key humanist concepts of autonomy and free subjectivity, and to place them in a new framework of intersubjectivity in order to adapt them to the requirements of the present age. To achieve this goal, the tradition of European Enlightenment must be placed in a fruitful dialog and dialectical relationship with similar and related intellectual heritages of non-European cultures. As a sinologist, I will attempt to sketch the foundations of such a dialog through an introduction and critical evaluation of the ethics of Sinic Confucianism, which represents a specific East Asian version of humanism, for it is based on a high valuation of interpersonal relationships, mutual empathy, and responsible autonomy. Within this dialectical framework, this chapter explores the ways in which specific Confucian notions of personhood and autonomy can contribute to a meaningful cross-cultural adaptation and revitalization of humanist values.

Nowadays, the prevailing view of Confucian ethics is based on a number of prejudices, for in today's world, it is usually seen as a strictly normative, hierarchical ethic, supposedly based on gerontocracy, patriarchy, and the oppression of subjects by the ruling elites who in this system supposedly demand absolute obedience from their people.

The vast majority of today's Western-trained philosophers are not too familiar with the deeper levels of Confucian ethical systems. The contemporary Berlin philosopher of Korean descent Byung-Chul Han, for example, sees the reasons for the more rapid establishment of pandemic control measures in the East Asian region as rooted in the autocratic traditions of those regions. Han writes,

> What advantages, compared to Europe, in the fight against the pandemic, can we find in the Asian system? Asian countries like Japan, Korea, China, Hong Kong, Taiwan and Singapore have an authoritarian mindset, originating from their cultural tradition (Confucianism). People are less rebellious and more docile than in Europe.
>
> (Han 2020, 2)

Such assertions are populist, generalizing, and without empirically provable basis. First of all, the thesis of the alleged "all-around obedience" of people throughout the Sinic region compared to Europe and America, where people are supposed to be more critical and less docile (as the statement implicitly implies), is completely ungrounded. It is based instead on the widespread assumption that Confucianism is a conservative normative ethic that advocates gerontocracy and the suppression of the individual in favor of the state. Few of those who blindly advocate such theses actually know the subject under discussion, and few know that the ethics of the original Confucianism was very progressive and critical of the social and political elites of the time for the period in which it arose.

The original Confucian teachings emphasized "humaneness (*ren* 仁)" and "rituality (*li* 禮)," advocated diversity and pluralism, and also contained many proto-democratic elements.

However, during the period of the first Confucian reform (i.e., the Han period, 206 BC–220 BC), there was an ideological misappropriation of Confucian teachings for the need for a new state-building doctrine. These processes led to an assimilation of many elements of autocratic legalism into the framework of the teachings and studies of Confucian ethics. In this way, a new state doctrine was formed out of proto-philosophical Confucianism (Bauer 1971, 117–140). Compared to the original philosophical ethics of Confucianism, which contained many pluralistic views and was highly contextual and based on flexibility and autonomy, it was a prescriptive, extremely rigid, and restrictive set of social rules that received its institutional foundation somewhat later with the introduction of the civil service examinations, which required all candidates for government positions to uncritically adopt the contents of Confucian classics, especially their formal rules (ibid.). While the latter became the basis not only of institutionalized Confucian state doctrine but also of constitutive social ethics characterized by strict vertical hierarchy; gerontocracy; discrimination against various marginalized groups, including women; social standardization; and suppression of individual autonomy, the former represents a dynamic and changeable framework of the constant reopening of diverse philosophical questions, appreciation of social diversity, and negation of dogmatism and autocratic rules.[4]

For at least a basic understanding of the respective traditional ideologies, therefore, we must first understand the differences between Confucianism as a humanistic philosophy, on the one hand, and Confucianism as a dogmatic state doctrine or conservative normative ethic, on the other. However, due to the complexity of the specific features that define Chinese political and ethical culture, these two currents have often overlapped throughout Chinese history: "Since rulers and scholar-officials joined themselves together to form an inseparable tie as members of the same community, culture and power existed in an unusually close relationship" (Huang 2014, 281). Nevertheless, for the sake of conceptual clarity and because of the many specific elements that define each of the two approaches, we must distinguish between political and philosophical Confucianism, and for the purposes of this chapter, we will focus on the latter. We will thus be concerned with the specific Confucian ethics, which in turn cannot be separated from its philosophical (or metaphysical) foundations.[5]

At the heart of such Confucian humanism[6] is the fundamental virtue of humaneness or co-humaneness (*ren*). The Chinese character with which this term is written consists of two parts; the left part denotes a human being, the right the number two, which also stands for the plural. So the term *ren* tells us, among other things, that no human being can exist alone, isolated from other human beings. We can all survive (and even come into existence) only through our vital connections with other people. No person is an island, and we can therefore only live in communities with our fellow human beings. This interconnectedness can only work if most people in a community are aware of its vital importance; therefore, ren also implies a mutual empathy, the ability to identify with other people, to feel their needs and fears, and to understand their situation.

Such mutual empathy is, of course, a foundation of social solidarity, which is of paramount importance, especially in times of widespread social crisis, such as the current COVID-19 pandemic. On the other hand, such solidarity based on mutual empathy is also the foundation of Confucian relational ethics, relics of which are still present, albeit often in a latent form, in most contemporary Sinic societies. This relational ethic, together with its elementary virtue of humaneness (*ren*), undoubtedly has much to do with promoting mutual interpersonal cooperation and solidarity among people. Therefore, such traditional ethical elements have, in my view, contributed much to the effective yet democratic containment of the pandemic in the Sinic region. In what follows, I will illuminate this conjecture through the lens of traditional Confucian relational ethics and its inherently humanistic values.

7.3 Relational self and independent individuality

With regard to the traditional structure of the relationship between the individual and society, there is a fundamental difference between the modern European (or "Western") and the traditional Chinese socio-political system. While the former is based on the idea of a free and abstract individual, the Sinic social order is founded on a network of relationships and could therefore be called "relational virtue ethics" (Li Zehou and Liu Yuedi 2014, 209). This fundamental distinction leads to major differences in the ethical thinking prevalent in these two discourses of cultural philosophy, not only in terms of their respective views on the relationship between the individual and society but also on the relationship between reason and emotion.

Traditional Sinic societies were structured as networks of relations that connected individuals who were not constituted as isolated and independent entities but as so-called relational Selves, meaning that people were essentially related to one another and their social relationships largely determined their identities. In Confucian ethics, the human Self is always located in particular concrete situations and social environments; therefore, all conceptions of the person focus on his or her relationships. This also implies that a person's chosen aspirations, failures, and achievements can only be understood in light of their interactions with others (Lai 2018, 64). Morality, then, is rooted in the harmonious interaction of different persons embedded in different social roles. Contemporary Chinese philosopher Li Zehou uses the term "relationalism" or (in his own translation) "*guanxi-ism*" (Li 2016, 1076) to refer to such particularities of Confucian ethics that grounds morality in social relations rather than in individualism.

Ancient Confucians defined the main structure of human social networks as consisting of five basic relationships (*wu lun* 五倫). This model can be regarded as a summary of the elementary human relationships in any civil society, as it consists of the familial, political, and comradely relationships. However, it also shows the Confucian emphasis on the family, as three of the five basic relationships are rooted in it. According to Li Zehou (ibid.), this is the basis of the relationalism mentioned earlier. This social system infuses emotions into interpersonal relationships, with the sincere emotion of parent-child love being the root, substance, and foundation (Jia 2018, 156). Thus, it is no coincidence that in this view, the family was linked to the state through the ideal of a good citizen; in Confucian ethics, a good citizen had to be a good family member first. The core idea behind such a view is that regulating relationships within one's family leads to a well-ordered state (see, e.g., *Mengzi*, n.d. Li Lou 1, 5[7]).

In their book *Confucian Role Ethics – A Moral Vision for the 21st Century*, Henry Rosemont and Roger Ames also emphasize that family reverence (*xiao* 孝) is the origin of virtuous social behavior and the source of humaneness (*ren*). They refer to the model that Li Zehou called "relationalism" as "role ethics" instead, emphasizing that it is a network of social roles that emerges from the roles of members within a family. In such roles, people's lives are embedded in meaningful contexts. Moreover, the network is dynamic and multi-layered, because no one takes only one role, but everyone plays many of them. Before modern society, Confucian individuals existed for the totality of their family, clan, tribe, or religion (Li 2016, 1118). But in the context of Western-type modernity, which emphasizes the values of subjective autonomy, the totality (e.g., society) exists for the individual.[8]

Moreover, within the framework of Western individualism, personal uniqueness is given central importance because it is a basis for human creativity and progress. And since personal uniqueness is also an important issue when it comes to the relationship between society and the individual in general, let us take a closer look at its place within traditional Confucian philosophy. This is all the more important because many people mistakenly believe that Confucianism does not allow for individual uniqueness, but rather tends to emphasize social unification and the merging of all individuals into an indiscriminate social whole.[9]

Many people see the Confucian Moral Self and the Western unique individual as posited in mutual contradiction. However, common Western arguments based on the belief that the Chinese notion of the Self does not have strong "individualistic" connotations are largely too generalized. Moreover, the Western notion of an isolated, detached, and completely independent individual is also, to a large extent, merely a product of the ideologies of modernization. Confucian ethics is based on the idea of self-cultivation and self-realization. However, people who have been socialized in modern Western societies tend to see these concepts as relating to individual existence. In fact, however, the Confucian Moral Self is a relational Self. It can therefore only be constituted and cultivated through one's fellow human beings, in community.

On the other hand, the term "individuality" has two different meanings (Hall and Ames 1998, 25). On the one hand, it refers to a concrete and indivisible entity with distinct characteristics that can be assigned to a particular class. As such, it is interchangeable and actually contradicts plurality. Such an individual has no discrete personality or distinct identity. As an element (or member) of a particular species or class, this "individuality" is replaceable and interchangeable. This concept of individuality represents the fundamental level of a human being since an individual belonging to this category is merely the product of his or her own effort to survive. As Hannah Arendt writes,

> To be sure, he too lives in the presence of and together with others, but this togetherness has none of the distinctive marks of true plurality. It does not consist in the purposeful combination of different skills and callings as in the case of workmanship (let alone in the relationships between unique persons), but exists in the multiplication of specimens which are fundamentally all alike because they are what they are as mere living organisms.
>
> (Arendt 1998, 212)

This solitude of any living creature struggling to survive is usually overlooked in Western literature, and the reason for this lies in the fact that the concrete organization of labor, necessary for survival and the social conditions that accompany it require the simultaneous presence of a large number of people engaged in a particular task. Therefore, it seems that there are no barriers between them (Arendt 1998, 212).

These individuals have no face, no definite, concrete personhood or identity. And yet it is precisely this concept of interchangeable, unitary individuality that forms the basis for the equality of all before the law, for the establishment of the concept of universal human rights, for equality of opportunity, and so on. This is the most generalized kind of equality, not pluralistic equality.[10] However, as Hall and Ames (1998, 25) point out, it is precisely this kind of understanding of the individual that provides the basis on which it is possible to form the ideas of autonomy, equal rights, free will, and similar concepts. This kind of Self belongs in the realm of the one-dimensional empirical Self, or, in Chinese terminology, in the realm of the "external king (*waiwang* 外王)."[11]

7.4 Personal uniqueness vs. faceless collectivism

The concept of the individual, however, can also be linked to the ideas of singularity and uniqueness that exist outside of any species or class. In such a conceptualization of the Self, the equality of individuals is rooted in the principle of parity (Hall and Ames 1998, 25). This notion of uniqueness inherent in each individual is something that also strongly defines the specific Confucian idea of the human Self. According to numerous Confucian scholars, this uniqueness that underlies such a traditional idea of the Self is a value in itself (Fang 2004, 259). But this kind of uniqueness is not constituted by an isolated position or a demarcation of an individual from his or her fellow human beings. As part of the relational paradigm, it is shaped by the uniqueness of one's position within the network of interpersonal and social relations.

However, due to the prevailing understanding of individualism, there is a pervasive bias in the Euro-American regions as regards the traditional Sinic view of the Self: people in Western countries generally still see East Asians as people who are fundamentally subordinate to collectivist requirements and therefore do not know how to fully develop their individuality, autonomy, and personal freedom. In the Western view, East Asian populations tend to think and act "collectively." The term "collectivism" is usually seen as the antithesis of individualism. Based on such a framework, many people believe that collectivism is essentially an autocratic or even totalitarian social system, as it supposedly does not take into account or value individual life. In a common view, such "collectivism" is typical of Sinic societies, which are often seen by Westerners as products of authoritarian and despotic traditions.

In fact, just the opposite is true, for collectivism is a system that also proceeds from the notion of an individual whose Self and existence are constituted in isolation from his or her fellow people. Therefore, collectivism is in fact a form of individualism and one in which all individuals are considered equal.

Collectivist social orders, in the common Western view, refer to the mechanistic systems of a group or society in which individuals are dehumanized and relate to each other only in the pragmatic sense of enabling the most efficient forms of production or for the benefit of the whole social system as such. In this context, the position and work of individuals are defined by their subordination to the system as well as by their isolation from other individuals since in a collectivist system people are related only by functions and objects and not by their personalities. In this sense, they are not only "equal" but practically the "same."[12] In such a system, individuals are a part of the faceless mass, comparable to small individual cogs functioning mechanistically within a large, all-encompassing machine. Hannah Arendt describes this system, which is only possible as a unity consisting of individuals deprived of their concrete identities, as follows:

> It is indeed in the nature of laboring to bring men together in the form of a labor gang where any number of individuals "labor together as though they were one," and in this sense togetherness may permeate laboring even more intimately than any other activity. But this "collective nature of labor," far from establishing a recognizable, identifiable reality for each member of the labor gang, requires on the contrary the actual loss of all awareness of individuality and identity.
> (Arendt 1998, 213)

The equality of all members of a collective is actually a form of conformism based on the somatic experience of common labor, where "the biological rhythm of labor unites the group of laborers to the point that each may feel that he is no longer an individual, but in fact one with all the others" (ibid., 214). Of course, this is precisely why certain systems of collectivism lend themselves well to autocratic, dictatorial, and totalitarian regimes, as they allow for effective centralized leadership and control over all individuals in society. Therefore, in the context of liberal modernization, which emphasizes human autonomy and freedom, it is sometimes difficult to understand that collectivism is actually the most typical system that emerges from the most emblematic forms of individualism, in which the relationship between the individual and society is such that all individuals are equal.

In this context, it is important to see that Confucian relationalism is not at all a form of such an ideological understanding of collectivism. In relational societies, people are aware of the fact that no human being can really survive alone, without other people. Therefore, they tend to develop a contextualized sense of self (ibid.). This specific type of individual personality is comparable to Jung's (1953, 1976, 301, 402, 433) idea of so-called individuation. In the context of individuation, each person is understood to have an inimitable, completely unique combination of characteristics that are in themselves universal. All human faces, for example, have two eyes, two eyebrows, a mouth, and a nose. All of these elements are universal. But the shape, color, size, and texture of these elements in each face are unique, special, and one of a kind. Individuation, then, is an ongoing process of culturalization that achieves the uniqueness of each person's individual qualities through her particular and specific consolidation of factors that are, as such, universal in nature.

Such self-realization is part of traditional Confucian self-cultivation, a process of human unfoldment that is central to Confucian ethics. It is within such a framework that (co)humaneness or *ren*, this specific type of Confucian empathy and solidarity, can be most efficiently developed: indeed, it is only through his or her uniqueness that a person can truly understand the significance and integral meaning of the social contexts and relationships of which he or she is a part.

Therefore, a relational view of the Self and the Other is more realistic than assumptions based on the idea of an abstract individual. A completely isolated and independent individual Self does not exist in the real world. No human being can be separated from her feelings, intentions, and relationships.

7.5 Individualism and relational models of social organization

In contrast to such a relational view, individualism, which is closely linked to the root of modern European values, turns out to be an egocentric and even selfish phenomenon because it focuses on how one is different from everyone else rather than on how one relates to others. This is why Henry Rosemont and Roger Ames wrote,

> It increasingly seemed to us that describing the proper performances of persons in their various roles and the appropriate attitude expressed in such roles in their relationship to others with whom they are engaged ... conform to our everyday experience much better than those abstract accounts reflected in the writings of the heroes of Western moral philosophy, past and present.
>
> (Rosemont and Ames 2016, 9)

These different ways of conceptualizing the relationship between "Self" and "society" have important consequences for understanding how communities function in different cultures and how they respond to different crises. Empirical studies in cultural and environmental psychology suggest that the interdependent, relational Self tends to care more about others and better control their own desires and behavior in favor of the collective social benefit (Silova et al. 2021, 3). The independent Self, on the other hand, is based on the assumption that "the individual comes before society" and therefore emphasizes individual autonomy and self-preservation. The independent Self, therefore, tends to exhibit values and attitudes that undermine collective efforts to solve problems of public interest (ibid.).

> Although the independent self has traditionally been a major cornerstone of Western civilization and further promoted as the key to achieving modernity from Descartes onward, its era of unthinking valorisation may now need to be brought to a close. To do so, we need to begin to recognize that self-construal manifests concretely in wider social arrangements and these arrangements, in turn, constitute the underlying driver of our current social trajectory. As such, rearticulating western Modernity's dominant concept of Self (i.e., independent Self) might be necessary to effect a departure from the present catastrophe trajectory and move – collectively – towards sustainability.
>
> (Komatsu et al. 2019, 11)

A large-scale comparison by the British polling institute *YouGov* (Sachs 2021, 96) also shows that the Sinic population – due to social norms and a better scientific understanding of the pandemic – shows a significantly higher willingness to engage in health-preserving behavior than people in Euro-American regions. Both factors, namely the belief in the importance and positive function of social norms and the emphasis on critical education, can also be linked to elementary Confucian values.

In several European and other Western countries, on the other hand, there have been public protests against even the most basic public health measures, such as the wearing of face masks, with agitators rejecting the mask requirement in the name of "freedom" (ibid.). However, these people seem to have forgotten that one of the most elementary principles of classical liberal political theories is that the right to liberty and freedom stops at the limit of potential harm to other people in society. In his famous and highly influential essay, *On Liberty*, John Stuart Mill wrote, "The only purpose for which power can be rightfully exercised over any member of a civilized community, against his will, is to prevent harm to others" (Mill 1998, 14).

In the context of the COVID-19 crisis, Mill would certainly approve of the government's request to wear face masks. And so would Confucius: while, as we saw in previous sections, Confucian relationism is in no way comparable to the so-called collectivism, the Confucian Moral Self may well be compared to a free individual acting in accordance with such elementary liberal values.[13]

It is therefore understandable that numerous scholars have been critical of Western discourses, accusing them of a one-dimensional emphasis on individual autonomy and on the notion of unlimited freedom of choice. Such paradigms are ultimately always based on the assumption that individuals can be separated and abstracted from their social contexts, relationships, and even from those elements of the human condition that are actually vital to human life, such as the capacity and need for interpersonal relationships and mutual care (Fan 2010, 13). Compared with such models, Confucian relationism seems to be a model composed of interdependent relational individuals. In this context, Li Zehou writes,

> That people are raised and cared for by their families and communities leaves them with duties and responsibilities to this relationality and even their "kind" (humankind). People do not belong to themselves alone. The very first passage of the *Classic of Filial Piety* (*Xiao jing*) tells us that as our bodies are received from our parents, we are not allowed to harm them. If even harming one's body is denounced, how could suicide possibly be allowed?
>
> (Li 2016, 1131)

Relational ethics, as we saw earlier, is deontological ethics. In moral life, duty is of paramount importance. And even more complicated is the fact that such a life is full of self-control, for one must overcome (almost) all immediate instincts and desires. In relational social systems, as we have seen, the individual is not supposed to act as an independent moral agent, separate from his fellows (Lai 2018, 6). But all this may not be as bad as it seems at first sight.

On the other hand, in relationalism, judgments about the individual are (almost) never defined in terms of an idealized standard of an independent Self. In such an understanding of the Self, it is the actual relationships and environments that define individual values, thoughts, motivations, behaviors, and actions in the first place. Moreover, in relationalism, relationships are always characterized by multiplicity, mutuality, and complementarity.

Ideally, not even the "unequal positions" that form the core of social ethics in all Confucian teachings, nor the strict hierarchy in which these positions are embedded, are as terrible as one is inclined to think. For somehow it is clear, for example, that the differences between a baby and his parent automatically lead to unequal positions. Over the course of a lifetime, of course, that position can change completely.[14] Even though relationalism contains unequal positions – both parties involved in a given relation are complementary and equal to each other, both in the metaphysical and moral sense, since together they form a part of the social whole that consists of these interpersonal relations.

This kind of ethics does not derive from the concept of normative justice, but from a tendency toward social harmony (*he* 和),[15] which appears in the relational network of interactions between individuals, whose individual identities – as we have seen in the description of individuation – are perceived as harmonies of different combinations of the unique, particular characteristics of each of them. The network of relationships is dynamic and diverse since no individual in it forms a fixed specific identity or entity. Each individual in it is the bearer of numerous roles that are interwoven and complement and perfect each other. Thus I myself am, say, a mother but also a daughter; I am a teacher but also a researcher; that is, I learn from the work of others. I am also a consumer, a singer, a driver, a citizen, a worker, etc. Analogously, my relationships with people are multi-layered and changeable. Therefore, in the network of relationality, I am never simply a fixed and unchanging entity defined by my role within the network.

As we have already indicated, Confucian relationism also contains a special kind of virtue ethics,[16] though it is – unlike the ancient Greek virtue ethics – not based on the concept of the isolated individual, but rather defined by relations, or relationships, which are emotional in their intrinsic nature. But many other authors point out that it is rational and even necessary to include, cultivate, and socialize emotions in visions of social systems, as they are rooted in biological instincts that need to be channeled into mechanisms of mutual aid (see Li Zehou 2016, 1097).

Another feature of relationism that is important for crisis situations, as in the COVID-19 pandemic, is the factor of inequality of younger and older persons, which is certainly related to the inequality of near and far, outer and inner,[17] etc. Confucianism emphasizes family relations in which people are automatically unequal. Therefore, relationism contains both a rational order and an emotional identification within conditions that are always concrete, unrepeatable, and connected with sensations and feelings. Concrete obligations, responsibilities, and actions in this context are different for each individual, depending on the concrete, changeable situation in which they find themselves.

7.6 Conclusion

Global crises, such as the COVID-19 pandemic, must be resolved through a process of global cooperation. Strategies to contain the spread of the viral disease cannot be confined to the narrow boundaries of individual nation-states. Within this framework, transcultural dialogs are not only possible but also necessary and important. This chapter proceeded from the assumption that different models of ethics and humanism that have emerged in various cultural traditions can help us to create a new global ethics that can respond to these burning issues and to the general social demands of today's globalized age. On this basis, I aimed to offer the readers a brief introduction and analysis of the specific features of Confucian relational ethics and the relational constitution of personhood. In this way, I hope to have provided some theoretical foundations for future crisis resolution strategies that can also serve for the future construction of a new global ethics.

The relational model of social composition is especially important in times of crises, such as that of the COVID-19 pandemic. Indeed, such times undoubtedly reinforce the need for cooperation that bridges the gap between the uniqueness of the individual on the one hand and his socio-relational Self on the other. It also poses a challenge to the artificially established dichotomies between the Self and the Other or between the specific and the general, the particular and the universal. This understanding is rooted in the paradigm of contrastive complementarity since the uniqueness of the individual can be measured not only by his or her individual achievements but also by his or her social influence. And the latter, in turn, can be measured by an individual's position within their contextual environment and their relationships with other individuals (Lai 2018, 88). From the perspective of ethics, such a web of relationships has several important implications, especially when compared to frames that postulate an individual's independent stability.

Both Confucian relationism and the corresponding role ethic represent a system in which people internalize the insight that they cannot survive alone, without their fellow human beings, and they, therefore, develop a contextual self-awareness. In China and most East Asian cultures, such self-awareness is more realistic precisely because each person, by virtue of his or her uniqueness, can actually understand the meaning and importance of the social contexts into which he or she is embedded. Based on such fundamental premises, it is much easier to understand the concept and basic structure of relationism and similar social systems rooted in the principles of original Confucianism. Since such a foundation of models of familial and social organization is rooted in mutual empathy and humaneness, it can doubtless better assure the preservation of group solidarity and responsibility. The specific kind of solidarity, which has been developed in the framework of traditional Confucian deontology, is a solid and forceful tool for the solving of epidemic, ecological, and political crises of contemporary times.

Notes

1 In this context, it is worth noting that many contemporary Confucians and numerous Western scholars of Confucianism, such as Tu Wei-ming and John A. Tucker, repeatedly stress the importance of reviving the Confucian tradition of ecological thought. Tucker, for instance, places it in constructive dialog with the concepts of "deep ecology" and "ecological egalitarianism" (Tucker 2013, 48), and Tu Wei-ming suggests (2001, 243) that such thinking has long been recognized by Confucians and manifests itself in the idea of the

"unity of heaven and humanity" (天人合一). Although this expression as such is actually a rather modern term, for it does not appear in this form in any work of classical Chinese philosophy, it refers to the holistic nature of the classical Chinese worldview inherent in most of the dominant currents of traditional Chinese philosophical history. In this context, the epistemological aspects of bodily recognition (*tiren* 體認) or the unity of body and mind, as developed, for example, by the Modern New Confucian scholar Xu Fuguan, were also of utmost importance (cf. Sernelj 2014, 86).

2 Let me here briefly explain and define the term Sinic regions. These are the regions that have historically been heavily influenced by Chinese writing and also by some crucial cultural discourses that originated in China, especially Confucian ethics and the Chan Buddhist religion. These cultural regions include but are not limited to Eastern Asian countries; thus, in addition to China, Korea, Japan, and Taiwan, they also include Vietnam, Hong Kong, parts of Laos, and even Singapore.

3 In this context, many sociologists point out that, according to empirical research, Sinic successes were "both top-down, in that governments imposed strong control policies, and bottom-up, in that the people supported governments and followed government-mandated health measures" (Sachs 2021, 93).

4 See, for instance, the following commentary from the Confucian *Chun Qiu Zuo zhuan*: "If the ruler says something is right, everyone says it is right. And if he claims something is wrong, then everyone will claim the same thing. But that's like adding more water to an already watery soup - who would want to eat it? Or as if the instruments in an orchestra all played the same musical line - who would want to hear it? Such sameness is not good" (君所謂可, 據亦曰可, 君所謂否, 據亦曰否, 若以水濟水, 誰能食之, 若琴瑟之專壹, 誰能聽之, 同之不可也如是; Chunqiu Zuo zhuan n.d. Shao Gong ershi nian, 2).

5 Huang Chun-chieh pointed out that this close relationship was already established before the second reform of Confucianism, as Zhu Xi, the most eminent neo-Confucian philosopher from the Song Dynasty, highlighted this dual axiological nature of Confucian teachings by interpreting the Confucian concept of "dao 道" as both a metaphysical principle and an ethical norm. (Huang 2011, 69)

6 Proponents of the Modern New Confucian movement have often emphasized that traditional Confucian teachings involve a "humanistic religion," implying the unity or fusion of humanism and religion. Lee Ming-huei, for example, states that according to Mou Zongsan, "the humanistic focus of Confucianism has a religious dimension as its essence" (Lee 2017, 26). Lee also notes that Mou's basic conception of the unity of morality and religion could be traced to the Modern Confucian "Manifesto on Chinese Culture for People All Over the World" (為中國文化敬告世界人士宣言). In this chapter, however, we will not discuss the possible transcendent elements of this specific type of humanism, but rather focus on its immanent ethics of relationships.

7 天下之本在國，國之本在家，家之本在身。

8 In this context, one is inclined to ask whether the relics of traditional ethics are still relevant in the social behaviour and attitudes of people in modern societies based on the rule of law, principles of normative-rational justice, and individual rights. It is true, of course, that modernization has been brought from the West to most regions of the world and that it is accordingly grounded upon the individual-based values of the European Enlightenment. However, in most regions of the so-called Sinic area, many Confucian elements still remain in contemporary social ethics. This is evidenced by many empirical studies; see, for example, my own transcultural survey (see Rošker 2012),

which found that over 80% of Taiwanese informants believed that society is more fundamental than the individual, and 78% of them believed that morality is more important and fundamental than laws. In contrast, over 90% of European informants believed the opposite.

9 One of the many passages of the Confucian Analects, in which this supposition is emphasized, is found, for example, in the well-known quotation (Lunyu n.d. Zi Lu, 23), in which Confucius sets forth that the morally conscious and cultured people know how to harmonize with others and are opposed to unification, while primitive and uneducated people prefer unification because they do not know how to harmonize (君子和而不同，小人同而不和).

10 This kind of equality is in fact a sameness, which is best expressed in collectivism. Actual equality, in the sense of an integral equal valuation of all human beings, is something quite different from sameness, and is possible only on the basis of a pluralistic conception of man, in which individuals are by no means all equal. It is also worth pointing out Arendt's differentiation between the two concepts (cf. Arendt 1998, 213).

11 This is the second part of the traditional Chinese distinction between the transcendental subject and the empirical Self (Kupke 2012, 1), which usually manifested itself in the Confucian tradition as the problem of the relationship between the "inner sage and the external ruler (*neisheng waiwang* 內聖外王)." Ideally, these two concepts have a complementary and interdependent relationship, constantly seeking to harmonize with each other through their mutual interactions.

12 We find a good illustration of this problem in Hannah Arendt's distinction between the concepts of "equality" and "sameness" (Arendt 1998, 213). In European culture, this understanding of equality, which is actually based on sameness, stems from the basic concept of Christian doctrine, within which we are all equal (and at the same time completely the same) before God and death (Ardent 1998, 235).

13 Although the former is both immanent and transcendent, while the latter is a merely a kind of "transcendental illusion," they can nevertheless be compared on the purely conceptual level.

14 This is not so readily true, for example, of the unequal relationship between ruler and subject, although in Confucianism, the former had to be benevolent, and the latter was often regarded as the "root of the state" (*minben*民本), but Confucian scholars were never motivated to change the formal structure of these hierarchical relationships. Rather, they were inclined to allow the modifications of the concrete contents of the two oppositional conceptualizations at issue. These consisted mainly of patterns of behaviour, norms, and possibilities. As mentioned earlier, however, in this chapter, we are not concerned with reformist Confucian political theory, but instead focus on its ethics as a way of learning some new possible forms of alternative social organization.

15 This concept of social harmony is, of course, not to be confused with the ideologically abused concept of harmony manifested in the patriotic propaganda of the Chinese leadership. For a more detailed description of this problem, see Rošker (2012).

16 At this point, it should be noted that all three types of ethics that are considered basic categories of this discipline – namely, virtue ethics, deontological ethics, and utilitarian ethics – are categories that emerged in the context of Western philosophy. Since the transfer of concepts and categories from one historical-cultural domain to another is a problematic process tied to different culturally conditioned frames of reference, we must take into account that none of the three aforementioned categorizations is entirely suitable to define

or describe the basic nature of Confucian ethics, which at the same time certainly belongs to the domain of deontological ethics (see, for example, Lee Ming-Huei 2017, 94).

17 The terms "outer" and "inner" in this context refer to positions of persons who are "inside" or "outside" certain social groups to which the subject associated with these persons belongs.

References

Arendt, Hannah. 1998. *The Human Condition*. Chicago: University of Chicago Press.

Bauer, Wolfgang. 1971. *Geschichte der chinesischen Philosophie: Konfuzianismus, Daoismus, Buddhismus*. München: Carl Hanser Verlag.

Chunqiu Zuo zhuan. n.d. 春秋左傳. In: Chinese Text Project. Pre-Qin and Han. https://ctext.org/chun-qiu-zuo-zhuan (Accessed 15.06.2020).

Fan, Ruiping. 2010. *Reconstructionist Confucianism – Rethinking Morality after the West*. Dordrecht: Springer.

Fang, Dongmei. 方東美. 2004. *Zhongguo zhexue jingshen jiqi fazhan* 中國哲學精神及其發展 [The Spirit of Chinese Philosophy and Its Development]. Taibei: Liming wenhua chuban she.

Hall, David L. and Roger T. Ames. 1998. *Thinking from the Han: Self, Truth, and Transcendence in Chinese and Western Culture*. Albany, New York: SUNY.

Han, Byung-Chul. 2020. "COVID-19 has reduced us to a 'society of survival.'" In: Carmen Sigüenza (int.) and Esther Rebollo (int). *Euractive*. 24.05.2020. pp. 1–4. https://www.euractiv.com/section/global-europe/interview/byung-chul-han-covid-19-has-reduced-us-to-a-society-of-survival/. (Accessed 08.06.2020).

Huang, Chun-Chieh. 黃俊傑. 2011. *Dongya wenhua jiaoliu zhongde rujia jingdian yu linian: hudong, zhuanhua yu ronghe* 東亞文化交流中的儒家經典與理念: 互動，轉化與融合 [Confucian Classics and Ideas in East Asian Cultural Exchanges: Interactions, Transformations and Integrations].

———. 2014. "Some observations and reflections." In: Frederick P. Brandauer and Chun-Chieh Huang (Eds.): *Imperial Rulership and Cultural Change in Traditional China*. Seattle and London: University of Washington Press. pp. 281–289.

Jia, Jinhua. 2018. "Li Zehou's Reconception of Confucian Ethics of Emotion." In: Roger T. Ames and Jia Jinhua (Eds.): *Li Zehou and Confucian Philosophy*. Honolulu: University of Hawai'i Press. pp 155–186.

Jung, Carl Gustav. 1953. *Psychological Types or the Psychology of Individuation* (Translated by H. Godwin Baynes). New York: Pantheon books.

———. 1976. *Symbols of Transformation* (Translated by R. F. C. Hull). Volume 5 of the *Collected Works of C.G. Jung*. Princeton, NJ: Princeton University Press.

Komatsu, Hikaru, Jeremy Rappleye, and Iveta Silova. 2019. "Culture and the independent self: Obstacles to environmental sustainability?" *Anthropocene* 26: 1–13, http://dx.doi.org/10.1016/j.ancene.2019.100198.

Kupke, Christian, 2012. "Subjekt und Individuum: zur Bedeutsamkeit ihres philosophischen Unterschieds in der psychiatrischen Praxis." *e-Journal Philosophie der Psychologie*: 1–11, http://www.jp.philo.at/texte/KupkeC2.pdf (Accessed 06.07.2012).

Lai, Karyn. 2018. "Global thinking: Karyn Lai's thoughts on new waves in Anglo-Chinese philosophy." *The Philosopher's Magazine* 1: 64–69.

Lee, Ming-Huei. 2017. *Confucianism: Its Roots and Global Significance.* Honolulu: University of Hawai'i Press.

Li, Zehou. 2016. "A response to Michael Sandel and other matters" (Translated by Paul D'Ambrosio and Robert A. Carleo). *Philosophy East and West* 66(4): 1068–1147.

Li, Zehou 李澤厚 and Liu Yuedi 劉悅笛. 2014. "Cong 'qing benti' fansi zhengzhi zhexue" 從「情本體」反思政治哲學 [Reflections on political philosophy on the basis of the concept of 'emotive substance']. *Kaifang shidai* 4: 194–215.

Lunyu 論語 n.d. (Analects). In: *Chinese Text Project. Pre-Qin and Han.* https://ctext.org/analects (Accessed 07.07.2020).

Mengzi 孟子. n.d. (Master Meng, Mencius). In: *Chinese Text Project. Pre-Qin and Han.* https://ctext.org/mengzi (Accessed 15.06.2020).

Mill, John Stuart. 1998. *On Liberty.* Pennsylvania: Penn State University Press.

Rosemont, Henry Jr., and Roger T. Ames. 2016. *Confucian Role-Ethics: A Moral Vision for the 21st Century?* Taibei: National Taiwan University Press.

Rošker, Jana S. 2012. "Cultural conditionality of comprehension: The perception of autonomy in China." In: Cao Qing et al. (Eds.): *Reinventing Identities: The Poetic of Language Use in Contemporary China (Dangdai Zhongguo shenfen chongjiande yuyan yunyong).* Tianjin: Nankai daxue chuban she. pp. 26–42.

Sachs, Jeffrey D. 2021. "Reasons for Asia-Pacific success in suppressing COVID-19." *World Happiness Report 2021.* pp. 91–106. https://worldhappiness.report/ed/2021/reasons-for-asia-pacific-success-in-suppressing-covid-19/ (Accessed 05.05.2021).

Sernelj, Tea. 2014. "The unity of body and mind in Xu Fuguan's theory." *Asian Studies* 2(1): 83–95.

Silova, Iveta, Hikaru Komatsu and Jeremy Rappleye. 2021. "Covid-19, climate, and culture: facing the crisis of (neo)liberal individualism." *Norrag-Blog.* https://www.norrag.org/covid-19-climate-and-culture-facing-the-crisis-of-neoliberal-individualism-by-iveta-silova-hikaru-komatsu-and-jeremy-rappleye/ (Accessed 01.06.2021).

Tu, Wei-Ming. 2001. "The ecological turn in new Confucian humanism: Implications for China and the world." *Daedalus* 130(4): 243–264.

Tucker, John A. 2013. "Dreams, nightmares, and green reflections on Kurosawa and Confucian humanism." In: Tsuyoshi Ishii and Lam Wing-Keung (Eds.): *Philosophizing in Asia.* Tokyo: UTCP (The University of Tokyo Center for Philosophy).

8 Danse macabre

Levity and morality in a plague year

Simone Gubler

8.1 Introduction

> After two weeks of multiple health screens and asking everyone to quarantine, I surprised my closest inner circle with a trip to a private island where we could pretend things were normal just for a brief moment in time. We danced, rode bikes, swam near whales, kayaked, watched a movie on the beach and so much more.
>
> – Kim Kardashian (2020)

> Even if they hadn't gotten caught or risked infecting others, there would still have been something 'off' about their behaviour. Intuitively, *they shouldn't have been having such good times in the first place.*
>
> – Ben Bramble (2020, 115)

In the statement above, Ben Bramble invokes an intuition (henceforth: "the Intuition"): even if our behavior presents no risk to others, we should not party during pandemics. But is it wrong to be publicly happy, or to engage in certain sorts of social leisure, when many members of one's community are sick and dying?

We might characterize this question as a matter of "onlooker" morality: having controlled for risk to others, how should a relatively unaffected person act and feel while they know that many of their compatriots are suffering? Is it true that (even private and safe) pandemic partiers "*shouldn't have been having such good times in the first place*"?

To the end of justifying the Intuition, I construct and consider a variety of plausible arguments in its defense. Some are inspired by public discourse about the propriety of feeling and behaving in overtly joyous ways during a pandemic, others by Bramble's discussion. I focus on arguments with a moral or political dimension – there may be something imprudent or inapt about experiencing or expressing joy during dark times – but my central concern here is with how we should relate to others, even incidentally, during times of great public suffering. These arguments are not comprehensive, but they cover much of the available ground. I consider whether they vindicate the Intuition.

DOI: 10.4324/9781003310129-10

Ultimately, I take the side of the good-times-havers. There's nothing inherently wrong with dancing while the world crashes down. While the arguments considered don't ultimately provide a defensible principled account of the Intuition, some could, under the right circumstances, warrant moral disapproval of "having such good times." But whether they do or not is an empirical question – and we shall have cause to note that circumstances allowing for such disapproval were not the norm in liberal societies during the COVID-19 pandemic.

In closing, I suggest that those who promote the Intuition as justified absent a compelling argument in its favor, are not just guilty of moral overreach, but of turpitude. Morality requires us to resist the urge to condemn the capacity of others to enjoy themselves during times of social crisis *where the target of criticism is simply the fact that a good time was had*.

8.2 Such good times

What does Bramble mean by "such good times"? His discussion fingers fun activities, like partying, as well as certain sorts of affective states, like pure or unadulterated joy. These states and activities often coincide, but I think that it is helpful to treat them as distinct. We may surmise on the basis of his discussion of onlooker morality, that Bramble would condemn ostentatious partying in the context of the pandemic, even if it failed to generate joy, and that he would look askance at unadulterated joy even if were generated by means other than partying.

What is important for Bramble's analysis is that partying and the experience of pure joy are undertaken against a background social context that is widely appreciated as *sad*. It is important that the activities and affect are incongruous with this context: in particular, that they fail to express (at least in a publicly discernable way) appreciation of the background cause for sadness. By way of analogy, Bramble says that to pursue such activities and states during a pandemic is like "watching cat videos during a funeral." The implication is that people in a context like a funeral *should not* (at least to the watchful observer) be engaged in having such a good time.

So, in what follows, let's adopt two target "good times" phenomena for investigation:

(1) an activity: partying – enjoying oneself at "a lively gathering, typically with drinking and music" (Oxford English Dictionary), and
(2) the pursuit and expression of an affective state: unadulterated joy.

We will take it as given that (1) and (2) take place against a background like the pandemic that is standardly acknowledged as sad, and that their pursuit fails to clearly communicate an appreciation of the sadness of the background circumstances. Since our ultimate object of inquiry is a matter of onlooker morality – a question of how a relatively unaffected person should act and feel while they know that many others are suffering – let's also abstract away from the worries about disease transmission that attended social behavior during the pandemic. Let's stipulate that *no direct risk* of infection attends (1) or (2).

Next, it might be helpful to have some illustrations in hand. The following cases illustrate behaviors of concern. One is adapted from an actual court's proceedings, the other from the court of public opinion.

8.2.1 Case one: Kim

> I know that none of them have had any release or break from their kids, from their life. And I thought it would just be so amazing for us all to have just a mental break, and got a private location… I've rented a plane, that can you know, fit all of us. And we'll do really intense quarantining process and Covid testing…but I am so excited!
>
> (Kim Kardashian, quoted in Stark 2021)

In the first case, a celebrity, Kim Kardashian, throws herself a 40th birthday party on a private island with 30 guests. It's October 2020, and the pandemic rages at home, but her party is planned in accordance with public health rules, and she is careful, when publicly discussing the event, to note the safety procedures followed. Assume, for the sake of argument, that these procedures are fail-safe, and no direct risk of harm to the public or participants attends the meeting. Assume too, that the party did not use funds that should otherwise have been dedicated to the commonweal. Was Kim wrong to throw a party during the pandemic?

8.2.2 Case two: Maria

MARIA GIOVANBATTISTA: They arrested me in the house belonging to my brother in Via S. Gallo, opposite the stables of the Signor Cardinale about ten days ago.

JUDGE: How were you found in the house of your brother?

MARIA GIOVANBATTISTA: Yesterday evening the door was open and in the house there was nobody else except for us, three sisters, and Domenico Fantini, our brother the priest, and in order to pass the time we dressed up our brother in a mask, and we were dancing among ourselves, and while he was mounted on the stairs dressed up like that, the corporal passed by and hearing us laughing he came closer to the door and saw what was going on inside the house.

(Henderson 2019, 260)

Maria's community in 15th-century Florence is in lockdown. The bubonic plague rages. She and her sisters are bored by their forced confinement and torment their older brother with games and dancing. A local official hears their laughter from the street and charges the sisters with breach of the quarantine. It is believed at the time that activities like dancing had the potential to spread bad air. But assume, for the sake of argument, that there is no risk to the public, and that this is known. The real offense is the expression of a degree of levity that is incongruous with the serious and sad public moment. Were Maria and her sisters wrong to engage in dancing and loud games during the plague?

There are various promising ways to proceed to the conclusion that Kim and Maria have done something wrong. Let's start with an argument from solidarity.

8.3 Solidarity

In the United Kingdom, public discourse concerning COVID-19 frequently invoked World War Two's Battle of Britain. The British were fighting on the "homefront." The National Health Service (NHS) workers were heroes of national defense, saluted nightly from the windows and doors of private homes by applause through the "Clap for Our Carers" movement (Stewart et al. 2022; Wicke and Bolognesi 2020). The moment even had its own uniformed World War Two hero, Captain Tom Moore. Moore was a 99-year-old veteran who pledged to walk 100 lengths of his garden to raise money for the NHS. He was wildly successful in his fundraising efforts and became a national icon. Moore was knighted by the Queen and featured in a new recording of "You'll Never Walk Alone," the 1945 Rogers and Hammerstein song that had become an anthem of support for essential workers and the quarantined. All this in 2020. In early 2021, Moore tested positive for COVID-19 and passed away. He asked that his tombstone read, "I told you I was old" (BBC 2021). He was a paragon of grit and derring-do, and an exemplar of solidarity.

Social scientists who studied the language used on NHS crowd-funding pages in the United Kingdom noted that many donor comments reflected an "intensely localized desire for normality and community," with invocations of aspirations for "togetherness." Themes of duty also figured prominently:

> We coded a range of related phrases across many of the pages as describing a sense of duty: 'we must all play our part,' 'give something back to the NHS', 'they deserve our support' and 'we owe so much'. The frequent use of 'we' and 'our' here mobilised a collective entity.
>
> (Stewart et al. 2022, 5)

Also prominent in the analysis was a sense that people were striving to help and wanted to galvanize others to do so, despite fears of impotence:

> Pages often expressed the need to 'do one's bit' in the context of relative helplessness: a wish to 'do what I can'.
> "To me and you, it may feel like we're not able to do anything, but we can still help from home too."
> "Everyone feels pretty helpless at the moment but it doesn't mean we can leave it to others."
> "Important that we try to help each other out in whatever way we can."
>
> Stewart et al. 2022, 5

Such responses communicate a desire for *solidarity*: the aspiration to participate in a collectivity whose members are interested in the well-being of each other, and/or stand in opposition to a common foe (such as disease, social instability, want). They express a relatively organic impetus, originating in small individual actions, and aimed at collectively rational ends like galvanizing an effective political response to the pandemic, preventing people from defecting from public health ordinances, and making the pandemic more bearable as a site of community connection.

Whether or not the solidarity pursued through fundraising campaigns and actions like "Clap for Our Carers" helped to promote public health or welfare goals, it is plausible that it might have. So, here's an argument against partying and unadulterated joy from a concern for solidarity.

8.3.1 *The argument from solidarity*

(1) At any given time, many people in the community cannot directly contribute to the official response to COVID-19 (as first responders, essential workers, the quarantined, etc.). Call these people the relatively helpless (RH).

(2) The RH nonetheless have a role to play: they should band together in solidarity to provide indirect support to the pandemic response (by reducing the incidence of illness through information and compliance/making charitable contributions/engaging in activities that alleviate social despair).

(3) Any collective activities or public expressions of affect that members of the RH engage in should support the solidarity described in (2).

(4) The RH should not engage in partying and public expressions of unadulterated joy that will not contribute to efforts to support solidarity.

Note that this does not rule out partying or the expression of unadulterated joy tout court – just instances of each that fail to buttress solidarity.

So, the argument gives us a nice result: the simple and joyful decisions of thousands of British schoolchildren to paint beautiful rainbows to display in their home windows in support of the NHS are not ruled out, but Kim and Maria's activities clearly fall afoul of the rule. Except that, perhaps they don't.

There are many problems with the argument from solidarity. It's illiberal. It's unclear what form the normative claim in (2) takes. But perhaps most striking is its failure to establish our goal – namely, the wrongness of Kim's party and Maria's good time. Take premise (4). Why suppose that Kim and Maria will fail through their activities to contribute to solidarity?

From a pragmatic perspective, apparent defectors – especially flagrant defectors – could be quite a good thing for the overall project of solidarity. After all, solidarity is standardly conceived as a volitional undertaking – part of its inspirational power comes from the fact that participants freely undertake to support the collective end, even at personal cost. The existence of defectors helps to insure a public appreciation of this. They demonstrate by example that the present atmosphere of solidarity is not attributable to global conditions of coercion, but rather, to common feeling. Having a few folks who don't clap undermines the case for cynicism about the spontaneity and authenticity of events like "Clap for Carers" – events that might otherwise look authoritarian and grim.

"But," someone might respond, "ultimately, solidarity relies on cohesion, and defectors cause division!" It's certainly true that where people were caught partying and enjoying themselves during the pandemic, it caused resentment and public outrage. But again, it's not clear that this was bad for the overall project of solidarity. Resentment can be a prosocial, pro-solidarity force. As Bishop Butler points out, shared resentment of deviant others is "one of the common bonds, by which society is held together, a fellow-feeling" (Butler 2017, VIII: 7). It's deeply satisfying to stand in common resentment with others. Defectors might galvanize solidarity.

There's also an interesting question about whether some perceived defectors are *required* to make standing in solidarity feel worthwhile for participants. Perhaps participants in solidarity movements can be more effectively motivated to feel good about the costs that they are shouldering if there's a clear comparison class of bad actors against whose example their virtue can blaze like a light. If this is the case, then Kim Kardashian arguably did the solidarity movement a great favor by deviating from public pandemic norms of behavior so spectacularly.

If any of the above suggestions about the value of defectors can be shown to hold – if they (a) helpfully illustrate the volitional character of solidarity, (b) inspire solidarity-galvanizing resentment, and (c) make participation in solidarity feel more creditable – then Kim and Maria, who acted *safely and ostentatiously* might have made real contributions to solidarity. Albeit, a contribution that turns on their playing a sacrificial role – for the contribution to be effective, a large portion of society must look askance at their behavior and engage in public shaming.

Of course, whether Kim and Maria ultimately buttress solidarity depends on empirical factors – how many defectors there are, what the social mood is like, and so forth. But we may observe that the argument from solidarity fails to preclude even those acts of partying and projects of joy that bear *no direct relation* to the pandemic effort.

8.4 Fairness

I've said that there's no reason to assume that defectors will undermine or compromise solidarity movements. But, even if defectors functionally support solidarity, they may still give members of solidarity movements (taken as members of solidarity movements) cause for complaint. After all, all members of society stand to benefit from the collective efforts of those working in solidarity to improve social conditions during crises like the pandemic. In a context of general solidarity, defectors inspire a free rider worry: they may be enjoying social benefits while failing to make a fair contribution to their production.

8.4.1 Free rider argument

(1) The members of the solidarity movement are engaged in providing shared resources (call these SR) that stand to benefit all members of society (in the form of positive public sentiment, effective political action, well-provisioned hospitals, etc.)

(2) Defectors from the solidarity movement could contribute to the provision of the SR, but they choose not to.

(3) Defectors nonetheless derive benefit from the SR.

(4) It is unfair to derive benefit from the SR if you choose not to contribute to their provision.

(5) So, defectors should contribute to the SR.

Now, we might resist the conclusion of this argument. Charity is standardly conceived as supererogatory. There are plenty of costly yet prosocial activities that we could imagine some people volunteering to perform, whose benefits will be enjoyed by a larger portion of the population, and where those beneficiaries have no concomitant obligation to contribute. If a group of idealists decides to spend an hour each morning cleaning carriages in the New York Subway, I might – as an ordinary metro-user – be happy to ride a cleaner train to work, but I don't have any special obligation to pitch in.

Free rider worries are most potent where free riders impose a burden that threatens the viability of a critical shared resource. Clean trains are nice but hardly essential. Now perhaps the failure of defectors to pitch in to the solidarity movement will imperil key resources (if my neighbors and I would just each just donate 5 cents, then our local council would have the funds to save the local hospital from bankruptcy – but we all choose not to, and the hospital fails). But whether the moral censure of defectors is justified will arguably still depend upon a complex calculus involving the nature of the shared resource, standing social expectations about responsibility for its maintenance (the council should arguably pay for the hospital with its own funds – it should not rely on private donations), the costs imposed on individuals (on the other hand, 5 cents isn't very much), and the extent of social need (we really need that hospital!).

But why assume that partiers and the exuberantly joyful are defectors from solidarity or the production of social benefits in the first place? Why class them as free riders? Ostentatious partying and joy might trigger the enforcers of fairness norms because they do not, at least *prima facie*, look like the sturdy business of "pulling together" or "doing one's bit." But of course, there's no reason why the jovial partier shouldn't also be making a fair contribution. No just norm of solidarity could demand that the relatively helpless spend all of their working hours on pandemic-related projects. Even the most virtuous keyboard warrior, who fights daily in the trenches of Twitter to bring emergent pandemic norms to public attention, will bake sourdough or watch Netflix from time to time. Making a fair contribution to the pandemic effort should not preclude leisure or rest. Would we really characterize someone who spent all day working to raise funds for the NHS, and all night safely drinking and carousing as a free rider? So, the free rider argument doesn't go through.

8.5 Influence

But perhaps focusing on individual acts of partying and joy expression, as if they were isolated acts of solidarity-defection or incidents of free-riding, elides a more serious threat to solidarity and its goals. Maybe what we should really be concerned about when it comes to *good times*, is their potential to inspire further, more dangerous, good times. Good times that threaten not just the fabric of the collective, but its ultimate goals (like public health). Even safe good times might, in short, create an adverse influence.

8.5.1 The argument from adverse influence

(1) Good times are inspirational.
(2) If a member of the public witnesses someone having a good time, they will often be inspired to initiate their own good time.
(3) Safety measures are often inconspicuous and less inspiring than the fun aspects of a good time.
(4) So, we may observe that safe good times will have a propensity to inspire progressively more reckless good times.

Kim and Maria might be frolicking safely, but others who see them will not appreciate this, and some of those others might take the frolicking as inspiration to much more unsafe behavior. Now, this isn't a devastating worry. It's easily dealt with by making sure that one's party or joy remains a private affair. It doesn't rule out good times, although it might rule out tweeting about them.

Indeed, to push back in defense of having an ostentatiously good time, we might note that whether a safe party or joyous activity inspires a reckless one will depend on background social norms. Is everyone in my society already habituated to testing, wearing masks, meeting outside? Then, if I am inspired by Maria to have a good time, I may reflexively ensure that it is a safe good time. The propensity of a specific act to have an adverse influence will also depend on its expressive content. Celebrities often function as norm-setters and so might in fact exercise a positive influence by advertising the safety measures they are taking. Kim publicly discussed her plans for a COVID-safe event. She followed public health rules. Perhaps, in doing so, she exercised positive rather than adverse influence on her followers.

But maybe what bothers us about Kim's partying is not its tendency to create an adverse influence, but the fact that it was only possible *qua* safe partying because she is so outrageously privileged. Perhaps the real worry here has to do with social inequality.

8.6 Inequality

Here, we may bring Ben Bramble back into the mix. Bramble says, "No one who properly understood and cared about what was happening in the world right now [during the pandemic] would be building luxury add-ons to their houses at the moment, or buying new ones" (Bramble 2020, 119). In a similar vein, he calls out wealthy New Yorkers and Rhode Islanders who built pools for themselves while citizens in those states were banned from swimming at public beaches (due to ordinances targeted at mass gatherings). To Bramble, there's something very wrong about luxury consumption during a pandemic. And the cases he focuses on are especially symbolically potent: they really dot the "i" in inequality. Appropriately moral onlookers, Bramble tells us, would not want to engage in activities like "ostentatious partying, building luxury add-ons to their homes, commissioning diamond-encrusted masks, etc." (Bramble 2020, 123).

One way to read the complaint from privilege is to observe that the economic, health, and social burdens of events like the pandemic are disproportionately borne by the socially disadvantaged. Pandemics aggravate existing circumstances of inequality. Perhaps, in the interest of reducing social inequality, those who are relatively unaffected by the crisis should refrain from activities and acts of consumption and enjoyment that express their relative privilege. This might include partying and the expression of unadulterated joy.

8.6.1 Leveling down argument

(1) Equality requires leveling down when leveling up is impossible.
(2) Many people are suffering significant harm as a result of the pandemic (call these SH), while others remain relatively unaffected (call these RU).
(3) The disparity in levels of pandemic-induced harm has resulted in significant social inequality between the SH and RU.
(4) This inequality is not just material, but emotional.
(5) We cannot make SH like the bereaved or illness-stricken happier.
(6) We cannot justly intervene to make the RU less happy.
(7) Nonetheless, to the end of equality, the RU can and should forgo nonessential activities and purchases that they know will increase their experience of joy and thereby their relative emotional advantage over the SH.
(8) So, the RU should not party or pursue joyous experiences.

Imagine that there is a planet on the other side of the Milky Way – call it Alpha Hedontauri. Surprisingly, it is peopled by human beings. Even more surprisingly, they live lives full of welfare. Illness, both mental and physical, is nonexistent. People are happy. They engage in lots of social leisure activities. By contrast, our condition on Earth remains relatively awful. We have no hope of improving our lives to any significant extent, no real prospect of attaining the collective level of joy that people experience on Alpha Hedontauri every day. Sadly, given the distances involved, the Alpha Hedontaurins cannot help us in any material way. Now, should individual Alpha Hedontaurins nonetheless commit to forgo the nonessential pursuit of joy and leisure, in recognition of the grotesque emotional inequality that obtains between our planets?

Perhaps some readers will think that the answer to this question is "Yes." But why? Leveling down is standardly a strategy of last recourse where ends of social justice are implicated. We might close schools like Eton, for example, so that the future leaders of Britain are schooled among the children of the middle and working classes, whom they will ultimately rule. Doing so could make Britons generally better off by reducing educational disparities and class distinctions that undermine social cohesion and the good function of democracy. But the policy might also lead to no good social consequences, and yet we might still think it justified, because it's just *unfair* that some children are so privileged in educational attainment. But what end of justice do we secure by asking that the inhabitants of Alpha Hedontauri pursue lives that are slightly less full of welfare? It certainly doesn't help or reassure me here on Earth, as I contemplate my miserable lot, to know that under the light of a distant star, someone skipped their skee-ball league. Nor does it seem to me unfair that someone else's life is, through no fault of their or my own, going better than mine.

Standard arguments for leveling down deal with areas of life in which the state is justifiably concerned with inequality and arguably licensed to engage in social engineering. They deal with public aspects of our lives, like employment, education, and economic status – aspects that are already highly regulated and mediated through social institutions whose features are determined by political decisions and can be adjusted to conduce to justice. And even so, many political theorists are loath to endorse any form of leveling down in these domains because of its potentially negative (if incidental and indirect) consequences for overall well-being. But the argument above demands a direct reduction in the pursuit of joy and social leisure – aspects of our experience that condition, and might even constitute, well-being. It *aims* at a reduction in global well-being. And it fails to supply a compelling reason of justice for doing so.

It is a mistake to approach relational disparities in emotion and the pursuit of harmless leisure activities in these political terms. What social entitlement are we protecting? What could be more justly distributed? It's nice to party, but there's no general right to be invited to party. It's nice to experience joy, but there's no general right to enjoyment. Even if such rights did exist, counseling people to avoid their exercise in order to secure equality with less fortunate others would be unjust. Our emotional lives and social pastimes are intimately connected to individual well-being and sense of self. Their maintenance is a matter continuous with the maintenance of one's body. As Kurt Vonnegut's heavy-handed but effective fable *Harrison Bergeron* illustrates, no righteous system of social normativity could ask us to mutilate our bodies, minds, and social pastimes to the end of relational equality (Vonnegut 1998, 7).

8.7 Flaunting it

But maybe the problem at hand isn't really one of injustice borne of relational inequality, but rather of how spectators are led to experience that inequality. Alpha Hedontauri is very far away. We don't think about it very often. But we have to live alongside people like Maria and share cyberspace with people like Kim Kardashian. Individual human beings may not know much about the people on the other side of the galaxy, but they are daily exposed to the lives of compatriots. And while the leveling-down argument also fails for compatriots for the reason that emotional well-being and harmless private leisure are not the sorts of things that can or should be justly targeted in pursuit of relational equality, it might still harm someone suffering during the pandemic to see evidence of Maria and Kim's relative well-being. And Kim and Maria might, under the right circumstances, be blameworthy for exposing their fellows to such evidence. For, even if good times are morally permissible, Kim and Maria arguably still shouldn't be "flaunting" their fun! They shouldn't be *showing off*. Nor, indeed, should the Alpha Hedontaurins. Imagine if the inhabitants of that far-off place decided to project an image of their relatively happy world onto our ozone layer. Forced to confront images of their joy daily, while suffering through a global pandemic, we might soon find real cause for moral complaint. Not with their happiness, but with their flaunting of it. A *flaunting* complaint could involve a couple of distinct moral worries – we'll deal with the first here and move to the second concern in the next section.

Where a person knows that an act of exhibitionism is liable to provoke envy – and where they seek to provoke envy by it, they arguably aim at the moral degradation of others. This is a generic worry that could be leveled at many of the Instagram activities of the rich and famous. It's not pandemic-specific, and indeed, as a moral critique, it arguably depends upon an appreciation of the propensity of the activity in question to provoke envy, and the desire that it do so. It's also a complaint that is somewhat complicated by the fact that there is a market for "flaunting" – people seem to want to feel jealousy and outrage and avarice, and contemporary celebrities appear happy to indulge this market. It's morally shabby to be prone to envy. And it's not good to cruise social media for a hit of jealousy or outrage. But the mere fact that many of us have poor moral hygiene and a propensity to envy doesn't indemnify those who exploit the situation. Nonetheless, leveling the flaunting critique at Maria and Kim will involve making complicated moral assessments that might also function to impugn those whom Maria and Kim are said to have wronged.

But here we should note that flaunting, construed as a moral worry about deliberately (or even negligently) inviting envy, fails to meet our target anyway. That is, it doesn't suffice to explain the wrongness of partying or unadulterated joy during a pandemic. For, it's not intrinsic to the activity of partying, or to the expression of joy, to seek to inspire envy in others. As for our protagonists: Maria is not trying to provoke envy in her neighbors – her exuberant horsing around is not aimed at spectators. Kim might be flaunting her party on Twitter to elicit envy. That would be bad. But it's still not the partying that is wrong, but its instrumentalization to the end of the moral degradation of others.

8.8 Disrespect

An onlooker who truly understands what is happening in the world right now, and is appropriately moved by it, and who happens to, say, live by a lovely beach in a remote location, might well take a stroll along that beach each day and take pleasure in that. But *it wouldn't be the same sort of fully relaxed or carefree pleasure they might feel in normal times*. It would be a mixed pleasure, one in some sense backgrounded by an awareness of the dire state of things elsewhere, pain at these far off events, and a sense of humility at themselves having been spared the worst of it.

(Bramble 2020, 117)

The phenomenon of *flaunting* prompts consideration of a second moral worry: a classic. For, under the right circumstances, certain actions function to express *disrespect*. And for such actions, when we complain about flaunting, what we might really be complaining about is the *amplification or aggravation of the expression of disrespect*.

It's possible that, in the context of a crisis like the pandemic, displays of partying and joy that seem unaltered by appreciation of the background darkness might be taken to express disrespect. Flaunting might aggravate or amplify that expression. But note that our partiers are *onlookers* – they are relatively unaffected by the pandemic. They are not sick, their intimates are not sick, they do not work with the ill and dying. So, toward whom, or what, are their good times supposed to be disrespectful? In what follows, we will consider a couple of plausible candidates. First, we will ask whether good times might be disrespectful in view of (1) important social norms and the compact that subserves them, and then we will consider whether (2) they might express disrespect for members of especially afflicted groups, like the ill and dying.

8.8.1 Argument from respect for shadow laws

It's disrespectful to sneeze in public without covering one's mouth. It's disrespectful to fail to wash one's hands after using the bathroom. There are activities that the state can't justifiably suppress (for fear of violating civil liberties, for example), but that the public still has a powerful safety interest in suppressing. In such cases, the public might develop and promulgate its own social norms to regulate behavior: call these the "Shadow Public Health Law" or "shadow law." Because the ultimate goal is public health, the norms of the shadow law are treated as weighty, and acts of disregard are liable to provoke outrage and disgust in spectators.

We have taken it as given that Maria and Kim are behaving in a way that is safe and in accordance with public health law and guidance. But we have not assumed their compliance with unofficial norms that govern behavior during the pandemic. If they can be shown to have flouted a shadow law, then their compatriots may have a justified social complaint against them. It may even be a justified *moral* complaint, if observing shadow law is widely deemed a matter of respect for the fundamental commitments of society, or for the general safety of its members. There's a kind of anarchic spirit that goes with licking bus poles that we may rightly view as disrespectful to the whole social project.

(1) The shadow law exists to protect us all from disease.

(2) The shadow law is promulgated by shadowy means, but we know that it is in force when a majority of members of society recognize its observance as *the done thing*.

(3) The shadow law is enforced by the informal mechanism of social shaming.

(4) Partying and other exuberant good times are associated with a heightened risk of disease transmission. They are "*risky activities.*"

(5) Given the pandemic, the shadow law strictly prohibits risky activities.

(6) Violating the shadow law, and/or being indifferent to the threat of shaming, expresses disrespect for key social norms and, by extension, for the social project.

Defenders of the shadow law will emphasize its softly coercive character, contrasting minor liberty costs with significant public safety gains. They will be untroubled by the claim that the ban in (5) captures all sorts of activities that present no real risk of disease transmission. In response, they will stress that many social activities that fall under the "good times" rubric *do prove risky* in practice, and they will say that we cannot afford to take a fine-grained approach to regulation where lethal risk to the public is involved – we need a clear and general norm.

Indeed, whether or not the prohibition on good times can be justified on public health grounds, we may observe that shadow laws, as significant social norms, *should* be followed. We may not agree with a particular rule, but compliance is still necessary to show due respect for the larger project of public health and societal well-being. For example, in many countries where food is eaten with the hands, there is a strict norm that only the right hand should be used to touch food. Eating with the left hand is taboo because the left hand is reserved for matters of personal hygiene. A left-handed person may think it a generally good rule to reserve one hand for eating and one hand for bathroom business but prefer to use their dominant hand to eat. But effecting the switch would violate the shadow law. Whether considerations of hygiene are observed or not, it is disrespectful to the generic other of society to eat with the left hand. Now social normativity is not moral normativity – but flouting a social norm, widely understood to support the common weal, may, if the norm is taken seriously enough, be construed as immorally disrespectful toward society. So here, perhaps is the sense in which our protagonists may be said to have acted immorally.

Note, however, that it's not the activity, not the partying or expression of joy, that's bad in itself. Rather it is the act of norm-flouting which – whether intentionally or not – functions to express disregard for the social project. If Kim and Maria were subject to a shadow law against good times, then their activities arguably expressed disrespect for society.

Of course, for this result to hold, we are required to accept the existence of the shadow law against good times (contentious), as well as the expressive significance ascribed to its violation (also contentious). But say that we do so. We might yet note that moral considerations can be outweighed by other moral considerations. Kim and Maria might have acted in a fashion that communicated an immoral form of disrespect for society, but perhaps their actions can be justified in light of a competing moral consideration. If the norm contained in the shadow law is a bad norm, then noncompliance – even at the cost of expressing disrespect to innocent others – might be the morally right choice. And indeed, a shadow law against good times might have quite oppressive and harmful implications.

Arguably, even in a democracy, the appropriate arbiters of public safety norms are public health officials. Public beliefs and superstitions about health may be one element in the calculus of public health, but we should be careful not to license norms that punish the individual exercise of hitherto standard freedoms without strong public health justification. Stigmatizing energetic outdoor activities such as jogging – activities that make a significant contribution to mental health and well-being and that pose little risk of disease transmission – arguably did more harm than good in the early days of the pandemic. Maria's exuberant activity with her family and Kim's legal adventures on the island might not meet the general public's standards for safe COVID-19 practice, but those standards are not necessarily scientifically informed or justified. Perhaps they should be challenged.

Let's move to our final argument – which will draw these considerations into sharper relief.

8.8.2 The argument that attention must be paid

(1) During crises like the pandemic, it is disrespectful to the sick and dying if an "unaffected person" (someone not sick or dying or intimately connected to those who are), knowing of the situation of the sick and dying, nonetheless engages in partying or the expression of unadulterated joy.

(2) During the pandemic, it was a standardly appreciated fact that many people were sick and dying.

(3) During the pandemic, it was wrong for unaffected people to party or express unadulterated joy.

Kim and Maria are connected to the sick and dying by membership in a community and the common experience of a social crisis. But they are still relative strangers to the sick and dying. Normal duties of care and relational standards of behavior proper to intimates do not apply. Nonetheless, if the argument above is correct, then witnesses to Kim and Maria's behavior might justifiably say, "That's very disrespectful to all those sick and dying today!"

Now, it's quite possible that a norm against good times – a norm that says "it's disrespectful to the sick and dying to have a good time during the present moment" could have arisen during the pandemic. Social norms concerning behavior in view of illness and death tend to be both highly mutable over time and cultural context, and strictly observed (often in a morally freighted fashion) in any given moment: we wear black and somber expressions to funerals, unless we are in New Orleans, in which case, we wear white and dance in the streets. Such norms can regulate a wide range of behaviors and even claim jurisdiction over those who are relative strangers: if a hearse passes on a public road, other cars must slow down or show disrespect to the deceased. Norms pertaining to onlooker behavior in cases of illness and death can also serve to significantly restrict our fun. When Queen Elizabeth II died, the United Kingdom observed ten days of public mourning, which meant, among other things, that comedy programming on public broadcast networks was suspended (Wilkins and Lane-Godfrey 2022). As onerous as this might seem, this was a relative improvement on the experience of the nation after the death of Elizabeth's father, when the official mourning period lasted for 16 weeks, and irritability became a conspicuous public companion to grief. As reported in the *Guardian*:

> After the death of George VI, in a society much more Christian and deferential than this one, a Mass Observation survey showed that people objected to the endless maudlin music, the forelock-tugging coverage. "Don't they think of old folk, sick people, invalids?" one 60-year old woman asked. "It's been terrible for them, all this gloom." In a bar in Notting Hill, one drinker said, "He's only shit and soil now like anyone else," which started a fight.
>
> (Knight 2017)

So, did a novel behavioral norm mandating a particular means of showing respect to the sick and dying arise during the pandemic? That's an empirical question. If it did, then violators like Kim and Maria might well have shown immoral disrespect to the sick and dying. But like the patron of the Notting Hill bar and the woman concerned with the well-being of the sick and invalid, we might yet think it stupid to adopt and observe such a norm. How does it help the sick if I am sad? How does it tend to the frayed bonds of the community if I avoid recreational socializing?

Indeed, we might, on reflection, decide upon joy as a means of moral revolution. It's a perilous affair to contest norms of respect in matters as emotionally charged as death, but *if we are successful* in shifting social normativity, then our previous sins are likely to be forgiven. Past failures to observe now-defunct norms are not going to figure prominently in the calculus of character that others assign to us. My sister's history of complaining loudly about gender-reveal parties, back when they were a thing to be piously enjoyed, has aged like a fine wine.

As important as they are, our practices with respect to the ill and dying are contingent and mutable. It may be that Maria and Kim violated standing norms and that their behavior accordingly functioned to express disrespect. It's certainly bad to disrespect others, perhaps especially when it comes to vulnerable and suffering others. But, as a society, we get to determine what actions function to express disrespect, and it's not necessary that good times during bad times should have this semiotic function. Indeed, since good times are things that add to the general store of human well-being, they arguably shouldn't have this function. Individuals might rightly fight the tendency to a dour propriety.

It's hard from inside a norm of somberness to see other more vital ways of life and of addressing death and suffering as preferable. But wouldn't it be better if, to hark back to the solidarity warriors, the pandemic became a site of social connection and even the mutual pursuit of joy? Not a joy that is *required* to be mixed, as Bramble would have it, with sadness. Such a joy will no doubt arise. But wouldn't it be nice to sometimes encounter a joy that escapes the sobriety of the moment? A joy that strikes cracks through the dour social mood. A joy that laughs and dances. That says: *la vita è bella*. A joy whose raucous sounds we are not required to resent, but that we may greet with a welcoming smile.

It may be that, for contingent reasons of culture and circumstance, we come to regard joy and partying as disrespectful or dangerous during times of great public suffering. But that doesn't render the pursuit of good times against a sad background necessarily immoral or bad-in-itself. And it remains an important consideration that, in the case of respect, we are the ultimate arbiters of what joy and partying function to express; just as, in the case of safety, we set the norms for safe behavior and determine what sort of provision is made for safe socializing by the general public.

8.9 Conclusion

According to the Census Bureau's American Time Use Survey, the amount of time the average American spent with friends was stable, at 6½ hours per week, between 2010 and 2013. Then, in 2014, time spent with friends began to decline. By 2019, the average American was spending only four hours per week with friends (a sharp, 37 percent decline from five years before). Social media, political polarization and new technologies all played a role in the drop. (It is notable that market penetration for smartphones crossed 50 percent in 2014.) Covid then deepened this trend. During the pandemic, time with friends fell further – in 2021, the average American spent only two hours and 45 minutes a week with close friends (a 58 percent decline relative to 2010–2013).

(Ward 2022)

In this chapter, we addressed a matter of onlooker morality: of how a relatively unaffected person should act and feel when they know that many of their compatriots are suffering. In particular, we asked whether it would be wrong to party or express unadulterated joy. Addressing case studies drawn from life during pandemics, we considered whether such behavior might unjustly violate standards of solidarity or fairness, aggravate inequality, immorally provoke envy, or express disrespect for social standards, the general weal, or the sick and dying. Several putatively plausible arguments were examined, but each failed to support the general conclusion that our protagonists were "wrong to have such good times." We were, as such, unable to discover support for the Intuition adopted at the outset of the chapter, whether as a general moral rule, or in the specific context of the COVID-19 pandemic.

So, what should we do now? Given the lack of a good argument in favor of the Intuition, we might opt to be cautious. We might say: we just don't have justification *yet*. Indeed, if online discourse during the pandemic was any indication, many people (and not just moral philosophers like Bramble) look askance at good times during dark times. The justification for their sentiment may be just around the corner. In light of this worry, we might adopt a wagering attitude.

8.9.1 *The wager*

> The Intuition is correct, or it is not. We cannot presently decide between the two alternatives. Nonetheless, the Intuition claims to govern us in matters of practical morality, so we must take a stance on its practical application – we must choose whether to follow it or not. Opting out is not an option. So, we weigh the potential gains and losses of acting as if the rule suggested by the Intuition is binding on behavior. If we follow the rule and the Intuition turns out not to be true, then we still have not harmed anyone or done anything immoral. We may have elected to have fewer good times, but importantly, we haven't done anything wrong. But if we don't follow the rule in some situations where it would apply, and the Intuition turns out to be true, then we have behaved immorally. Therefore, if our ultimate concern is to behave morally, caution should be the watchword of the hour! We should assume the Intuition is true until it has been decisively falsified.

But this is no way to live. Joy is hugely important for human flourishing. So is fun in company. The cautious approach of the wager is flawed because it fails to acknowledge that it is standardly good to enjoy oneself and to socialize with others. Reducing the amount of human well-being in the world *is* a real cost, one that is not appropriately assessed. And although the wagering agent only claims to abstain for themselves, it is often the case that our subjective experience of joy and engagement in social life is a boon to others as well. Indeed, whether or not the conclusion of the wager is supportable, we have good reason to be highly suspicious of its starting premise, of the possible truth of the Intuition. A morality worth observing – a morality appropriately concerned with human well-being – would not wantonly license reductions in joy and sociality, especially during times of great suffering and isolation. So, absent a compelling argument, we should ignore the Intuition. It will always be tempting to condemn the capacity of others to enjoy themselves during times of social crisis. But we must resist the urge where the target of criticism *is simply the fact that a good time was had.*

References

Bramble, Ben. 2020. *Pandemic Ethics: 8 Big Questions of COVID-19*. Sydney: Bartleby Books.

BBC News. 2021. "Captain Sir Tom laid to rest in hometown of Keighley," (July 5), sec. Leeds & West Yorkshire. https://www.bbc.com/news/uk-england-leeds-57725373.

Butler, Joseph (edited by David McNaughton). 2017. *Fifteen Sermons and Other Writings on Ethics*. Oxford: Oxford University Press.

Kardashian, Kim [@KimKardashian]. 2020. "After 2 weeks of multiple health screens…" Tweet. *Twitter*, (October 27). https://twitter.com/KimKardashian/status/1321151217482014726.

Henderson, John. 2019. *Florence Under Siege: Surviving Plague in an Early Modern City*. 1st edition. New Haven, Conn: Yale University Press.

Knight, Sam. 2017. "'London bridge is down': The secret plan for the days after the queen's death." *The Guardian* (March 17) sec. UK news. https://www.theguardian.com/uk-news/2017/mar/16/what-happens-when-queen-elizabeth-dies-london-bridge.

Stark, George. 2021. "Kim Kardashian plans THAT controversial 'tone deaf' 40th birthday." *Mail* Online (May 27). https://www.dailymail.co.uk/tvshowbiz/article-9627369/Kim-Kardashian-plans-controversial-tone-deaf-40th-birthday-holiday-KUWTK-episode.html.

Stewart, Ellen, Anna Nonhebel, Christian Möller, and Kath Bassett. 2022. "Doing 'our bit': solidarity, inequality, and COVID-19 crowdfunding for the UK National Health Service." *Social Science & Medicine* 308 (September 1): 115214. https://doi.org/10.1016/j.socscimed.2022.115214.

Ward, Bryce. 2022. "Opinion Americans are choosing to be alone. Here's why we should reverse that." *Washington Post* (November 24). https://www.washingtonpost.com/opinions/2022/11/23/americans-alone-thanksgiving-friends/.

Wicke, Philipp, and Marianna M. Bolognesi. 2020. "Framing COVID-19: How we conceptualize and discuss the pandemic on Twitter." *PLOS ONE* 15, no. 9 (September 30): e0240010. https://doi.org/10.1371/journal.pone.0240010.

Wilkins, Bridie, and Georgie Lane-Godfrey. 2022. "What happens during the mourning period for the queen? EYNTK about gyms, schools, sport events and more." *Women's Health* (September 11). https://www.womenshealthmag.com/uk/health/a41121947/what-happens-during-the-12-day-mourning-period-for-the-queen/.

Vonnegut Jr., Kurt. 1998. *Welcome to the Monkey House: A Collection of Short Works*. New York: Dial Press.

9 Well-being in the time of COVID-19

Mauro Rossi

9.1 Introduction

Over the past two years, the world has been hit by a dramatic pandemic, which has brought death, suffering, and hardships of many sorts to millions of people. For some, however, the pandemic has brought happiness and a better life. In some cases, this contrast does not present a puzzle. Some individuals have simply been spared by the COVID-19 virus and by the waves of suffering that it has generated. In this chapter, however, I am interested in those individuals whose well-being has increased despite the direct or indirect experience of the virus and some of its negative consequences, and, in some ways, as a result of this experience. How can we make sense of their situation? In what follows, I propose an explanation that is based on the fitting happiness theory of well-being that I have recently developed with Christine Tappolet (Rossi and Tappolet 2022, n.d.-a). Our theory holds that an individual's life goes well when the individual is fittingly happy – that is, when the individual affectively experiences items, situations, and activities that are of genuine value and that match the individual's deepest evaluative attitudes. I argue that, for some individuals, the pandemic has been the occasion to revise their most fundamental evaluative attitudes and has created opportunities for fitting affective experiences that better align with these attitudes. For those individuals, the pandemic has brought personal flourishing despite the suffering.

I proceed as follows. In Section 9.2, I present some empirical evidence about how COVID-19 has affected people's well-being. In Section 9.3, I briefly consider how the main traditional theories of well-being can explain the favourable changes in well-being that some individuals underwent and express some doubts about the plausibility of these explanations. In Section 9.4, I present the fitting happiness theory of well-being (Subsection 9.4.1) and use it to shed light on the phenomenon at stake (Subsection 9.4.2).

DOI: 10.4324/9781003310129-11

9.2 The impact of COVID-19 on people's well-being

At the time of this writing, there have been 623,605,879 reported cases of COVID-19 and 6,551,200 deaths all over the world.[1] In order to limit the spread of the virus, many governments have imposed various restrictions, oftentimes quite strict. People's lives have been upended and their well-being significantly affected. The consequences of the pandemic have, of course, been different in different countries. Here, however, I will present a general picture of these consequences, primarily referring to the OECD[2] report, *COVID-19 and Well-Being: Life in the Pandemic* (2021), which tracked the evolution of people's well-being through data collected during the initial 12–15 months of the pandemic.

The OECD report is based on the OECD Well-Being Framework for understanding and measuring well-being. This framework includes two main variables: "Current well-being," which tracks the present state of well-being, and "Resources for the future," which considers the sustainability of well-being across time and countries. What matters for the present purpose is "Current well-being." To assess it, the OECD framework considers 11 dimensions: Income and wealth, Housing, Work and job quality (grouped together as "Material conditions"), Health, Subjective well-being, Knowledge and skills, Environmental quality (grouped together as "Quality-of-life"), Social connections, Work-life balance, Safety and civic engagement (grouped together as "Community relations"). These dimensions constitute a somewhat motley crew. Most of them seem to be *sources* of well-being, but some (such as Housing and Safety) are most likely characterized as (pre-)*conditions* for enjoying well-being, while others (such as the elements of Subjective well-being) are, arguably, *constituents* of well-being. Be that as it may, these dimensions are robustly correlated with well-being so that collecting data about them can reveal important information about current well-being.

A quick look reveals the far-reaching, and unequal, effects that COVID-19 has had. Thanks to government measures, household disposable income increased on average by 2.19% from 2019 to 2020, yet close to one-third of people reported experiencing financial difficulties by the end of the same year. Unemployment rose by 1.7% from 2019 to 2020, and labour underutilization doubled in the first two-quarters of 2020. Remote work partly mitigated the impact of the pandemic, but it was possible only for some workers and in some sectors. In fact, job losses affected especially already vulnerable population groups, such as less-educated individuals, women, racialized minorities, and members of the LGBTQ+ communities, who were more likely to work in industries hit by governments' containment measures. This created work-related anxiety, as evidenced by the 14% of workers in ten OECD European countries who felt "likely" that they would lose their jobs in the next three months.

"Quality-of-life" also decreased across the OECD area, with one-third of individuals reporting that their life has been greatly affected by COVID-19. Deaths have been on average 16% higher than in the period 2015–2019, and life expectancy fell by 0.6 years. Reduced physical activity and increased alcohol consumption, amongst other things, created the conditions for future health problems. Mental health dramatically worsened, the decline being sharper and longer for already disadvantaged groups. One-quarter of the population in 15 OECD countries was at risk of depression or anxiety by the end of 2020. Physical distancing and lockdowns produced increased loneliness, with one in five individuals in 22 European OECD countries feeling lonely most or all the time in early 2021. Changes in the work conditions left many workers exhausted, with one in three people feeling too tired to perform the necessary household chores. Not surprisingly, women's work-life balance was particularly affected by the restrictions, as they took on the highest share of childcare and domestic responsibilities.

Subjective well-being deserves a separate word, considering its role for well-being more generally. Subjective well-being is typically measured in a rather coarse-grained way by considering three indicators: "Life evaluation," as reported by the respondents on a scale from 0 to 10; "Positive emotions," which gathers information about three positive emotions (i.e., laughter, enjoyment, and interest) experienced by the respondents the previous day; and "Negative emotions," which gathers information about three negative emotions (i.e., worry, sadness, and anger) experienced by the respondents the previous day (see Helliwell et al. 2022, chapter 2). Somewhat surprisingly, average life evaluations remained quite stable during the two years of the pandemic. Similarly, positive emotions remained twice as prevalent as negative emotions, in conformity with pre-pandemic levels. By contrast, negative emotions (particularly worry and sadness) increased by 8% in 2020 and by 3% in 2021 compared to pre-pandemic levels.

As expected, these data show an overall decline in the dimensions relevant to well-being. Since the data give us only an average picture, they suggest that for some individuals, particularly those belonging to already marginalized and underprivileged groups, the conditions during the pandemic were especially bleak. As I mentioned in the introduction, however, this was not true across the board. In fact, for some individuals – and not just the rich and the privileged – the pandemic brought an increase in well-being. This happened not always *despite* the pandemic, but oftentimes *because* of it, in as much as the pandemic forced them to adapt their outlook and behaviours.

In part, the change was driven by the attitudes the individuals took in response to the pandemic or that were fostered by the environment where they were fortunate to live. One effect of the pandemic was to lead some people to appreciate more what they had. Some studies have shown that "gratitude" experienced in this context was associated with increased well-being and resilience (see Helliwell et al. 2021, 134). Another response to the pandemic, particularly in the early stages, was to adopt an optimistic outlook in the face of adversity. For instance, during the first lockdown, many Italians displayed in their windows hand-drawn rainbows with the slogan *Andrà tutto bene!* ("Everything will be all right!"), a response that was later adopted in other countries. Such "positivity resonance, or shared feelings of positivity" (Helliwell et al. 2021, 134) have been associated with better mental health. More generally, the sense of social connectedness that many people actively sought by reconnecting with friends offered protection against the direness of the situation. Trust was an especially important attitude. The World Happiness Reports (WHR) in 2021 and 2022 showed that trust towards one's government and one's fellow citizens was consistently associated both with lower death rates and increased happiness (see Helliwell et al. 2021, chapter 2; Helliwell et al. 2022, chapter 2).

In large part, however, changes in well-being have been the result of deliberate decisions that people took about how to live their lives. In the immediate, many reacted by helping others, either via donations, volunteering, or other forms of help. Measures of prosocial behaviour indeed increased by one-quarter in 2021. Generosity, benevolence, and kindness created "a positive feedback loop with happiness, with the benevolent more likely to be happy and the happy more likely to act benevolently" (see Helliwell et al. 2022, 45). Perhaps, however, the most significant impact of the pandemic on people's life choices is that it led many to *redefine their goals* and to *shift their priorities*. This stance has taken many forms. For some, the pandemic has been the catalyst for a more robust commitment to self-care, which manifested through the adoption of a healthier diet, a more active lifestyle, and increased attention to one's mental health. By disrupting established routines, the pandemic forced others to re-examine the purpose and quality of their jobs. This has led to what is now known as the "Great Resignation" or, perhaps more aptly, the "Great Reshuffle," where several individuals quit their employment and looked for better paid or more meaningful jobs as well as for better working conditions. Alternatively, the pandemic led some individuals to downplay the centrality of work in their lives and to favour a more multidimensional lifestyle. On the one hand, purpose, achievement, and learning at work became less important for happiness, whereas flexibility and supportive management became more important (see Helliwell et al. 2021, chapter 7). On the other hand, in a phenomenon labelled "Quiet Quitting," some adopted a policy of fulfilling the minimum job requirements while investing themselves in other activities outside work. For some, this meant cultivating new hobbies, which contributed to their subjective well-being. The WHR 2021 lists the experience of flow, an emotion of enjoyment felt in relation to a challenge that matches the individual's skills (Tappolet 2022), as "protective" of people's well-being during the pandemic (Helliwell et al. 2021, chapter 6). For others, it meant spending more time with their families and developing stronger bonds with their friends. Finally, and more generally, the pandemic led many individuals to a "rediscovery" of nature. People used green spaces and were on trails more than before. A recent study shows that the appreciation of nature and the awareness of its emotional and spiritual benefits increased during the pandemic (Park et al. 2022). Consistently with previous findings, data also show that being in nature increased people's happiness and that people who spent more time outdoors were happier than those who did less (Natural England 2020).

To sum up, in a context characterized by so many premature deaths and intense sufferings, some individuals found a way to be happier and increase their well-being. Now, I have so far used these terms in a broad sense, drawing especially on social-scientific usage. It is clear, however, that these terms also have a philosophical pedigree and have been conceptualized in specific ways by different philosophical theories. The question that I want to consider in the next two sections is how these theories can explain the positive changes in well-being that some individuals underwent during the pandemic and whether these explanations are plausible.

9.3 COVID-19 and traditional theories of well-being

Let me start with a caveat. To some extent, all the philosophical theories of well-being *can* explain the phenomenon under consideration. No *gotcha!* moment is possible here. And indeed, none of the arguments developed in this section is meant to be a decisive objection against the competing theories of well-being that I will discuss. Nonetheless, I think that it is possible to raise some doubts about the explanations that they provide. Ultimately, my claim will be comparative. I will argue that the fitting happiness theory of well-being offers a more convincing explanation than the traditional theories of well-being. Besides shedding light on life during the pandemic, I take this to bring additional support to the theory to which I adhere.

Before proceeding, let me remind the reader of an important distinction. While the terms "well-being" and "happiness" are often treated as synonyms in everyday life as well as, occasionally, in the social-scientific literature, it is more and more common in philosophy to distinguish the two. "Well-being" is used as an evaluative term, designating the life that is *good for* the individual living it. It refers to a distinctive kind of value, i.e., *prudential* value, that a life may have to various degrees. By contrast, "happiness" is used as a psychological term, designating a favourable mental state (or a combination of favourable mental states) that an individual may undergo. According to the mainstream view, then well-being and happiness are conceptually distinct. This does not mean that they are not related but simply that their relation is, if there is any, a *substantive* one.[3]

In fact, one of the historically most popular well-being theories, hedonism, holds that well-being entirely consists in happiness, which is conceived as a positive balance of pleasures and displeasures.[4] More specifically, hedonism has it that an individual's well-being in a given interval of time is a function of the number, intensity, and duration of the pleasures and displeasures that the individual experiences during that period. Hedonism has a straightforward explanation of why some individuals increased their well-being during the pandemic. The changes they made in their lives and the attitudes they adopted were such that they experienced, on balance, pleasures that were more numerous, intense, and longer than displeasures.

The simplicity of this explanation is also its main defect. Hedonism does not seem to fully capture one of the main features of these individuals' well-being increase – namely, that the latter was often the result of a profound change in these people's outlook, which went beyond the states they experienced. As suggested earlier, it was a change in priorities and a redefinition of their objectives that drove their well-being increase. A hedonist may insist that changes of this sort contributed to increases in well-being *only by virtue of* having an impact on the pleasantness of the states that the individuals experienced. But I think there are reasons to resist this thought. An important one is that, in some cases, what made people's lives go better was the experience of mental states such as calm, feelings of peace, a sense of life balance, and harmony, which are typically regarded as positively valenced, yet low-arousal, affective states.[5] Although these states have a positive phenomenology, they do not seem to always have a pleasant phenomenology (more on this in the next section). Moreover, they do not seem to be experienced with the level of phenomenal intensity required to account for the relevant changes in the individuals' well-being. If this is true, then hedonism cannot adequately capture their contribution to well-being.

The desire fulfilment theory appears to perform better than hedonism.[6] According to it, well-being consists in the satisfaction of the individual's desires. More specifically, well-being is a function of the number and strength of the desires that are satisfied.[7] The desire fulfilment theory appears to easily account for the effect that redefining their goals had on some people's well-being. On a common reading, having a goal involves having a desire-like state that motivates the subject to pursue some objective. During the pandemic, some individuals changed their desire structure and adopted certain goals, such as having a healthier diet, physical exercise, and mental care, whose attainment increased their well-being.

I think the problem with this account is a general one. It gives the wrong account of degrees of well-being. On the traditional understanding, a desire's strength is simply the desire's motivational force, that is, the strength with which it pushes an individual to act in one way or another. Accordingly, an individual's life goes well to the extent that the desires that are satisfied are motivationally strong in this sense. But this generates various problems, which have been well documented.[8] One that is relevant for the present purpose is that it cannot account for the contribution to well-being of states like calm, tranquillity, and peace of mind, which typically are neither caused by attitudes with strong motivational force nor come with such a motivational character. One possibility is to adopt an alternative account of desire strength, according to which the latter is the extent to which an individual is phenomenally attracted to the object of their desire (see Heathwood 2019). It seems to me, however, that this move brings back some of the problems that we examined with respect to hedonism, most notably, the fact that it reduces the relative contribution to well-being of the changes in people's states of mind to the effects that these had on the phenomenology of people's desires.

A close cousin of the desire fulfilment theory, the value fulfilment theory seems to provide some improvements. According to it, an individual's well-being consists in the fulfilment of their valuings – that is, in the attainment of what the individual values.[9] There are various ways to understand the notion of valuings, but according to a prominent one, "to value something is to have a stable pattern of affective, conative, and doxastic attitudes towards that object" (Tiberius 2018, 35; see also Raibley 2010). This characterization avoids the problems faced by the desire fulfilment theory. Valuings are stable mental states that involve desires, but that are not reducible to them. As such, degrees of valuings are, arguably, neither a matter of motivational strength nor a matter of degrees of attraction. At the same time, the value fulfilment theory seems to be well positioned to explain how people's changes in their outlook drove changes in their well-being during the pandemic. The direct and indirect experience of COVID-19 led some individuals to modify their valuing structure, by either adopting new valuings or changing the relative importance of their valuings.

I think there are three potential problems with this account. The first is that fulfilling values requires time, more time than fulfilling simple, short-term desires. Depending on how value fulfilment is conceived, then the theory may open a gap between the time the individuals appeared to undergo a change in well-being during the pandemic and the time the theory suggests as the temporal locus of the individual's well-being variation. A second, related problem – in fact, a general problem for the theory – is that the theory seems incapable of recognizing the *direct* contribution that the individuals' affective states make to their well-being. Arguably, states like gratitude, flow, positivity resonance, the feeling of social connectedness, calm, and harmony increased the well-being of the individuals who experienced these states simply in virtue of how they felt. But unless degrees of value fulfilment are conceived, at least in part, as a function of the phenomenological character of these states – which would seem to involve an equivocate use of the term "fulfilment" – then the theory cannot vindicate this intuitive idea. Finally, it also appears that it is not necessary that a positive affective state be an object, or a manifestation, of an individual's valuings for it to contribute to the individual's well-being. During the pandemic, shared feelings of positivity improved people's conditions not because they were previously valued, but because they brought some "light" in a rather dark and scary moment.

I want to conclude my analysis of traditional theories of well-being by considering perfectionism.[10] According to the standard version, well-being consists in the development and exercise of distinctively human capacities.[11] Insofar as rational deliberation is one of the most important prudentially relevant capacities, perfectionism can explain how decisions concerning one's objectives, values, priorities, and behaviours adopted in response to the pandemic led some people to increase their well-being. Similarly, perfectionism can account for the prudential contribution made by the cultivation of new hobbies and the strengthening of social bonds, both of which appear to fulfil some important dimensions of human nature.

That said, I think that the explanation offered by perfectionism is problematic in other respects. To put it bluntly, I find it hard to believe that the reason why certain people's lives improved during the pandemic is that they all became more "virtuous," as perfectionism suggests. This is certainly true of some of them, perhaps those who committed to a better lifestyle and who invested themselves in helping others. However, it does not seem to be true as a general explanation of well-being increase. In particular, as we have seen, it seems that in many cases, changes in well-being were the result of the individuals' attitudes towards the situation, including calm, peace of mind, and appreciation of nature, which do not seem to necessarily involve virtue. Perfectionism, like other traditional theories of well-being, does not have the resources to capture the direct contribution of these states to well-being.

9.4 COVID-19 and the fitting happiness theory of well-being

To explain increases in well-being during the pandemic, we need to look elsewhere. In this section, I argue that the fitting happiness theory of well-being provides a good framework for understanding these changes.

9.4.1 The fitting happiness theory

As its very name suggests, the basic idea underlying the theory is simple: well-being consists in fitting happiness. There are, however, several important details that need to be specified to get a full grasp of the theory and that are important for explaining well-being variations during the pandemic. Since Tappolet and I have spelt out these details at length else-where (see Rossi and Tappolet 2022, forthcoming, n.d.-a), here I will simply summarize them.

The first crucial notion for understanding the theory is that of "happi-ness." The fitting happiness theory (FHT, henceforth) adopts an affective theory of happiness.[12] According to it, happiness consists in a positive balance of occurrent affective states such as emotions, moods, and sensory pleasures and displeasures. More specifically, on our account, positive emotions and moods, as well as sensory pleasures, are happiness-constituting states; negative emotions and moods, as well as sensory displeasures, are unhappiness-constituting states. For simplicity, in what follows, I will pri-marily focus on the former states.

There are two main differences with respect to the theory of happiness endorsed by standard hedonism. The first concerns the nature of the states that constitute happiness. According to the FHT, emotions, moods, and sensory pleasures are different kinds of perceptual experiences of evaluative properties. Consider, for example, an emotion of joy at the birth of one's child. In our view, this emotional episode consists in a per-ceptual experience that (non-conceptually[13]) represents the birth of one's child as joyful. Likewise, an emotion of admiration of a musician consists in a perceptual experience that represents that musician as admirable. A similar account holds for moods and sensory pleasures. Consider a mood of elation. In our view, an episode of elation consists in a perceptual experience of the joyful. In this respect, elation is similar to joy: they both target the same evaluative property, i.e., the joyful. The difference between the two is that joy (like other emotions) has a specific object (e.g., the birth of one's child, in the previous example), whereas elation (like other moods) has a non-specific object.[14] Consider, finally, the sensory pleasure of drinking a tasty coffee in the morning. In our view, this episode con-sists in a perceptual experience that represents the coffee being tasty as pleasurable. The difference with emotions and moods is that, by essence, sensory pleasures have a particular kind of "sensory" object, i.e., an object having some sensory quality, and target a particular evaluative property, i.e., the pleasurable.

Putting all this together, we can say that all the happiness-constituting states are kinds of phenomenal evaluations – that is, evaluations with a phenomenal dimension. By presenting their objects as possessing specific evaluative properties, they provide the individual experiencing them with an evaluation of these objects. Moreover, they provide an evaluation that is distinctively "felt" since affective states typically come with a distinctive phenomenology.[15] While sensory pleasures have, by definition, a *pleasant* phenomenology – after all, this is what makes them (sensory) "pleasures" – this is not the case for all positive emotions and moods.[16] In our view, the phenomenology of these states depends on their evaluative content – that is, on the evaluative properties that they represent. As we have seen, each emotion and mood token represents an evaluative property that belongs to a given type (e.g., the joyful, the admirable). These types can be seen as different specifications of the general evaluative property of being good. Thus, emotion and mood tokens represent their objects as *being* good in specific ways. Insofar as the phenomenology of these states depends on their evaluative content, it is then plausible to say that different emotion and mood tokens *feel* good in specific ways. However, in the same way as there are different ways of *being* good, not all of which are ways of being pleasurable, so are there different ways of *feeling* good, not all of which are ways of feeling pleasant.[17] This implies that, although all positive emotions and moods have a positive phenomenology – they all feel good, insofar as they all represent ways of being good – they do not all have a pleasant phenomenology. As such, not all happiness-constituting states are "pleasures." This is the first difference with respect to the theory of happiness adopted by standard hedonism about well-being.

The second difference concerns the dimensions of the happiness- and unhappiness-constituting states that determine the overall level of an individual's happiness. Recall that according to standard hedonism, happiness is a function of the number, phenomenal intensity, and duration of pleasures and displeasures. According to the FHT, an additional dimension is relevant – namely, the centrality of the happiness- and unhappiness-constituting states. By centrality, we mean the extent to which these states are connected to the individual's *valuings*.[18] The idea is that two equally phenomenally intense affective states may contribute differently to happiness to the extent that they differ in centrality. For example, your excitement at having a paper accepted by a prestigious journal may increase your happiness more than your equally intense joy at your national team's soccer world cup victory if you value academic success more than your national team's sportive achievements. As this example shows, centrality is independent from phenomenal intensity. Thus, an affective state may be highly central in our sense even if it is not phenomenally intense, and vice-versa. What matters is the connection to the individual's valuings.

Earlier on, I mentioned that a prominent view conceives of valuings as involving conative, doxastic, and affective elements. The FHT adopts a different account, according to which to value something is to have a sentiment towards that thing (such as love, care, like). In a nutshell: valuings are sentiments.[19] We conceive of sentiments as standing evaluations. They are "evaluations" insofar as they represent their objects as possessing specific evaluative properties. For example, when you have a sentiment of love for your partner, your love represents your partner as possessing the property of being lovable. In this respect, sentiments are just like emotions. They differ from emotions insofar as sentiments are dispositional states. This is what makes them "standing" evaluations. More specifically, sentiments are multi-track emotional dispositions – that is, dispositions to experience different types of affective states related to the object of one's sentiment. For example, your love may manifest in episodes of joy at your partner's success, sadness at your partner's illness, admiration at your partner's accomplishment, and so on.

Let me sum up: according to the FHT, happiness consists in a broadly positive balance of affective states such as emotions, moods, and sensory pleasures, where the balance depends, amongst other things, on the relation between these states and the individual's sentiments. Emotions, moods, and sensory pleasures are kinds of phenomenal evaluations, whereas sentiments are standing evaluations. It follows that according to the FHT, happiness can be conceived, at the same time, as a global affective experience of evaluative properties (or, more simply, "values") and as a global affective evaluation of the individual's situation, which takes into account the individual's more general evaluative stance.

The FHT holds that well-being consists in happiness thus conceived, provided that happiness is *fitting*. This brings us to the second notion that is crucial for understanding the FHT of well-being, that of "fittingness." As we have seen, happiness is constituted by phenomenal and standing evaluative states. *Qua* "evaluations," these states can be assessed as correct or incorrect. They are correct when the world is as they say it is – i.e., when their objects possess the evaluative properties that these states represent them to possess. They are incorrect otherwise. For example, an emotion of joy at the birth of one's child is correct if and only if that event is really joyful. Similarly, a sentiment of love towards one's partner is correct if and only if one's partner is really lovable. We use the term "fitting" to characterize an affective state that is "representationally correct" in this sense.[20]

Insofar as it is constituted by states that have fittingness conditions, it is plausible to think that happiness too can be assessed as fitting or unfitting. According to the FHT, happiness is fitting to the extent that (a) its constituent states are fitting and (b) they are based on fitting sentiments. Clearly, happiness can be more or less fitting during a given interval of time, since its constituent states and the states on which they are based may be fitting to various degrees. In light of what we have seen before, we can say that when happiness is fitting, it provides the individual, at the same time with a global affective experience of *genuinely* valuable items, and with a *correct* global evaluation of their life. This is what it is to be in a state of well-being, according to the FHT.

9.4.2 Explaining well-being increases

In this subsection, I want to do two things. First, I want to advance a general hypothesis about the mechanisms by which some people increased their well-being during the pandemic and as a result of it. Second, I want to argue that the FHT provides a good explanation of *why* these mechanisms positively changed people's well-being.

My hypothesis is quite simple. People increased their well-being during the pandemic in two ways. On the one hand, they appreciated or engaged with things *of* value. Sometimes, these were things already present in these individuals' lives, but for which the individuals had a new or redis-covered appreciation; other times, they were things that the individuals introduced in their lives in response to the pandemic. On the other hand, people increased their well-being by changing *what* they valued. Once again, in some cases, people discovered "new" values, in other cases, they simply revised the relative importance of "old" values.

Here is how the FHT can explain the role of these mechanisms. One lesson that we can learn from the empirical evidence discussed above is that positive affects played a crucial role in people's happiness. Gratitude, grit, resilience, flow, a sense of social connectedness, care for oneself and towards others, positivity resonance, shared feelings of positivity, calm, and trust were protective of people's subjective well-being and active drivers of happiness. In fact, the WHR 2022 states, more strongly, that "[m]uch of the impact of social support, freedom [to make choices] and generosity on life evaluations" – that is, much of the impact of three of the six variables that the WHR uses to explain life evaluations – "is chan-nelled through their influence on positive emotions" (see Helliwell et al. 2022, 23). Positive emotions, more than the absence of negative emo-tions, played a central role in happiness. This is not a surprise for the FHT. According to it, positive affective states are not just sources of hap-piness, they are constituents of it. By experiencing these states during the pandemic, then, the individuals increased their happiness.

There is more. The FHT conceives of affective states as perceptual expe-riences of evaluative properties. In other words, according to the FHT, in experiencing certain affective states, an individual apprehends certain things as valuable in specific ways. Thus, for instance, in experiencing gratitude during the pandemic, some individuals experienced what they already had as deserving recognition, appreciation, and thankfulness. In adopting new hobbies and experiencing flow, they experienced these activ-ities as enjoyable insofar as they presented new challenges that matched their skills. Generalizing, positive emotions presented certain things to the subjects as being valuable. As such, they counted as ways of appreciating and engaging with things that *seemed* of value to the subject. Of course, as we have seen in the previous subsection, in order to contribute to well-being, and not just to happiness, positive emotions must be fitting. That is, they must be ways of appreciating and engaging with things that genu-inely *are* of value. But arguably, many of the emotions that the individuals experienced during the pandemic were fitting in this sense.

According to my hypothesis, the first mechanism by which some indi-viduals increased their well-being is that they appreciated or engaged with things *of* value. The FHT gives an interpretation of this hypothesis and an explanation of why it holds. By experiencing fitting positive emotions, the individuals *affectively* engaged with items that were of genuine value. This increased their well-being *because* well-being consists in such fitting affective experiences.

As we have seen, another key driver of people's changes in well-being was a revision of their goals and priorities. As I hinted in Section 9.3, I think that such a revision is best interpreted as a change in people's valuing structure. Accordingly, part of what led some individuals to have a prudentially better life during the pandemic was their valuing new things or assigning a different relative importance to the things they already valued. Arguably, following a new healthier diet or beginning to do some physical activities are instances of the former phenomenon, whereas reconnecting with friends and spending more time with one's family are instances of the latter. This interpretation of the empirical evidence is nothing but the second mechanism which, I hypothesized, contributed to increasing people's well-being during the pandemic. How did it do so?

The FHT offers the following explanation. Changes in valuings led some individuals to adopt attitudes, develop habits, and perform actions that generated positive affective experiences. Reconnecting with one's friends and family generated a higher sense of connectedness; physical activity typically has a rewarding and satisfying effect; self-care generated an increased sense of balance. According to the FHT, these experiences increased happiness because they are constitutive of it.

Most importantly, changes in the valuing structure had an impact on the centrality of these affects. The development of new valuings led to newly central affective experiences, while shifts in priorities made some affective experiences more central than before. As we have seen, the FHT holds that centrality is one of the dimensions that determine the relative contribution to happiness of different affective states. Thus, by increasing the centrality of some of these states, changes in the valuing structure increased happiness.

Of course, by now we know that to increase well-being in this way, changes in valuings must be fitting. And indeed, it seems that many were during the pandemic. It certainly seems appropriate to increase the relative weight of social relations compared to work or to develop a healthier lifestyle.[21] My hypothesis was that the second mechanism by which people increased their well-being during the pandemic was by changing what they valued. According to the FHT, these changes had positive prudential effects because they led the individuals to experience fittingly central positive affects.

To sum up: for some individuals, the pandemic has created opportunities to appreciate, or engage with, things of value and to revise the things they value. This increased their well-being, according to the FHT, because well-being consists in a positive balance of affective experiences of genuinely valuable items, whose contribution depends, amongst other things, on their connection with the individual's deepest evaluative attitudes.

I want to conclude this subsection by showing that the explanation offered by the FHT is immune from the objections faced by the traditional theories of well-being. The objections raised against hedonism were two. The first was that it offers an inadequate account of how the depth of internal changes affected the individuals' well-being during the pandemic. The FHT avoids this objection because it assigns valuings an important role in determining happiness and well-being. Valuings are some of the deepest evaluative attitudes of an individual. Changes in valuings affect the centrality of the affects that they dispose the individual to experience. Since centrality is independent of phenomenal intensity, the FHT can explain how these changes increased some individuals' well-being during the pandemic in a way that is not reducible to their effects on the phenomenal character of their occurrent manifestations.

The second objection was that hedonism does not adequately recognize the contribution to happiness and well-being of low-arousal affective states. The problem is that, while there is evidence that states such as calm, peace of mind, and tranquillity significantly contribute to happiness and well-being, they do not seem to be very intensely pleasant states. The FHT avoids this objection in two ways. On the one hand, it denies that these states are, by essence, "pleasures." They are positive affective states and, as such, have a positive phenomenology. However, they do not always have a pleasant phenomenology. On the other hand, the FHT holds that low-arousal positive affects contribute to happiness and well-being not just as a function of their phenomenal intensity but also of their centrality. When they are connected to the individual's valuings, as they typically are, these states are highly central. Hence, they have a significant impact on happiness and well-being even if they are not intensely felt.[22]

The main objections against the value fulfilment theory were that it potentially misplaces the timing of the benefits accrued to the individuals during the pandemic and that it offers an inadequate account of what makes positive affective states well-being-enhancing. Let us start from the latter problem. The FHT holds that positive affective states do not contribute to well-being in virtue of their being objects, or manifestations, of the individual's valuings. Rather, they do so, when they are fitting, in virtue of their being positively valenced experiences of the good. Valuings do play a role, insofar as they determine the centrality of these states. However, it is not necessary that these affects are connected to valuings for them to contribute to well-being. Positive affective experiences increase well-being even when they are not objects, or manifestations, of previously held valuings. This also helps address the issue of timing. The well-being benefits accrued to the individuals during the pandemic at the time when they experienced positive affective states, even if the valuings to which these affective states were possibly connected were not fully fulfilled yet. More generally, according to the FHT, valuings require affective experiences in order to make a contribution to well-being. They enhance well-being by causing these experiences and by affecting their centrality.

Finally, against perfectionism, the FHT denies that all the individuals who increased their well-being did so by becoming more virtuous. What explained the change is the fact that the pandemic offered them some opportunities to affectively engage with value. This claim must be correctly understood. We should not think of value in a grandiose way. Some of the genuinely valuable items that the individuals experienced were pretty ordinary: friends, family, nature, hobbies, physical activities. But they still contributed to making those individuals' lives better for them at a time that looked darker than most in recent history. Well-being does not require virtue, but it does require fitting happiness.[23]

Acknowledgements

I would like to thank Joshua Preiss for his helpful comments on a previous draft of this chapter.

Notes

1 See https://www.worldometers.info/coronavirus/. Retrieved on October 3, 2022.
2 The OECD is the *Organisation for Economic Co-operation and Development*, an international organisation including 38 countries, founded in 1961 to promote economic progress and implement better socio-economic policies.
3 See also Wayne Sumner, *Welfare, Happiness, and Ethics* (Oxford: Oxford University Press, 1996) and Guy Fletcher, *The Philosophy of Well-Being: An Introduction* (New York: Routledge, 2016b).
4 For a classic statement, see Jeremy Bentham, *An Introduction to the Principles of Morals and Legislation* (Garden City: Doubleday, 1789/1961). For an overview, see Alex Gregory, "Hedonism," in *The Routledge Handbook of Philosophy of Well-Being*, ed. Guy Fletcher (London: Routledge, 2016), 113–123. In some versions (e.g., Ben Bramble, "A New Defense of Hedonism about Well-Being," *Ergo* 3, no. 4 (2016): 85–112), reference to happiness is eliminated. Well-being is taken to consist simply in a favorable balance of pleasures and displeasures, where this holds independently of whether happiness should also be conceived hedonistically.
5 The WHR 2022 reports indeed that these states strongly contributed to life satisfaction in all regions of the world. See John F. Helliwell, Richard Layard, Jeffrey D. Sachs, Jan-Emmanuel De Neve, Lara B. Aknin, and Shun Wang, eds. *World Happiness Report 2022* (New York: Sustainable Development Solutions Network, 2022), chapter 6.
6 For an overview of desire fulfilment theories, see Chris Heathwood, "Desire-Fulfilment Theory," in *The Routledge Handbook of Philosophy of Well-Being*, ed. Guy Fletcher (London: Routledge, 2016), 135–147.
7 As far as ill-being is concerned, the idea is that some desires may have negative strength – in which case they are aversions – and their satisfaction can thus detract from an individual's well-being.
8 See, e.g., Chris Heathwood, "Which Desires are Relevant to Well-Being?" *Noûs* 53, no. 3 (2019): 664–688.

9   See Jason Raibley, "Well-Being and the Priority of Values," *Social Theory and Practice* 36, no. 4 (2010): 593–620 and Valerie Tiberius, *Well-Being as Value Fulfillment: How We Can Help Each Other to Live Well* (New York: Oxford University Press, 2018).

10   For reasons of space, I will not consider objective list theories here. For an overview, see Guy Fletcher, "Objective List Theories," in *The Routledge Handbook of Philosophy of Well-Being*, ed. Guy Fletcher (London: Routledge, 2016a), 148–160.

11   For an overview of perfectionist theories, see Gwen Bradford, "Perfectionism," in *The Routledge Handbook of Philosophy of Well-Being*, ed. Guy Fletcher (London: Routledge, 2016), 124–134.

12   See Daniel Haybron, *The Pursuit of Unhappiness: The Elusive Psychology of Well-Being* (New York: Oxford University Press, 2008) and Antti Kauppinen, "Meaning and Happiness," *Philosophical Topics* 41, no. 1 (2013): 161–185, for alternative affective accounts of happiness.

13   The qualification "non-conceptual" is important. It allows for the possibility that individuals who do not possess evaluative concepts (e.g., the concept of the joyful), such as young children and non-human animals, can also experience emotions. For simplicity, however, I will omit this qualification in what follows. For further details on the non-conceptual content of emotions, see Christine Tappolet, "Emotions Inside Out: The Nonconceptual Content of Emotions," in *Concepts in Thought, Action, and Emotion: New Essays*, ed. Christoph Demmerling and Dirk Schroeder (New York: Routledge, 2020), 257–276.

14   This idea has been elaborated in different ways in the literature. For instance, I argued elsewhere that moods have undetermined objects – that is, objects that the individual is unable to identify (see Mauro Rossi, "A Perceptual Theory of Moods," *Synthese* 198, no. 8 (2021): 7119–7147). Alternatively, moods can be conceived as having generalized (Robert Solomon, *The Passions: Emotions and the Meaning of Life* (Indianapolis: Hackett Publishing Company, 1976/1993); Jesse Prinz, *Gut Reactions: A Perceptual Theory of the Emotions* (New York: Oxford University Press, 2004)), plural (Matthias Siemer, "Mood Experience: Implications of a Dispositional Theory of Moods," *Emotion Review* 1, no. 3 (2009): 256–263), or modal (Carolyn Price, "Affect Without Object: Moods and Objectless Emotions," *European Journal of Analytic Philosophy* 2, no. 1 (2006): 49–68; Christine Tappolet, "The Metaphysics of Moods," in *The Ontology of Emotions*, ed. Hichem Naar and Fabrice Teroni (Cambridge: Cambridge University Press, 2018), 169–186) intentional objects. For the present purpose, it is not necessary to take a stance on this debate.

15   Tappolet and I leave the question open of whether emotions, moods, and sensory pleasures can sometimes be unconscious. For simplicity, I will omit the qualification "typically" in what follows.

16   I developed the argument that follows at greater length in Mauro Rossi, "An Evaluativist Theory of Pleasure," n.d.

17   Note the distinction between the property of being pleasurable and the property of being pleasant. The former is an evaluative property, which sensory pleasures represent their *objects* to have; the latter is a phenomenal property that sensory *experiences* may possess and whose character depends on the representation of the pleasurable.

18   This is what Tappolet and I have elsewhere called "input- (or source-) centrality" (see Mauro Rossi and Christine Tappolet, "Well-Being as Fitting Happiness," in *Fittingness: Essays in the Philosophy of Normativity*, ed. Christopher Howard and Richard Rowland (Oxford: Oxford University

Press, 2022), 267–289). It differs from Daniel Haybron's understanding of centrality as the extent to which an affective state is productive of other mental states and behaviors (see Haybron, *The Pursuit of Unhappiness*), which we call "output-centrality."

19 We presented and defended this account at length in Mauro Rossi and Christine Tappolet, "Valuings as Sentiments," n.d.-b

20 For criticisms of this understanding of fittingness, see Sigrun Svavarsdóttir, "Having Value and Being Worth Valuing," *Journal of Philosophy* 111, no. 2 (2014): 84–109, and Christopher Howard, "Fittingness," *Philosophy Compass* 12 (2018): e12542.

21 In many cases, these changes were deliberate. But it seems to me descriptively inadequate to think that in *all* cases people changed what they valued by means of conscious value judgments. Instead, these changes seem primarily the effect of a more profound, sentimental shift, which occurred in the individuals' minds. This is consistent with the account of valuings endorsed by the FHT.

22 *Mutatis mutandis*, these considerations are also relevant to explain how the FHT can avoid the objections raised against the desire fulfillment theory of well-being.

23 In fact, Tappolet and I have argued elsewhere that virtue is neither necessary nor sufficient for well-being. It *can* affect well-being, via the intermediary of the fitting affective states that are partly constitutive of virtue, but only when the external circumstances are favourable, so that the individual experiences *positive* fitting affective states. See Mauro Rossi and Christine Tappolet, "Virtues, Happiness, and Wellbeing," *The Monist*, 99, no. 2 (2016): 112–127, for more details.

Bibliography

Bentham, Jeremy. 1789/1961. *An Introduction to the Principles of Morals and Legislation*. Garden City: Doubleday.

Bradford, Gwen. 2016. "Perfectionism." In *The Routledge Handbook of Philosophy of Well-Being*, edited by Guy Fletcher, 124–134. London: Routledge.

Bramble, Ben. 2016. "A new defense of hedonism about well-being." *Ergo* 3, no. 4: 85–112.

Fletcher, Guy. 2016a. "Objective list theories." In *The Routledge Handbook of Philosophy of Well-Being*, edited by Guy Fletcher, 148–160. London: Routledge.

Fletcher, Guy. 2016b. *The Philosophy of Well-Being: An Introduction*. New York: Routledge.

Gregory, Alex. 2016. "Hedonism." In *The Routledge Handbook of Philosophy of Well-Being*, edited by Guy Fletcher, 113–123. London: Routledge.

Haybron, Daniel. 2008. *The Pursuit of Unhappiness: The Elusive Psychology of Well-Being*. New York: Oxford University Press.

Heathwood, Chris. 2016. "Desire-fulfilment theory." In *The Routledge Handbook of Philosophy of Well-Being*, edited by Guy Fletcher, 135–147. London: Routledge.

Heathwood, Chris. 2019. "Which desires are relevant to well-being?" *Noûs* 53, no. 3: 664–688.

Helliwell, John F., Richard Layard, Jeffrey D. Sachs, and Jan-Emmanuel De Neve, eds. 2021. *World Happiness Report 2021*. New York: Sustainable Development Solutions Network.

Helliwell, John F., Richard Layard, Jeffrey D. Sachs, Jan-Emmanuel De Neve, Lara B. Aknin, and Shun Wang, eds. 2022. *World Happiness Report 2022*. New York: Sustainable Development Solutions Network.

Howard, Christopher. 2018. "Fittingness." *Philosophy Compass* 12: e12542.

Kauppinen, Antti. 2013. "Meaning and happiness." *Philosophical Topics* 41, no. 1: 161–185.

Natural England. 2020. *The people and nature survey for England: Adult data Y1Q1 (April–June 2020) (experimental statistics)*. Natural England. https://www.gov.uk/government/statistics/the-people-and-nature-survey-for-england-adult-data-y1q1-april-june-2020-experimental-statistics/the-people-and-nature-survey-for-england-adult-data-y1q1-april-june-2020-experimental-statistics (accessed on October 3, 2022).

OECD. 2021. *COVID-19 and Well-Being: Life in the Pandemic*. Paris: OECD Publishing. https://doi.org/10.1787/1e1ecb53-en.

Park, Sohyun, Seungman Kim, Jaehoon Lee, and Biyoung Heo. 2022. "Evolving norms: social media data analysis on parks and greenspaces perception changes before and after the COVID 19 pandemic using a machine learning approach." *Scientific Reports* 12: 13246. doi.org/10.1038/s41598-022-17077-3.

Price, Carolyn. 2016. "Affect without object: moods and objectless emotions." *European Journal of Analytic Philosophy* 2, no. 1: 49–68.

Prinz, Jesse. 2004. *Gut Reactions: A Perceptual Theory of the Emotions*. New York: Oxford University Press.

Raibley, Jason. 2010. "Well-being and the priority of values." *Social Theory and Practice* 36, no. 4: 593–620.

Rossi, Mauro. 2021. "A perceptual theory of moods." *Synthese* 198, no. 8: 7119–7147.

Rossi, Mauro, and Christine Tappolet. 2016. "Virtues, happiness, and wellbeing." *The Monist*, 99, no. 2: 112–127.

Rossi, Mauro, and Christine Tappolet (2022). "Well-being as fitting happiness." In *Fittingness: Essays in the Philosophy of Normativity*, edited by Christopher Howard and Richard Rowland, 267–289. Oxford: Oxford University Press.

Rossi, Mauro, and Christine Tappolet. Forthcoming. "Ill-being and fitting unhappiness." In *Ill-Being: Philosophical Perspectives*, edited by Mauro Rossi and Christine Tappolet. Oxford: Oxford University Press.

Siemer, Matthias. 2009. "Mood experience: Implications of a dispositional theory of moods." *Emotion Review* 1, no. 3: 256–263.

Solomon, Robert. 1976/1993. *The Passions: Emotions and the Meaning of Life*. Indianapolis, Indiana: Hackett Publishing Company.

Sumner, Wayne. 1996. *Welfare, Happiness, and Ethics*. Oxford: Oxford University Press.

Svavarsdóttir, Sigrun. 2014. "Having value and being worth valuing." *Journal of Philosophy* 111, no. 2: 84–109.

Tappolet, Christine. 2000. *Emotions et valeurs*. Paris: Presses Universitaires de France.

Tappolet, Christine. 2016. *Emotions, Values, and Agency*. Oxford: Oxford University Press.

Tappolet, Christine. 2018. "The metaphysics of moods." In *The Ontology of Emotions*, edited by Hichem Naar and Fabrice Teroni, 169–186. Cambridge: Cambridge University Press.

Tappolet, Christine. 2020. "Emotions inside out: The nonconceptual content of emotions." In *Concepts in Thought, Action, and Emotion: New Essays*, edited by Christoph Demmerling and Dirk Schroeder, 257–276. New York: Routledge.

Tappolet, Christine. 2022. "Sailing, flow and happiness." In *The Sailing Mind*, edited by Roberto Casati, 17–29. Cham: Springer.

Tiberius, Valerie. 2018. *Well-Being as Value Fulfillment: How We Can Help Each Other to Live Well*. New York: Oxford University Press.

Part III

Social arrangements and moral conflicts

10 Delving into denialism

Rationality, emotion, value, and trust in social context

Leonardo de Mello Ribeiro

10.1 Introduction

It is a well-known thesis that the conditions of modern sociality require the development of trusting relations as one of its distinctive features (Gambetta 1988; Giddens 1990; Misztal 1996; Seligman 1997). Sztompka (2000, 11), for example, argues that those conditions include great differentiation of roles in the division of labour (making our lives both more interdependent and less predictable to one another), opacity of large segments of society (institutions, organizations, expert systems), a growing sense of anonymity and impersonality, new and expanding threats and hazards of our own making. Although Sztompka and others draw our attention to the development of trust as a social necessity, we should notice that those same conditions can create, in case of failure of that development, pressure for *distrust*. Further multifarious ongoing social processes in our modern times seem to reinforce this: multiple ways of information transmission; media fragmentation, the impact of technological advances on daily life and forms of social organization, high-level of specialization of scientific knowledge affecting its communication and public reception, pervasive social, economic, and political inequalities.

Indeed, authors from a variety of perspectives and concerns (Cook 2001; Misztal 1996; Seligman 1997) have identified a generalized crisis of trust in our modern societies (especially in Western liberal democracies). Contrary to what we may socially need, we seem to be living in a world of increasing and pervasive *distrust* among social peers. We will take this diagnosis as an assumption here. However, many things we will say in this chapter about trust can be understood as providing support for it.

That complex social scenario has substantial implications for the ways people gather and weigh evidence to justify their beliefs and actions. A current phenomenon that can arguably be traced to it (at least partly) as an outcome is a form of *denialism* regarding official public health measures and scientific discourse in the context of the COVID-19 pandemic. Denialism involves a variety of forms of resistance, scepticism, and

DOI: 10.4324/9781003310129-13

rejection of those measures and discourse. Although denialism comes in varying forms, degrees, and particularities concerning the phenomenon it aims to be a denial of,[1] it can be understood in a broad sense as a standpoint of rejection of scientific consensus (and associated official public discourse) about a given phenomenon and the adoption of alternative explanations at variance with scientific evidence. Typically, denialist views are expressed in *social* terms, alleging that scientific consensus is unreliable because it is part of a conspiracy or hoax, ideologically biased, politically threatening.

Denialism invites us to ask: what kinds of epistemological and practical processes lead people to adhere to denialism in spite of scientific evidence to the contrary? Is denialism irrational? To what extent, if any, can it be rational?

Our main aim here is to argue that it would be too fast to say simply that denialism is altogether irrational. Given an appropriate explanation of its context of occurrence and conditions of development, some expressions of denialism might be considered rational in a specific sense: according to a *social-psychological* meaning of rationality, the way we gather information, weigh evidence, and identify reasons to believe and act is part of social processes, mediated by socially embedded evaluations and emotional reactions. So, although a denialist attitude may be individually irrational when it comes to *epistemic* standards (denialists often fall into fallacies and cognitive biases) it can be rational in a social-psychologically "adaptive" sense. This is explained, as we will see in this chapter, by the restrictions of information and cognitive limitations that denialists experience and the social conditions under which they form beliefs and deliberation.

Trust as an attitude involving, as we will argue, both a cognitive and an emotional-evaluative dimension plays a crucial role in information-gathering processes of belief-formation and decision-making. In an uncertain and potentially threatening world, where conflicting information abounds, there seems to be no option but to get advice from those you *trust* in social context. This is a pervasive phenomenon in the individual-society relation. But what distinguishes the epistemological and practical processes of denialists is arguably the way reality is contextually perceived by them, in particular through the social sources of information they take as trustworthy. So, in order to better understand denialism, we should recognize the role of trust in mediating social epistemological processes.

Before proceeding, two clarifications are worth making. Firstly, it is far beyond our aim to attempt to provide a full-blown analysis of denialism. We are focusing on one feature of it – namely, the role of trust for the development of COVID-19 denialism. Secondly, we should acknowledge that many statements that compose the general hypothesis advanced here would need empirical confirmation (including data to turn it finer-grained vis-à-vis cultural and social differences). Nevertheless, the hypothesis put forward here can (and should) be empirically tested.

The text is divided as follows. In Section 10.2, we will provide a characterization of denialism and its conflicting relation with scientific discourse. Our task will be twofold. Firstly, we will argue that in order to understand denialism, we should focus on science as a *social institution* and source of information. Secondly, drawing on some empirical studies we will find that denialism seems closely associated with a series of social-psychological factors. Following Neil Levy's (2019a, 2019b, 2022) account of the social dimension of epistemology, we will argue that denialists' reactions can be understood as a form of "adaptive" social rationalization.

In Section 10.3, we will argue that a crucial feature of that "adaptive" denialist reaction can be explained by drawing on the role of trust in social relations. To do this, we will get involved in some conceptual issues. We will advance an account of trust according to which trust is a socially contextualized sort of *emotional-evaluative* projection that goes beyond evidence of a social partner's trustworthiness (understood as a rational calculus of costs and benefits).

Finally, in Section 10.4, we will argue that our account of trust offers adequate conceptual resources to better understand denialism. We will then be able to explain more thoroughly (psychologically and socially) denialists' assessment of scientific discourse as untrustworthy. Trust is a social phenomenon, and denialists are *socially* rational to the extent that they get informed through trust (and despite the fact that their trusting relations can make them *epistemically* irrational). As a general conclusion, we hold that denialism is more an overall social problem (about the social conditions for trust) than a problem that can be ascribed to individuals concerning the rationality of their epistemic capacities. A series of social, economic, and political factors decisively influence people's psychologies and perception of social reality, having a deep impact on how they make decisions and establish trusting relations.

10.2 Denialism, scientific discourse, and rationality

10.2.1 Denialism and the social dimension of science

First of all, we should distinguish two senses of "denialism" as this term has been used. According to one common use of the term, denialism involves a series of articulated and intentionally coordinated processes, spread among many spheres of society, motivated by political and ideological purposes, including strategies of manipulation and control of public discourse. In this sense, denialism is a sort of politically constructed *instrumental* standpoint and might be better called "ideological denialism" (Lewandowsky et al. 2016). But this is not the sense that will be our focus here. Here we are interested in discussing denialism as a social phenomenon that reveals the *sincere* expression, shared by significant portions of society, of people's (particularly laypeople) views and reactions to the pandemic. These include denying either the existence of the virus or the associated disease or the effectiveness of the public health measures of control, etc. This latter sense might be called "genuine denialism," and we will be assuming it throughout here.

COVID-19 denialism is striking because even after millions of cases of infections and deaths, a significant number of people among many societies still deny the seriousness or even the existence of the virus. This raises a challenge of how to interpret it. What can possibly justify those beliefs? What sorts of social and psychological mechanisms might explain them? This is especially challenging when we reflect on the fact that one clear feature of denialism is resistance and dismissal of *scientific discourse*. Throughout the COVID-19 pandemic, denialism has taken many forms and expressions against public health measures informed by specialized science: denying the need of social distancing and lockdown measures of control, denying the efficacy of prevention strategies (like the use of masks), rejecting the necessity and safety of the vaccine, etc. This is particularly noteworthy in a world increasingly organized around technological and scientific expertise.

One way of trying to explain denialism would be to characterize it as an expression of sheer *epistemic irrationality* of individuals. People might be interpreted as exhibiting unjustified resistance to overwhelming evidence, incurring in a series of formal and informal fallacies as well as cognitive bias. There is surely truth in this hypothesis. But its truth seems to be only part of the story and, as far as it goes, it lacks substance when not coupled with a convincing explanation about *why* people incur in such irrational moves. Thus, a "complementary" explanation seems as important as detecting individual epistemic irrationalities – at least if we want a broader picture of denialism as a *social* phenomenon. It is very likely that the phenomenon as a whole is probably much more complex and finer-grained than the sheer irrationality hypothesis seems to convey. It is part of our aim here to try to unpack part of the complexity of the phenomenon.

A promising first step in trying to understand denialism from a broader social perspective would be to trace it to well-established literature on the public uptake of science. This topic has been a concern of social scientists for decades. One trend in that literature claims that scientific discourse often fails to communicate successfully its results to the public mostly because it often clashes with laypeople's practices, social relations, and values. But we need to understand why this is so beyond the mere surface of things. To do this, we need to firstly focus on the sense in which scientific discourse is a *social institution*. As such, it is one among many available sources of information, practices, and values in society (Wynne 1991, 113).

As Wynne (1996; 1993; 1991) claims, scientific discourse as a social institution is, in a sense, "socially grounded, conditional and value-laden" as any other (although it obviously bears significant differences to other social sources of knowledge and information). From a concrete social perspective, its credibility is "influenced not so much by what it says directly and explicitly, as in the way it is institutionally and intellectually organised" (Wynne 1996, 38) and, we could add, its knowledge socially transmitted. So, scientific knowledge is never perceived "free of imputed social interests" (Wynne 1993, 327). The public understanding of scientific discourse is always an epistemological issue related to its social purposes and impacts on its contexts of application.

Thus, the socially situated and contextualized reception of scientific discourse by laypeople needs to involve, as any other social relation, "negotiation," projected risks, and unavoidable assessments of trustworthiness. But these projected risks and assessments are not perceived as "objectively neutral" (entirely exhausted by the standards of scientific knowledge); they are always mediated by laypeople's experience of science as part of social arrangements and institutional structures. So, it should be recognized that

> trust and credibility are themselves analytically derivative of social relations and identity-negotiation; thus, like risk, they too should not be treated as if they have an objective existence which can be unambiguously measured and manipulated.
>
> (Wynne 1996, 42)

This is Wynne reminding us that scientific discourse often gets incorporated into public policy and administration without "social negotiation" in that it imposes or gets translated into social prescriptions in a way that frequently neglects social identities. As a result, science as a social institution will be often experienced as a *threat* to these identities (especially when it affects the ways lives are organized around a core of values, practices, and relationships). In this sense, the reception of science will frequently be ambivalent and sometimes assimilated through inconsistent hypotheses, beliefs, and reactions. But, as Wynne (1996, 27) advises us, ambivalence or inconsistency in laypeople's reactions at the surface level of discourse and behaviour will often be followed by coherence "at a deeper level, of the defence and negotiation of social identities."

Now, that overall sociological theoretical picture seems to find echo in the phenomenon of COVID-19 denialism. Firstly, statistics indicate that over the last decades, public distrust in science has increased (Goldenberg 2021).[2] This is probably related to what Engdahl and Lidskog (2014) identify as a complex social scenario involving contextual factors, shortcomings of science as a social institution, and associated risks. For example, science as a social institution has been an object of suspicion when related to "regulatory failures," "the new character of industrial risks," "the technical framing of public issues," "involvement with companies and nation-states at the expense of wider social concerns" (Engdahl and Lidskog 2014, 703).

Besides, it should be noticed that the general conditions under which the COVID-19 pandemic has evolved have significantly contributed to the sort of negative reaction to scientific discourse characteristic of denialism. The pandemic has evolved very rapidly and under a cloud of uncertainty. It has been met with mixed messages and sometimes inconsistencies in public health recommendations. People have been subject to a large amount of changing information updated almost on a daily basis. Scientific research has been called upon to develop concomitantly with the spreading of the pandemic, issuing a series of provisional and tentative results.

Finally, several empirical studies about the pandemic suggest that Wynne's sociological picture is applicable to denialism (Bicchieri et al. 2021; Freeman et al. 2020; Freeman et al. 2021; Jaspal and Nerlich 2022; Jennings et al. 2021; Lewandowsky 2021; Rutjens et al. 2021; van Mulukom et al. 2022). They show a consistent relation among people's values, worldviews, social identities, political tendencies, social conditions of living, and the grasping of scientific discourse as threatening, uncertain, and untrustworthy. In a case study about attacks on scientific discourse during the pandemic, Lee et al. (2021) have found that some people "mistrust the scientific establishment ("Science") because they believe that the institution has been corrupted by profit motives and politics" (Lee et al. 2021, 14). In addition, they believe that science as an institution is not unquestionable in that "valid science must be a process they can critically engage for themselves in an unmediated way. *Increased* doubt, not consensus, is the marker of scientific certitude" (ibid.).

Those studies suggest that it would be a mistake to infer from the denialists' resistance to scientific discourse that they reject science altogether or are expressing, as it were, an "anti-scientific" social identity. This may well be the case with some individuals, but the general point seems to be a form of resistance directed specifically to scientific discourse as *a social institution* (and its reproduction by governments, legal systems, mass media, etc.). What seems at stake in those studies is a question about the *social reliability* of *sources*, where to get information from. Indeed, as we will suggest in the following section, given that our lives and societies are deeply organized around scientific and technological knowledge, it seems almost impossible to get on without relying on it. So, denialists seem to be somehow disputing with science (as an institution) the same social space. In this sense, if denialists are accusing scientists' consensus of something like a hoax or a conspiracy (as studies like Lee et al. suggest), it seems to reveal not a rejection of science *per se*, but a question about how to *socially* interpret scientific discourse.

This hypothesis seems further explained by another pattern that abounds in the empirical literature on denialism – namely, *conspiracy beliefs* (Allington et al. 2021; Constantinou et al. 2021; Freeman et al. 2020; Freeman et al. 2021; Jennings et al. 2021; Rutjens et al. 2021; Soveri et al. 2021; Uscinski et al. 2020; van Mulukom et al. 2022). Several studies show a correlation between conspiracy beliefs, diminished trust in scientific discourse, and non-compliance with official guidelines to tackle the pandemic. Although conspiracy beliefs vary significantly in scope and verisimilitude, many conspiracy beliefs do not seem to carry an outright rejection of science per se. They seem to be related to a complex interplay of socio-psychological contextual factors that lead to suspicion, scepticism, or rejection of official scientific discourse. Dramatic scenarios like the pandemic, which involve significant restrictions, changes, and impacts on lifestyles and social organization, are the most favourable to the spring of conspiracy beliefs. Let us ask now what all this can show specifically about *rationality*.

10.2.2 Denialism, conspiracy beliefs, and rationality

There is a vast literature on the social and psychological nature of conspiracy beliefs (Douglas et al. 2019). As Levy (2019b) reports, conspiracy beliefs are associated with lower levels of analytic thinking and education, are more likely to be accepted by those who feel a lack control over their social lives, more appealing to those of low socio-economic status (and historical records of vulnerability to social exploitation due, for example, to income or ethnicity). Douglas (2021) tells us that studies have found data suggesting that people are drawn to conspiracy beliefs when important epistemic and social-psychological needs are not being met. Some of these needs are associated with avoidance of uncertainty, which leads people to search and identify patterns and meaning where there is none. Others involve a "desire to restore a threatened sense of security and control" (which may be related to anxiety and a feeling of powerlessness). From a social perspective, people more prone to conspiracy beliefs exhibit "a desire to hold one's self and one's groups in positive regard" (for example, when they "feel that their group is under-appreciated or under threat") (Douglas 2021, 271). Studies have also found association with "low political trust" and factors like "being on the losing end of a power asymmetry" (Douglas et al. 2019, 10–12).

From an epistemic point of view, Levy (2019b, 2007) points out that conspiracy believers are more prone to commit a series of formal and informal fallacies and be guided by cognitive bias. They tend to develop a disposition to detect patterns in random noise and be prone to the clustering illusion, are more likely to commit the attribution error, the confirmation bias, as well as tend to be biased towards pattern-seeking and hypersensitivity of agency detection.

However, as Levy contends, despite all that, it would be too fast to conclude that conspiracy believers are simply altogether irrational. Any plausible explanatory hypothesis here should appreciate the complex interplay of social and psychological factors *in context*. Accordingly, conspiracy believers may be interpreted as responding "adaptively" to their environments and background conditions of assessment and deliberation, which may involve multiple significant restrictions (personal, social, economic, political). In this sense, Levy holds that

> we might argue that conspiratorial ideation arises from dispositions that are psychologically, and perhaps socially, adaptive. If one is a member of a low status group or is otherwise at the mercy of forces that one cannot control and which cannot be expected to have your best interests at heart, hypervigilance with regard to threats might be adaptive. Whether people are intentionally conspiring against one or one's group or not, institutions may be structured, and individuals may act, in ways that reinforce inequalities, and it may be adaptive to be alert for these possibilities.
>
> (Levy 2019b, 68)

So, if one sees oneself immersed in a threatening environment, under a series of social and psychological restrictions, deciding and acting heuristically may be the adequate response. Some psychologists hold that in dramatic scenarios (involving threatening events, change, instability, contradictory information, compromised communication) people's "crafting" of their own explanations makes them "feel less uncertain and more in control" (DiFonzo 2019, 259). As Levy (2019b, 68) puts it, in such scenarios, "false positives may be a small price to pay for protection against genuine plots"; "accepting bizarre conspiracies is the price agents pay for being alert to real dangers."

This now introduces another meaning for "rational." Levy's proposal not only explains the spring of conspiracy beliefs but also *rationalizes* it. That is to say, although conspiracy beliefs can be typically formed on the basis of a series of intellectual vices and defective inquiry procedures, they can be the adequate response available to those people under the restrictions of their environments and background conditions of deliberation. (For a contrary interpretation, see Lewandowsky, Kozyreva, and Ladyman 2020.) True, under ideal, abstract, or fully informed conditions of belief-formation and decision-making, there may not be "objective" reasons for forming conspiracy beliefs. But in *real-world, socially concrete* conditions of belief-formation and decision-making, people may have no option other than adhering to conspiracy ideation. There is a meaning of "rationality" which is related to how to cope with circumstances in the face of restrictions or make best use of limited information. We might call this a *psychological* or *subjective* sense of rationality. One might object that, in the case of denialism, people have available a reliable and qualified source of information to rely on: scientific expertise. However, as we have seen, this is exactly what is at stake when scientific discourse gets socially contextualized.

This is now very useful to help us explain the distinction between most of us and denialists. Just like denialists, most of us also grasp scientific knowledge only through its socially mediated role. As Levy (2022, 2019a, 2007) and others have defended, scientific knowledge (arguably, knowledge in general) is a robust social enterprise which observes a complex (and historically inherited) division of labour. Not only most of us, non-specialists, but also the scientific specialists themselves, are intertwined in complex networks of testimony and trusting relations (scientists need to trust each other as well as the whole technical apparatus their work depends on). This is inescapable in that it is vital for our very survival, for our need to organize our ordinary lives and social engagement. As Levy says (2007, 188), detaching ourselves from those networks and means of production of scientific knowledge is to deny to ourselves "access to the cognitive landscapes that they open up for us." Thus, the production and transmission of scientific knowledge are the result of complex networks of division of labour from which we largely benefit but over which we have only limited control.

So, just like denialists, most of us have access to scientific knowledge through science as a social institution. But denialists arguably have that access under different social and psychological conditions of perception of reality. As a result, the difference comes to the *social sources* we rely on to have that access. Whereas most of us believe in societal official statements and scientific discourse, denialists tend to rely on alternative sources. Thus, it should be no surprise to find denialists preferring to rely on people or institutions who are similar to or like them in terms of their social identities; who share their beliefs, values, and worldviews; who have the same political sympathies.

In sum, although denialists' beliefs can surely be deemed rationally defective or irrational from an "objective" *epistemic* point of view, for their belief-forming processes lead them away from truth, they do not seem to be psychologically or subjectively criticizable for that, given that they do not have better cognitive resources for rationally coping with their situation. Besides, their cognitive resources and the way they perceive reality are to a significant extent shaped by their social environments in which trust plays a crucial role. It is through trust that denialists get access to information and knowledge. As we will see in the following section, it is the social background conditions under which denialists establish trusting relations that make them trust unreliable sources of information and hold false beliefs. But the question about *who to trust* is primarily a sort of practical (not epistemic) question, and its criteria are social. In this practical and social sense, denialists do not seem to be irrational (although their trusting relations can provide them with information that makes them epistemically defective or irrational).[3]

All the discussion so far has explicitly referred to *trust* as a pivotal explanatory concept. But we have been assuming only an intuitive grasp of it. So, in the next section, we will discuss more thoroughly the general nature of trust. Then, in the final section, we will explore our account of trust in connection with denialism.

10.3 Trust

10.3.1 The general nature of trust

Discussing trust in more detail is particularly important for our purposes here for two reasons. Firstly, it is through a better understanding of trust that we will be able to highlight the role of emotions and values in the denialist attitude. Secondly, given that some rationalist accounts tend to reject a relevant role for emotions in trusting relations, they raise a challenge to our account that has epistemological bearings on our previous discussion. So, let us go through this.

Trust is commonly understood as having both social and psychological dimensions. Socially speaking, trust is a relation of presupposed reliability between agents that makes their social cooperation possible. As Baier (1986, 232) once said, "[A]ny form of cooperative activity, including the division of labor, requires the co-operators to trust one another to do their bit." In the same vein, Lewis and Weigert (1985, 968) claim that trust is "a functional prerequisite for the possibility of society" the alternative to which is "chaos and paralysing fear."

Psychologically speaking, trust involves positive expectations regarding others' behaviour with whom one interacts in an *asymmetric* way: to trust someone is to put oneself in a relation of dependence on another's choice and action, for whom there is always the possibility of defection. Trust is, then, as Giddens (1990, 32) holds, "a particular type of confidence," but one that never excludes the possibility of frustration. Möllering calls this the *ambivalence* of trust because

> actors trust *despite* their vulnerability and uncertainty, *although* they cannot be absolutely sure what will happen. They act *as if the* situation they face was unproblematic and, although they recognize their own limitations, they trust *nevertheless*.
>
> (Möllering 2006, 6)

The ambivalence lies in the fact that trust is an "as if" solution to a problem of social interaction: as to how to face uncertainty in cooperation that never removes completely its risks. This is nicely formulated by Luhmann (1979, 26) when he says that "no decisive grounds can be offered for trusting; trust always extrapolates from available evidence; it is (…) a blending of knowledge and ignorance." As should be clear, the social and psychological dimensions of trust are interdependent. Trust is a solution to a problem of social cooperation (in concrete social contexts) dependent on the psychological dispositions of the actors at stake.

There is a long-standing tradition that interprets those features of trust as amenable to rational theorizing about decision-making and modelled on Bayesian/expected utility maximization, game-theoretic/prisoner's dilemma frameworks. In this sense, trusting someone involves a *cognitive* task of assessing how *trustworthy* agents are through a rational decision procedure in which the (would-be trustor) agent subjectively ascribes probabilities (on the basis of available evidence) to the expected choices and actions of others (would-be trustees). So, for example, Hardin (2002), one of the most prominent advocates of such account, says that trust can be explained by the trustor's probabilistic prediction of potential social partners' (trustees) encapsulating her (trustor's) interests so that they would act to satisfy her (trustor's) interests and expectations. Trustees have incentives and interests to be trustworthy because they can individually benefit from the trusting relation and because there are institutional and social constraints against defection (e.g., sanctions, social ostracization, loss of reputation). Hardin thinks that we should not understand this account as modelled on abstract scenarios and laboratory-controlled experiments. He thinks we need a "street-level epistemology" of trust, which takes into account the restrictions (of information, time, cognition, etc.) we face in concrete situations. Still, he thinks the account must be "pure" rationalist.

There have been many criticisms of those "pure" rationalist accounts, and here is not the place to pursue them in detail (Barbalet 2009; Giddens 1990; Lewis and Weigert 1985; Luhmann 1979; Möllering 2006). But it might be instructive for our discussion to at least remind us that all such criticisms tend to agree that rationalist accounts seem to simply explain away the problem of trust without really giving it its due weight. Rationalist accounts see the problem of trust as simply a problem about being rationally justified in believing someone *trustworthy*. In this sense, as Hardin (2002, 10) claims, "trust is in the cognitive category with knowledge and belief." Indeed, for him, there is nothing in trust that adds to trustworthiness. The mental state of trusting is simply the (rationally justified) cognitive grasping of trustworthiness. In this sense, even though rationalist accounts may maintain that there is always an element of risk and uncertainty in acting on trust, this element is, as it were, "calculated risk" in that it is integral to the ascribed probabilities.

However, such an account seems to leave unexplained exactly what seems to be the most distinctive features of trust: uncertainty, risk, and social vulnerability. This is not only related to the cognitive limitations (of information, time, etc.) in concrete situations, which make the trustor's expectations always incomplete and uncertain. It is also related to a deeper feature of the very nature of human agency in concrete social interaction: *time* and *contingency*. After all, as Luhmann (1979, 25) holds, "whether action on the basis of trust has been right, therefore, in the final, retrospective, reckoning, depends on whether the trust has been honoured or been broken." Thus, the "real" criterion of justification of trust is ultimately *retrospective*, one which does not seem to be fully available to the typical "objective and timeless perspective" of rational decision theory. The relevant meaning of 'uncertainty' in a temporally unfolding process of concrete contingent interaction cannot be exhausted by rational ascriptions of probabilities.

Now, before advancing an alternative account, two comments are in order. The first is the fact that "distrust" or "mistrust" usually do not merely mean "absence or lack of trust" but "the existence of considerations or reasons for *not* trusting." The second is that, although trust is commonly modelled on relations between individuals, there seems to be nothing that precludes its usage as directed to what Giddens calls "abstract systems." *Expert systems* are one type of abstract system. They are "systems of technical accomplishment or professional expertise that organise large areas of the material and social environments" (Giddens 1990, 27). Scientific and technological knowledge, for example, are expert systems. The influence of these on many aspects of our lives is pervasive and inescapable. Here we will simply follow Giddens in assuming that trust may occur also between individuals and abstract systems.

A final qualification about the general nature of trust concerns its *social dimension*. Trust never occurs simply as the interaction between two individuals detached from their social contexts and backgrounds. The supposition that it does occur is another illusion of the pure rationalist interpretation of trust. As Möllering says (2006, 9), "[T]here is usually always a context and a history, and there are also other actors that matter." So, trustor and trustee are always embedded in complex concrete social contexts (involving networks of social relations and identities, public uptake of institutional rules, social history records, economic and political structures, etc.) which influence how agents see themselves vis-à-vis other agents. As Wynne (1996, 40–41) claims, "trust" is "a function of the complex web of social relations and identities."

10.3.2 *Emotional-evaluative trust*

Now that we have seen the limitations of the rationalist account, we should ask what kind of alternative to it might be available. Authors have attempted this by characterizing the psychological state of trust variously: as involving an emotional component (Barbalet 2009; Engdahl and Lidskog 2014; Lewis and Weigert 1985) or a non-cognitive/affective state (Jones 1996) or an attitude of faith (Giddens 1990; Möllering 2006) or a mild rationalistic practical commitment (Gambetta 1988). We will explore one of those attempts here – namely, the one that finds an essential *emotional* component in trust (although our account differs from other emotional accounts in significant ways).

An influential emotional account of trust is put forward by Lewis and Weigert (1985). They propose that trust involves interdependent cognitive, emotional, and behavioural dimensions (1985, 969). The emotional and cognitive dimensions are complementary to each other in that "if *all* cognitive content were removed from emotional trust, we would be left with blind faith or fixed hope"; "if all emotional content were removed from cognitive trust, we would be left with nothing more than a cold-blooded prediction or rationally calculated risk" (1985, 972). So, trust must be a mixture of them.

What is particularly interesting about Lewis and Weigert's account is that they preserve the cognitive component of trust as essential. This seems to be the right thing to do because, firstly, we want to understand the emotional dimension of trust as related to its cognitive dimension. Secondly, we also need to understand emotion as directed towards the world. Let us develop this further.

This is not the place to discuss the astonishingly vast literature on emotion. So, whatever we will say here about the nature of emotion will be incomplete and based on minimal common ground among the majority of theories. In order to make sense of the relation between emotion and the world (or the object of perception or belief),[4] we need only to assume, firstly, that emotions have *intentional objects* – i.e., that they are about the world or directed towards the world – and, secondly, that emotions are inextricably related to *evaluations* as their *formal objects* (Kenny 1963). Thus, as commonly said, fear is directed towards something in the world (its object) seen as *dangerous*; anger is related to *harm*; grief is related to *losses*; indignation is related to *unfairness*, etc.[5]

So, if there is an emotional dimension in trust, it had better be composed of its directness towards the world and associated evaluations. It would now be tempting simply to call *trust* an emotion that has *trustworthiness* as its formal object. This may be right as far as it goes. But it needs qualification and, as will become clear, it does not seem to be the appropriate way of explaining the nature of trust.

There is an obvious cognitive dimension in assessments of trustworthiness. Believing or perceiving an agent as trustworthy involves accessing or gathering information or considerations that support such assessments about an agent. Such information or considerations should reveal that the trustworthy agents have behaved as expected on past occasions, have taken to heart the interests of those whom they interact with, have proven to be truthful, competent, etc. Thus, *beliefs* or *perceptions* of trustworthiness may be said to give rise to an emotion of *confidence* in those (the potential "trustors") who are interacting with the believed or perceived trustworthy agents. Thus, insofar as assessments of *trustworthiness* involve the emotion of confidence, trust may indeed be a mixture of emotion and cognition.

But this cannot be the whole story. We have provided so far an account of assessments of trustworthiness, but not yet of *trust*. Understanding trust as conceptually linked to assessments of trustworthiness, but going beyond it, helps us see a common mistake in emotional accounts. Some authors who think of trust as an emotional state also think it has no relevant relation to *trustworthiness* (e.g., Barbalet 2009; Jones 1996). But this sounds odd. This would make trust a blatant non-rational reaction or literally blind faith. This would leave unexplained exactly what trust is a reaction to. Without a connection with information about the world and assessments of trustworthiness, we would seem to relegate trust and its emotional dimension to an obscure corner of our minds or make our social dispositions to trust sound like a miracle. So, preserving the tenet that trust is conceptually linked to trustworthiness is essential to make trust intelligible.

Does it now mean that, as rationalists claim, trust is nothing over and above belief in trustworthiness? No. We should preserve the "risking" dimension of the attitude of trust in the face of uncertainty – uncertainty which, as we have seen, is not surmounted by any form of rational calculation and evidence-gathering. Now, this ineliminable risking dimension of trust may well be understood as an expression of a *further* emotion. It should be a *higher-order* emotional reaction connected with assessments of trustworthiness and its accompanying emotion of confidence. But such a higher-order emotional state should also *go beyond* the assessments of trustworthiness (all the information cognitively gathered and emotionally infused with confidence): it should involve a sort of *optimism* and *openness* (as a further emotion) towards (socially cooperative) relations with the potential partner (perceived or believed trustworthy). This risking attitude, infused with openness and optimism, *amplifies* the evidence gathered in assessments of trustworthiness. So, trust should be a complex two-level psychological state that is, at the lower level, an emotionally infused response (of confidence) to assessments of trustworthiness and, besides, a higher-order emotional reaction (of *optimism* and *openness*) that goes beyond those assessments. Trust is, then, an *emotional-evaluative projection*.

The emotional reaction of trust should not, however, be understood as being *against* evidence of trustworthiness. That evidence "counts in favour" of the risking emotional reaction constitutive of trust, but without "warranting" it. The reaction is an *amplification*, not a disregard of evidence of trustworthiness. The relation here is a sort of "rationalizing support." This means that we could claim that someone who trusts someone else without evidence of their trustworthiness is trusting without rationalizing support and, as such, criticizable for that. In this way, we can make trust intelligible.

Now, the same framework can be applied to *distrust*. Distrust, we have said, is not merely absence of trust, but involves considerations for not trusting someone. So, just as in trust, there should be two levels of explanation in distrust. Distrust should be understood, firstly, as involving assessments of untrustworthiness of potential social partners, which get emotionally infused. The relevant emotion here could be *insecurity*. But, beyond this level of explanation, distrust also should involve a higher-order emotional reaction to such assessments of untrustworthiness. At this level, we should find the emotional reaction going beyond evidence provided by the emotionally infused assessments of untrustworthiness and taking a species of "precautionary" attitude, which *amplifies* the risks evidenced by the assessment of untrustworthiness, and express *pessimism* and *closeness* (as a further emotion) towards the potential relationship.

10.4 Trust, denialism, and society

Our socially embedded emotional-evaluative account of trust can shed light on denialism in the following way. Firstly, it seems apt to explain how denialists can be more susceptible to biases and experience persistent (dis)trust. Secondly, it shows that the main problem with denialists lies not in their trusting capacities, but in their background social and psychological conditions for assessments of trustworthiness. So, let us take these in turn.

Our account of trust provides conceptual resources to explain why denialists seem to be more susceptible to misinformation in their environment. The emotional component of trust seems fit to explain this. As we have learnt from the specialized literature, many biases are influenced by emotional reactions (Slovic 2020). Denialists, as we have seen, tend to be more hypervigilant, finding patterns of meaning where there isn't, making attribution errors, etc. These biases are probably (at least partly) explained, as empirical studies have suggested (van Mulukom et al. 2022), by the fact that denialists typically feel threatened, uncertain, anxious, powerless, as well as experience a series of cognitive limitations. All this makes them more susceptible to the complex environmental pressures of information-gathering in the context of the pandemic. If trusting others is inevitable to help one cope with those pressures, and if trust is partly emotional, trust can be part of the explanation of those biases. One's source of trust can reinforce those patterns of psychological and environmental pressures (by turning them emotionally loaded) and, as a result, likely increase the tendency to those biases. Actually, this relation can be even more direct: those biases can get transmitted and reproduced directly from the patterns of thinking of one's sources of trust. One's sources of trust can be directly responsible for making one perceive social reality as threatening, uncertain, politically oriented.

Another distinctive feature of emotions that can also further explain denialists' tendency to those biases is their making objects in our environment *salient* by drawing our *attention* to them (Brady 2013, 20). In so doing, emotions can select something for us to focus on within the complexity of information in our environment. Also related to this, the emotional component of trust can explain why denialists' (dis)trust can be particularly persistent even when confronted with contrary information. Emotions have a "feel" and a practical output that make them *recalcitrant* in the face of contrary evidence (D'Arms and Jacobson 2003). Sometimes this is self-consciously experienced: people can continue experiencing fear of flying even when they believe the statistics on aviation safety. But sometimes the disregard of evidence is not transparent to our minds: emotions can blind us to evidence or reframe our perception of reality.

Having specified the ways in which our account of trust can help in explaining some distinctive features of denialism, we should now ask in which sense, if any, denialism can be considered *rational* according to our account. The answer to this question brings us back to the point where the emotional dimension of trust meets its *social* dimension.

Since trust is always socially situated and, we have emphasized, should not be understood as a dyadic relation between individuals detached from social context, trusting relations are socially *shaped*. This means that, when it comes to trust, there is no perception of reality – of the trustworthiness attached to potential social partners – without mediation of social relations and structures. Given that people gather information about potential partners in socially embedded contexts of interaction, no one trusts another without getting information from third parties, some social historical record, being already part of a social identity and a network of social relations, considering its risks on social attachments, being influenced by social, economic, political conditions. In sum, (dis)trust is a deeply social phenomenon, also framed by division of labour, involving a complex interplay of psychological and social factors. An answer to the question "who do you trust?" is a sort of social good.

Now, that means that the standards for trust are primarily practical and social, not epistemic. Surely, if someone trust another and gets systematically frustrated because, say, the trustee only holds false beliefs that lead the trustor to fail to achieve her ends, then the trustor has an epistemic reason for believing the trustee untrustworthy. But, even in such cases, depending on the trustee's social role, position, and status, the trustee's continuous failure to deliver true beliefs may be minimized. When it comes to trust, the social criterion tends to have precedence over the epistemic. Getting back to denialists, even if they are systematically deceived or led away from truth by their trusting sources, they can still justifiably stick to these sources given the social contexts in which their trusting relations are established and maintained. This is a social-psychological practical sense of rationality that is preserved in denialists, despite their epistemic failures and irrationalities. In this sense, one may be social-psychologically rational although epistemically irrational.[6]

So, we might draw as an overall conclusion that there seems to be nothing amiss with denialists' (dis)trusting attitude as a response to their assessments of (un)trustworthiness regarding scientific discourse in the context of the pandemic. The way they perceive reality is part of a social process. Their assessments of trustworthiness occur in socially embedded and constrained conditions for inquiry and decision-making. Some evidence from empirical research seems to endorse this interpretation. To conclude our discussion, let us have a brief look at it.

Researchers have empirically found that the degree of trust people confer on public authorities and scientific discourse is consistently related to the degree people are willing to comply with public health measures during the pandemic (Bicchieri et al. 2021; Jennings et al. 2021; Soveri et al. 2021; van Mulukom et al. 2022). Data also strongly suggest that scepticism towards scientific discourse is associated with worldviews and political ideologies, which, in turn, indicates a connection with social identity protection (Lewandowsky et al. 2013; Lewandowsky and Oberauer 2016; Lewandowsky and van der Linden 2021; Rutjens et al. 2021; Uscinski et al. 2020). Furthermore, studies provide evidence that conspiracy beliefs predict reliably denialist views on the COVID-19 pandemic (Freeman et al. 2021; Jennings et al. 2021; van Mulukom et al. 2022).

When it comes specifically to conspiracy beliefs about the pandemic, although the findings are mixed, sometimes conflicting, and inconclusive, van Mulukom et al. (2022), in a systematic review of the literature, report that "broad individual differences, such as socio-demographic factors including age, gender, ethnicity, income, and education levels, are related to the endorsement of COVID-19 conspiracy beliefs." We also learn from those studies some correlation between lower income, lower levels of education (including scientific literacy), and stronger beliefs in COVID-19 conspiracy theories. All that very likely contributes to making the individuals "less able to distinguish between true and false information regarding COVID-19 and more likely to share misinformation" (van Mulukum et al. 2022, 5).

Those empirical studies suggest that relevant social, economic, and political inequalities not only affect the exercise and development of people's psychological capacities but also directly influence their content. And this seems to happen in complex diverse ways, at multiple levels of society. On the one hand, denialism seems associated to a significant extent with groups of people whose features fall under traditional sociological indicators of vulnerability to manipulation and exploitation which typically coincide with the least-privileged groups of society. This may explain many of the negative reactions and limitations we have seen associated with denialists' profiles. But, on the other hand, denialism is also found among groups of people who strive to maintain the status quo or are representative of the Establishment. For example, researchers have found that conspiracy beliefs about the pandemic have been closely associated with right-wing ideology and free-market moral values, involving influential politicians, companies, private organizations (Lewandowsky 2021; Rutjens et al. 2021; Uscinski et al. 2020). This is evidence of the highly heterogeneous social nature of the phenomenon.

Our account of trust and trustworthiness as socially mediated and emotionally loaded seems to do justice to that complex interplay of factors of which denialism is part. Denialism should be seen more as a problem of socially embedded environmental pressures and conditions for decision-making than a problem about individuals' failures in the exercise of their rational capacities. We have argued that social, economic, and political conditions and inequalities have a decisive impact on people's psychologies as to how they perceive social reality and make decisions. In all that, *trust* is a crucial explanatory concept. It is through trust that people organize to a significant extent their social lives and elect their sources of information, practices, and values.[7]

Notes

1 Denialism has been associated with denial of scientific consensus about climate change, tobacco carcinogenicity, vaccines, HIV/AIDS.
2 Recent figures (from the 2020 Welcome Global Monitor) show an increase of trust in science and scientists. This is probably related to people's expectations (and possibly hopes) regarding the pandemic. However, it seems yet too early to know what those figures mean.
3 Here we seem to depart from Levy's proposal, given that Levy (2019b) holds that conspiracy ideation can be not only subjectively rational but also *objectively* rational. Although it is not entirely clear what Levy means by "objective rationality," he seems to have in mind an *epistemic* sense (in addition to a social one). But our account does not find room for understanding denialism as "objectively rational" in any epistemic sense.
4 We are simply assuming that emotion bears a "cognitive" relation to the world in two possible senses: involving either judgment/belief or perception. But it is likely that a complete account of emotion will need to find room for *both* senses, for emotions seem to vary in the way they are manifest in our psychologies: some are fast, reflex, automatic; others slow, reflective and thought-responsive.
5 Varieties of versions of judgmentalism, perceptual or feeling theories of emotion can accept that. Even "revisionary" theories about the formal objects of emotions (e.g., projectivism) could accept that assumption as far as it goes.
6 Here, again, we seem to depart from Levy's (2022) account. According to Levy, testimony is second-order epistemic evidence (that is, evidence about first-order evidence) and trust in it is a *direct* epistemic rational response. Although interpreting testimony as second-order evidence is compatible with our account here, we have emphasized that trusting testimony (at least in the case of a social phenomenon like denialism) is primarily related to a practical and social meaning of rationality, not an epistemic one.

7 I thank Evandro Barbosa, Flavio Williges, Matheus Mesquita Silveira and Lisa Bortolotti for many helpful comments on earlier versions of this chapter.

References

Allington, Daniel; McAndrew, Siobhan; Moxham-Hall, Vivienne; Duffy, Bobby. 2021. "Coronavirus conspiracy suspicions, general vaccine attitudes, trust and coronavirus information source as predictors of vaccine hesitancy among UK residents during the COVID-19 pandemic." *Psychological Medicine*: 1–12. https://doi.org/10.1017/S0033291721001434

Baier, Annette. 1986. "Trust and antitrust." *Ethics* 96: 231–260. https://doi.org/10.1086/292745

Barbalet, Jack. 2009. "A characterization of trust, and its consequences." *Theory and Society* 38, no. 4: 367–382. https://doi.org/10.1007/s11186-009-9087-3

Bicchieri, Cristina et al. 2021. "In science we (should) trust: Expectations and compliance across nine countries during the COVID-19 pandemic." *PLoS ONE* 16, no. 6: 1–17. https://doi.org/10.1371/journal.pone.0252892

Brady, Michael. 2013. *Emotional Insight: The Epistemic Role of Emotional Experience*. Oxford: Oxford University Press.

Constantinou, Marios; Kagialis, Antonios; Karekla, Maria. 2021. "COVID-19 scientific facts vs. conspiracy theories: Is science failing to pass its message?" *International Journal of Environmental Research and Public Health* 18, no. 12: 1–10. https://doi.org/10.3390/ijerph18126343

Cook, Karen S., ed. 2001. *Trust in Society*. New York: Russell Sage Foundation.

D'Arms, Justin; Jacobson, Daniel. 2003. "VIII. The significance of recalcitrant Emotion (or anti-quasijudgmentalism)." *Royal Institute of Philosophy Supplement* 52: 127–145. https://doi.org/10.1017/S1358246100007931

DiFonzo, Nicholas. 2019. "Conspiracy rumor psychology." In *Conspiracy Theories and the People Who Believe Them*, edited by Joseph E. Uscinski, 257–268. Oxford: Oxford University Press. https://doi.org/10.1093/oso/9780190844073.003.0017

Douglas, Karen M. 2021. "COVID-19 conspiracy theories." *Group Processes & Intergroup Relations* 24, no. 2: 270–275. https://doi.org/10.1177/1368430220982068

Douglas, Karen M. et al. 2019. "Understanding conspiracy theories." *Political Psychology* 40: 3–35. https://doi.org/10.1111/pops.12568

Engdahl, Emma; Lidskog, Rolf. 2014. "Risk, communication and trust: Towards an emotional understanding of trust." *Public Understanding of Science* 23, no. 6: 703–717. https://doi.org/10.1177/0963662512460953

Freeman, Daniel et al. 2020. "Coronavirus conspiracy beliefs, mistrust, and Compliance with government guidelines in England." *Psychological Medicine* 52, no. 2: 251–263. https://doi.org/10.1017/S0033291720001890

Freeman, Daniel et al. 2021. "COVID-19 vaccine hesitancy in the UK: The Oxford coronavirus explanations, attitudes, and narratives survey (oceans) II." *Psychological Medicine*: 1–15. https://doi.org/10.1017/S0033291720005188

Gambetta, Diego. 1988. "Can we trust trust?" In *Trust: Making and Breaking Cooperative Relations*, edited by Diego Gambetta, 213–237. Oxford: Blackwell.

Giddens, Anthony. 1990. *The Consequences of Modernity*. Cambridge: Polity Press.

Goldenberg, Maya J. 2021. *Vaccine Hesitancy: Public Trust, Expertise, and the War on Science*. Pittsburgh: University of Pittsburgh Press.

Hardin, Russell. 2002. *Trust and Trustworthiness*. New York: Russell Sage Foundation.

Jaspal, Rusi; Nerlich, Brigitte. 2022. "Social representations of COVID-19 skeptics: denigration, demonization, and disenfranchisement." *Politics, Groups, and Identities*: 1–21. https://doi.org/10.1080/21565503.2022.2041443

Jennings, Will et al. 2021. "Lack of trust, conspiracy beliefs, and social media use predict COVID-19 vaccine hesitancy." *Vaccines* 9, no. 6: 1–14. https://doi.org/10.3390/vaccines9060593

Jones, Karen. 1996. "Trust as an affective attitude." *Ethics* 107, no. 1: 4–25. https://doi.org/10.1086/233694

Kenny, Anthony. 1963. *Action, Emotion and Will*. London: Routledge.

Lee, Crystal et al. 2021. "Viral visualizations: How coronavirus skeptics use orthodox data practices to promote unorthodox science online." *Proceedings of the 2021 CHI Conference on Human Factors in Computing Systems (CHI '21)*. Article no. 607: 1–18. https://doi.org/10.1145/3411764.3445211

Levy, Neil. 2007. "Radically socialized knowledge and conspiracy theories." *Episteme* 4, no. 2: 181–192. https://doi.org/10.3366/epi.2007.4.2.181

Levy, Neil. 2019a. "Due deference to denialism: Explaining ordinary people's rejection of established scientific findings." *Synthese* 196: 313–327. https://doi.org/10.1007/s11229-017-1477-x

Levy, Neil. 2019b. "Is conspiracy theorising irrational?" *Social Epistemology Review and Reply Collective* 10, no. 8: 65–76. https://wp.me/p1Bfg0-4wW

Levy, Neil. 2022. *Bad Beliefs: Why They Happen to Good People*. Oxford: Oxford University Press. https://doi.org/10.1093/oso/9780192895325.001.0001

Lewandowsky, Stephan; Kozyreva, Anastasia; Ladyman, James. 2020. "What rationality? A comment on Levy's 'is conspiracy theorising irrational?'" *Social Epistemology Review and Reply Collective* 9, no. 2: 25–31. https://wp.me/p1Bfg0-4Oc

Lewandowsky, Stephan; Oberauer, Klaus. 2016. "Motivated rejection of science." *Current Directions in Psychological Science* 25, no. 4: 217–222. https://doi.org/10.1177/0963721416654436

Lewandowsky, Stephen. 2021. "Liberty and the pursuit of science denial." *Current Opinion in Behavioral Sciences* 42: 65–69. https://doi.org/10.1016/j.cobeha.2021.02.024

Lewandowsky, Stephen; Gignac, Gilles E.; Oberauer, Klaus. 2013. "The role of conspiracist ideation and worldviews in predicting rejection of science." *PLoS ONE* 8, no. 10: e75637. https://doi.org/10.1371/journal.pone.0075637

Lewandowsky, Stephen; Mann, Michael E.; Brown, Nicholas J. L.; Friedman, Harris. 2016. "Science and the public: Debate, denial, and skepticism." *Journal of Social and Political Psychology* 4, no. 2: 537–553. https://doi.org/10.5964/jspp.v4i2.604

Lewandowsky, Stephen; van der Linden, Sander. 2021. "Countering misinformation and fake news through inoculation and prebunking." *European Review of Social Psychology* 32, no. 2: 348–384. https://doi.org/10.1080/10463283.2021.1876983

Lewis, J. David; Weigert, Andrew. 1985. "Trust as a social reality." *Social Forces* 63, no. 4: 967–985. https://doi.org/10.1093/sf/63.4.967

Luhmann, Niklas. 1979. *Trust and Power*. Chichester: John Wiley & Sons.

Misztal, Barbara A. 1996. *Trust in Modern Societies: The Search for the Basis of Social Order*. Cambridge: Polity Press.

Möllering, Guido. 2006. *Trust: Reason, Routine, Reflexivity*. Amsterdam: Elsevier.

Rutjens, Bastiaan T.; van der Linden, Sander; van der Lee, Romy. 2021. "Science skepticism in times of COVID-19." *Group Processes & Intergroup Relations* 24, no. 2: 276–283. https://doi.org/10.1177/1368430220981415

Seligman, Adam B. 1997. *The Problem of Trust*. Princeton: Princeton University Press.

Slovic, Paul. 2020. *The Perception of Risk*. New York: Routledge. https://doi.org/10.4324/9781315661773

Soveri, Anna et al. 2021. "Unwillingness to engage in behaviors that protect against COVID-19: The role of conspiracy beliefs, trust, and endorsement of complementary and alternative medicine." *BMC Public Health* 21, 684: 2–12. https://doi.org/10.1186/s12889-021-10643-w

Sztompka, Piotr. 2000. *Trust: A Sociological Theory*: Cambridge: Cambridge University Press.

Uscinski, Joseph E et al. 2020. "Why do people believe COVID-19 conspiracy theories?" *The Harvard Kennedy School (HKS) Misinformation Review* 1, Special Issue on COVID-19 and Misinformation: 1–12.

van Mulukom, Valerie et al. 2022. "Antecedents and consequences of COVID-19 conspiracy beliefs: A systematic review." *Social Science & Medicine* 301: 1–14. https://doi.org/10.1016/j.socscimed.2022.114912

Wynne, Brian. 1991. "Knowledges in context." *Science, Technology, & Human Values* 16, no. 1: 111–121. https://doi.org/10.1177/016224399101600108

Wynne, Brian. 1993. "Public uptake of science: A case for institutional reflexivity." *Public Understanding of Science* 2, no. 4: 321–337. https://doi.org/10.1088/0963-6625/2/4/003

Wynne, Brian. 1996. "Misunderstood misunderstandings: Social identities and public uptake of science." In *Misunderstanding Science? The Public Reconstruction of Science and Technology*, edited by Wynne, Brian; Irwin, Alan, 19–46. Cambridge: Cambridge University Press. https://doi.org/10.1017/CBO9780511563737

11 COVID rule breakers and the social contract

Peter R. Anstey

11.1 Introduction

The urgent need for government interventions brought the issue of the social contract to the fore during the COVID-19 pandemic. Indeed, as early as July 2020 the secretary-general of the United Nations, António Guterres (2020), entitled his Nelson Mandela Lecture "Tackling the Inequality Pandemic: A New Social Contract for a New Era." Whether it be city-wide lockdowns, mask-wearing mandates, or stringent social distancing rules, governments in many parts of the world imposed snap restrictions on their citizens in a manner rarely experienced in living memory. It is hardly surprising that many people objected. In any society, there's a delicate balancing act between individual liberties and community needs, and in my own country, in pre-COVID Australia, we probably had the settings about right. But the pandemic changed all that, and the recalibration was not to everyone's liking. At various periods throughout the height of the pandemic, individual liberties were dramatically curtailed in order to bring an invisible enemy under control and to protect the community's health. As a result, many citizens not only protested but defied the health orders of their governments. So, what is the social contract? And how should we respond to these rule breakers? Are their actions justified, and if so, on what grounds? This chapter examines three different types of COVID rule breakers within the context of the social contract: the conspiracy theorist, the generic dissenter, and the free rider.

11.2 What is the social contract?

When people live together in societies they engage in all sorts of agreements. The social contract is one such agreement. It is the agreement between each and every individual in any particular society that determines who the authorities of that society are and provides the grounds for the obligations that each citizen has to those authorities. A helpful way to characterise the way social obligations arise in a social contract is in terms of the following conditional:

DOI: 10.4324/9781003310129-14

If an *agreement* of all *citizens* in a collective social arrangement is the *source* of *authority* to exercise power over any of the individuals – including the power to limit their freedom – then that *agreement* is the grounds of *normative relations* between the individuals and *those with authority*.

When a group of citizens enters into such an agreement, it is a social contract. However, each of the italicised terms in this conditional needs to be unpacked in order for us to understand the nature and scope of a social contract; once this is done, even in a summary way, the idea seems fairly intuitive.

Let's take *citizens* first. It is natural to think that the citizen participants in a social contract are both rational agents and adults. Of course, we also need to explain how children and visitors from other societies fit in, but it's best to focus on the central cases in the first instance. Next, consider the nature of the *agreement*. It belongs to everyone in the society in so far as every citizen is a participant in the agreement, and the agreement is the source or basis upon which the authority of the rulers – *those with authority* – rests. Another way of putting this is: the authority of the rulers derives from and exists in virtue of the agreement of all citizens that make up the society. It is analogous to the way the members of a sports team elect a captain and then submit to the captain's authority and even allow the captain to make decisions on their behalf. There are many social arrangements where the authority of the rulers does not derive from the agreement of the citizens. The situation in contemporary Myanmar is a clear example; there the military currently rules by might and not by agreement.

We also need to get clear on the nature of the *normative relations* between the citizens and their rulers. In a society with a social contract, those with *authority* can exercise power over others. These power relations are normative because they involve norms or rules, and they entail obligations and duties on the part of both citizens and rulers. Furthermore, normally many of the rules imply limits to the freedoms of citizens, limits that are worth putting up with because the results of compliance are better either for the individual, or the society, or both. Speed limits for car drivers limit our freedom to drive as fast as we would like but have a big payoff for ourselves in terms of safety, and a payoff for everybody else.

Already we can see that in any social contract, there is a need for a balance between the freedoms that citizens can enjoy and the needs of the community as a whole. High-functioning societies generally have an equilibrium between restrictions on individual freedoms and concomitant societal benefits: an equilibrium that is satisfactory for both the citizens and those with authority who have responsibilities to the society. Clearly, the COVID pandemic in many societies upset this equilibrium.

Furthermore, if a social contract is to be viable and to endure, certain powers of the citizens need to be retained and cannot be handed over to the rulers. These include the power to protest against the authorities or against other citizens or citizen groups, the power to speak publicly about one's beliefs, and the power to resist authorities if they violate the terms of the contract. Normally, these powers are spoken of in terms of rights; so, the right to protest, the right to freedom of speech, and the right of resistance are constitutive of any liberal democracy. There is no doubt that the COVID pandemic prompted, indeed compelled, many people to exercise these powers, but the nature of the pandemic itself has made the exercising of these powers difficult and constrained. How, for example, can groups of citizens effectively protest when public gatherings are prohibited for public health reasons and all citizens in public spaces must conform to social distancing rules, such as standing 1.5 metres apart?

Finally, it is important to address one of the leading arguments against the social contract, namely, the claim that, in fact, such contracts do not actually exist and are mere fictions or useful models for explaining the nature of political obligation and the powers of rulers. It would be unnecessarily digressive for me to respond in detail to this argument here; however, two points are worth making. First, there are many instances in the actual debate over the impact and rationale of government-based COVID interventions that have been framed in terms of the social contract, so it is clear that the social contract *is* providing the terms of reference for evaluating and responding to government interventions (see Madgavkar et al. 2020; Atlani-Duault et al. 2021; Wolff 2022). And second, there is a case for the claim that the social contract is not merely a conception that is explained by analogical reasoning, but rather that it is a *sui generis* contract in its own right, a contract that in many ways is disanalogous with other types of contracts in which we regularly participate, such as marriage, property leases, or business agreements. The social contract can be considered as a peculiar kind of contract quite unlike any other contracts we engage in but a contract, nonetheless.

Instead of focusing on the ontological status of the social contract in any particular society, there is a far more interesting issue to examine – namely, the different types of COVID dissenters and their responses to the social contract, especially those who defy the public health orders with regard to assembly, the wearing of face masks, social distancing, isolating, travel restrictions, and so on. There seem to be at least three different types of COVID rule breakers: the conspiracy theorist, the generic dissenter, and the free rider. Understanding their motivations and their reasoning opens up some fascinating philosophical issues, so let us examine each in turn.

11.3 Conspiracy theorists

First, there are the conspiracy theorists. The COVID pandemic has given rise to a host of new conspiracy theories, theories such as that COVID-19 is caused by the 5G mobile network or that the virus was created by Bill

Gates, the founder of Microsoft. This phenomenon is now the subject of an increasing body of research. (For a literature review, see van Mulukom et al. 2022. For a sampling, see, for example, Ball and Maxmen 2020; De Coninck et al. 2021; Douglas 2021; Hartman et al. 2021). One key finding of this research is that COVID conspiracy theorists are less likely to abide by government health orders and less likely to get vaccinated against COVID (De Coninck et al. 2021, 2).

This leads us to consider who are the COVID conspiracy theorists. They are not merely COVID deniers but those who hold conspiratorial beliefs about COVID-19. I spoke to one on a Sydney train in the early months of the pandemic. He was a conspiracy theorist who didn't believe that there was a virus circulating in the community and that it was all government propaganda. A second encounter was in the local supermarket. At the cheese counter, another customer gave me a knowing smile. He and I were the only customers in the store not wearing face masks, which seemed to be a cue for him to tell me that he didn't believe in viruses: not just COVID-19 but viruses full stop! He believed that it was a scientific conspiracy. These are not cases of denialism; they are proponents of conspiracy theories. How should one respond?

The first question to ask is, What is a conspiracy theory (Räikkä and Ritola 2020, 56–58)? There is a debate in the philosophical literature over this central question. Some philosophers claim that all beliefs about conspiracies start off as speculative theories and only some of these theories are true; they are made true by the conspirators who implement their conspiratorial plans. As Charles Pigden (2007) urges, there's nothing intrinsically wrong with conspiracy theories: after all, some conspiracy theories turn out to be true. The main problem with this view is that the term "conspiracy theory" in popular usage, really does seem to refer to an explanation that is wacky, out there, or completely unbelievable. The conspiracy to assassinate Julius Caesar does not seem to be a conspiracy theory in this sense.

On the other hand, some philosophers claim that there are theories about actual conspiracies, and these are to be differentiated from Conspiracy theories – with a capital "c" – which are intrinsically implausible explanations of events based upon beliefs that violate widely accepted norms for evaluating evidence. The main problem for the latter view is that it is very difficult to set out demarcation criteria that will enable us to distinguish between theories about conspiracies and Conspiracy theories.

It all comes down to the nature of the evidence and how one evaluates that evidence. Three philosophical notions are worth considering here. First, there are our epistemic duties; second, there is the role of testimony; and third, there is the notion of trust. Each of these notions can be considered in relation to the causal histories of beliefs and their transmission.

If a public figure or influencer who has the aura of being informed concocts a conspiracy theory about COVID and backs it up, say, with some scanty anecdotal evidence, and then disseminates this theory through social media, some adult consumers will take it on trust and share it with their friends and children. The influencer has almost certainly transgressed some epistemic duties, the adults have adopted the theory because they have taken it on trust, and they have spread it to their friends and children by testimony. Such causal belief chains need not be very long, but they have proliferated and mutated such that for the duration of the pandemic so far, there are numerous different conspiracy theories about the nature, origin, and cure of COVID-19. Let us examine the sorts of belief chains that characterise COVID conspiracy theorists.

One common distal (remote) cause of belief in conspiracy theories is mistrust in government. If an individual's trust in government is low, then they are more prone to accept claims that imply the government is at best incompetent and at worst covering up, lying, or systematically deceiving the populace. A common proximate (near) cause of belief in conspiracy theories is a prior belief that one has special access to certain knowledge that is not widely available. Here is one such belief chain that I have encountered in conversation about the pandemic:

1   The government is beholden to Big Pharma and over-inclined to endorse the policy settings of its major international allies (in the case of Australia, the USA, and the United Kingdom).
2   These are the primary reasons why it wants us to believe in the efficacy of COVID vaccines.
3   There is ample scientific evidence to support the claim that COVID vaccines lack efficacy.
4   Given 1 and 2, the government has suppressed this evidence, and it is very difficult to access.
5   Happily, I have access to this evidence through covert sources.
6   *Therefore*, there are strong grounds for not trusting the government's position on COVID vaccines and for resisting calls to get vaccinated.

One enticing psychological feature of this scenario is the sense arising from 5 – the belief that one is privy to special knowledge that is not available to others – that one is in an epistemically superior state or privileged position – that one is "in the know." (For secret knowledge and the need for uniqueness among conspiracy theorists, see Lantian et al. 2017. For a survey of the epistemic motives that motivate beliefs in conspiracy theories, see Douglas et al. 2017 and Douglas et al. 2019.) Perhaps this is how I should have interpreted that wink in the supermarket at the cheese counter: what we might call the conspiracy theorist's wink of common knowledge. How should a reasonable person respond?

There is no doubt that sometimes we are too inclined to take the authorities' word on trust, but during the COVID pandemic, the quantitative evidence for the efficacy of the leading vaccinations is compelling. If the COVID conspiracy theorists will not seek out and reasonably evaluate this evidence, then there's not much we can do. If they use their conspiratorial beliefs as a pretext for violating COVID-related public health directives, then they may be morally culpable. Furthermore, there are persuasive reasons for believing that COVID conspiracy theorists who violate public health orders may be morally culpable, even if, *per impossibile*, their particular theory turns out to be true. Their situation is analogous to military personnel who disobeyed orders to fight in the second Iraq War because they didn't believe that Saddam Hussain was in possession of weapons of mass destruction. Of course, the Australian government has not enforced vaccinations for COVID for the population at large, but the various state governments did enforce strict social distancing rules, severe restrictions on movement beyond prescribed borders, rules prohibiting public gatherings, and rules requiring the wearing of face masks in many settings, and many COVID conspiracy theorists disobeyed these health orders on the grounds of their conspiratorial beliefs. (For the World Health Organisation's information on COVID-19 vaccine efficacy as early as July 2021, see https://www.who.int/news-room/feature-stories/detail/vaccine-efficacy-effectiveness-and-protection. For a summary of early research on vaccine efficacy in July 2021, see Olliaro, Torreele, and Vaillant 2021. For a study of the waning of vaccine efficacy, see Feikin et al. 2022.)

11.4 Generic dissenters

A second, very interesting, type of rule breaker is what I call the generic dissenter. This form of dissenter is easy to describe but difficult to locate in the literature on civil disobedience and conscientious objection. Initially, generic dissent presents as a form of civil disobedience, for these dissenters break the law by not conforming to COVID health orders. However, they are not primarily motivated by conscience in the manner of, say, the pacifist, nor are they motivated by a sense of obligation or even specific considerations pertaining to the law itself. (On the moral motivations for civil disobedience, see Cooke 2021.) Their protest is more generic; it is against the very presumption on the government's part of curtailing their civil liberties without due process. Their common refrains are, "We were never asked," and "Why did we have no say in this?" As such, it seems their objection is to the recalibration of the delicate balance of civil liberties and constraints that characterised pre-COVID times. Thus, they are practising a form of civil disobedience, but civil disobedience based not on particular principles within the social contract itself but on its manner of implementation. It is the phenomena of new constraints on civil liberties which are the catalyst for their civil disobedience rather than any particular health order or set of health orders. Nor do their actions represent the majority; indeed, during the height of the pandemic, the majority of Australian citizens may well have regarded their acts of protest as misguided or even foolish in so far as they might put the whole society at risk. These were not acts intended to be catalysts for public reasoning about the nature of our democracy, nor were they considered to be acts of courage or acts worth emulating.

The criticisms of the generic dissenter pertain to failures of representation, failures of consultation, failures of due process in implementation of COVID-related health orders, and not necessarily objections to the content of the health orders themselves, though often particular health orders are singled out as examples. Thus, a generic dissenter might complain about not being able to walk in the open with a friend without social distancing or having to wear a face mask in certain contexts, but it is the imposition of this kind of law rather than the specific law itself that is the cause of contention. In some cases, generic dissenters misunderstand the nature of a state of emergency, the nature and legal status of health orders, and the legal constraints on government. While it is difficult to find empirical data on this, the generic dissenter seems to be relatively uninformed about the legal context and checks and balances on the COVID-related public health orders. Nevertheless, throughout the pandemic in Australia, information about civil rights and the content and legislation of COVID health orders has been easily accessible online. (See, for example, the Australian Human Rights Commission website https://humanrights.gov.au/about/covid19-and-human-rights/what-commissions-view-limiting-human-rights-during-covid-19 and the Human Rights Law Centre website:https://www.hrlc.org.au/factsheets/2021/8/30/explainer-protecting-human-rights-and-democracy-in-victorias-pandemic-laws.)

It is worth reflecting on this phenomenon as it occurred in Australia for, in spite of the negative side of this form of protest, there is a silver lining. First, the absence of such generic forms of civil disobedience pre-COVID is an indicator that the government's settings on civil liberties were, more or less, right. We might say they were in the Goldilocks Zone for promoting the well-being of the majority of its citizens. Of course, things were far from perfect, but the absence of sustained and high-profile civil protests can reasonably be taken as an indicator of a healthy social equilibrium around civil liberties.

Second, and more importantly, the recalibrations of civil liberties and the concomitant civil unrest and disobedience are perhaps the first time that many Australians have had to consider the nature of the social contract itself, including the role of political representation and the government's power to declare a state of emergency and to limit civil liberties. To be sure, there are precedents in living memory for the exercise of these powers in times of war, such as the Vietnam War or region-specific catastrophic natural disasters. Nevertheless, the COVID pandemic has presented many scenarios not experienced in Australia since the Spanish Flu pandemic in 1918–1919, which is effectively beyond living memory for all Australians. For the first time in over 100 years, Australians had constraints put on their movements, their ability to assemble, to cross state borders, and to leave the country. This has forced many citizens to think through the nature of the social contract, including their civil liberties and the powers of the executives of governments for the first time. And this is a good thing. Change rarely comes without pushback, and some, perhaps many, generic dissenters are now more aware of normative relations in which they stood and about which until now they only exercised a kind of tacit consent.

11.5 Free riders and sensible knaves

The third rule breaker is more dangerous than the conspiracy theorist and the dissenter. This is the free rider. If everyone pays their taxes, surely it doesn't hurt society if one of us gets away with cheating on their tax return? If everyone drives up to the speed limit, surely it won't hurt anyone if I drive as fast as I want? There will always be free riders in society. Whether we evaluate their behaviour in terms of duties or consequences, either way, they present a threshold problem. If one person cheats on their taxes, there's virtually no impact to society, and the free rider is better off, but if, say, one in three people cheat on their tax returns, then the government won't be able to fund the roads on which the free riders want to speed or to fund the hospitals that sufferers of severe COVID-19 need.

However, free riders present an acute problem in a pandemic. If I cheat on my tax return, the impacts are negligible, but if I break the health directives while infected and become a super-spreader the impact can be devastating. The actions of just one careless free rider can create a threshold problem very quickly, and it may well be that the cause of some of the waves of infection that we experienced across Australia since early 2020 was a small group of free riders, free riders who might not even have known that they had the virus. Of course, hosting parties and leaving lockdown areas when taken out of context seem like harmless acts, but in a pandemic, the consequences may be far-reaching.

Free riders come in all shapes and sizes. Some are blissfully unaware that they are free riding, some are ashamed of their free riding and hope to correct it in the future – "When I get my first pay cheque, I'll start buying tickets and stop traveling on the train for free" – and some are crafty and intentional in their behaviour, living by the code "if you can get away with it, do it." However, there is a particularly insidious type of free rider, the sensible knave.

The conspiracy theorist and generic objector object to the new COVID restrictions on individual liberties but can grudgingly comply. The benign free rider might not even know that they are violating certain health orders. By contrast, the sensible knave agrees with the health orders entirely. "Bring them on," says the sensible knave, "everyone should stay at home during lockdown and keep to the rules"; everyone, that is, except the sensible knave. The name "sensible knave" derives from the English philosopher Shaftesbury and was popularised by David Hume. (See Shaftesbury 2001; Hume 1998, 81–82. For interpretations of the role of Hume's sensible knave in his moral theory, see Gautier 1990, 129–149, including a discussion of Gyges' ring, and Crisp 2019, 154–157.) Literature and film abound with sensible knaves. (For examples in Jane Austen, see Pigden 2012). Indeed, the idea goes back at least to Plato's *Republic* and the story of Gyges' ring. In that story, a shepherd using an invisibility ring (think Frodo Baggins), seduces the Lydian queen, murders the king, and takes the kingdom for himself (Plato, *The Republic*, book II, 1989, 359^a–360^d). The suggestion is that if you yourself can break the law without anyone seeing you do it, then breaking the law is a rational course of action: it's the "sensible" thing to do even if you are fully "sensible" (aware) of the fact that you are a lawbreaker.

Of course, the behaviour of sensible knaves is easily dealt with by those who evaluate moral actions in terms of duties: knaves violate their duties and are therefore morally culpable. However, knaves are more difficult for the consequentialist to deal with. What if everyone hated the king and wished him dead and, moreover, the shepherd turns out to be a just and compassionate ruler? By the consequentialist's reckoning, the knave's actions seem to be the morally right course of action.

In the context of the pandemic, however, sensible knaves potentially present a grave risk to society. Sensible knaves are experts in risk assessment; they are intuitively able to calculate their chances of no one seeing them doing it and to weigh the benefits of rule breaking, whether those rules be civil laws or unwritten social conventions. Their rule-breaking behaviour is calculated, covert, and intentional. They are the ones who slip out under the cover of darkness across COVID boundaries and state borders to holiday and party in regions where COVID health orders don't yet apply. As such, they have posed the greatest risk as super-spreaders of the virus.

How should we respond to sensible knaves? One approach is to say that we don't have anything to worry about at all; sensible knaves are experts at risk assessment and wouldn't be foolish enough to run the gauntlet. It's not the danger of being caught crossing borders that presents a risk to the knave; that sort of rule breaking is child's play. It's the accuracy and speed of genomic sequencing which is, in effect, a trail of breadcrumbs that leads to patient zero. Any sensible knave is canny enough to know that in a 21st-century pandemic, one cannot cover one's tracks entirely; in the COVID pandemic, there are no invisibility rings.

A second response is to question the status of the sensible knave as a free rider. To be sure, sensible knaves free ride when it suits them and make a grand show of conformity when there is a guaranteed payoff. However, to conflate the sensible knave with the free rider is to misunderstand the knave's true fiendishness. For, free riding is just one ruse in their bag of knavish tricks. Deceit, betrayal, hypocrisy, scheming, duplicity, and disingenuousness are the currency of knavery. And, more than anything else, the sensible knave is adept at navigating complex and subtle social conventions to their advantage and much of this has nothing at all to do with free riding. The talented Mr Ripley would be justifiably insulted should he be called a mere free rider!

But perhaps this is conceding too much to the sensible knave; perhaps for all their sophistication, the tricks of knavery are all reducible to instances of free riding. After all, getting away with lying is just free riding on a principle of charity – namely, the presumption that almost everyone in this social circle tells the truth. To be branded a hypocrite or duplicitous is simply to have one's free riding exposed. Disloyalty and betrayal are easily covered up by gaslighting and subtle truth twisting, which can, in turn, be analysed in terms of free riding. Whatever the case, we will always have knavery among us, and it may be that deep down there is a knave in each one of us.

11.6 Conclusion

One positive benefit is that the COVID pandemic has got us thinking about the social contact and about individual versus communal rights again. Moreover, in spite of the proliferation of Conspiracy theories and disinformation across the globe, empirical evidence is emerging suggesting that the pandemic has led to an increased trust in science and scientists (see Wellcome Global Monitor 2020). This is hardly surprising given that our dependence on medical research has never been higher. And if we cast the net more widely, we can see that the pandemic has brought other social issues into sharper relief, and this too has led to widespread discussion of the need for a new social contract. This brings us back to António Guterres' Nelson Mandela Lecture on "a new social contract for a new era" in which he argues the COVID pandemic has highlighted a host of unacceptable inequalities across the globe. Guterres' lecture is a passionate call for a new "global deal," cashed out in terms of the social contract, in the face of the gross inequalities that have come to the fore during the COVID pandemic, such as access to medical supplies and technology. These are issues that transcend our own individual responses to our governments' interventions during the pandemic. Whether or not you and I are rule breakers in some shape or form, these large-scale inequalities highlighted by the pandemic should be cause for positive action, action that can be taken by those of us who are privileged to live in societies with effective social contracts.

Acknowledgements

David Braddon-Mitchell, Mark Colyvan, Fred D'Agostino, Karen Douglas, Charles Pigden all provided helpful advice.

References

Atlani-Duault, Laetitia et al. 2021, April. "Immune evasion means we need a COVID-19 social contract," *The Lancet: Public Health*, 6: doi: 10.1016/S2468-2667(21)00036-0

Ball, Philip and Maxmen, Amy. 2020, May 28. "Battling the infodemic," *Nature*, 581, pp. 371–374.

Cooke, Maeve. 2021. "The ethical dimension of civil disobedience." In ed. William E. Scheuerman, *The Cambridge Companion to Civil Disobedience*, Cambridge: Cambridge University Press, pp. 231–253.

Crisp, Roger. 2019. *Sacrifice Regained: Morality and Self-Interest in British Moral Philosophy from Hobbes to Bentham*, Oxford: Oxford University Press.

De Coninck, David, et al. 2021. "Beliefs in conspiracy theories and misinformation about COVID-19: comparative perspectives on the role of anxiety, depression and exposure to and trust in information sources," *Frontiers in Psychology*, 12, pp. 1–13: doi: 10.3389/fpsyg.2021.646394

Douglas, Karen M. 2021. "COVID-19 conspiracy theories," *Group Processes & Intergroup Relations*, 24, pp. 270–275. doi: 10.1177/1368430220982068

Douglas, Karen M. et al. 2017. "The psychology of conspiracy theories," *Current Directions in Psychological Science*, 26, pp. 538–542: doi: 10.1177/0963721417718261.1177

Douglas, Karen M. et al. 2019. "Understanding conspiracy theories," *Political Psychology*, 40, Supplement 1, pp. 3–35: doi: 10.1111/pops.12568

Feikin, Daniel R. et al. 2022. "Duration of effectiveness of vaccines against SARS-CoV-2 infection and COVID-19 disease: results of a systematic review and meta-regression," *The Lancet*, 399, pp. 924–944: doi: 10.1016/S0140-6736(22)00152-0

Gautier, David. 1990. *Moral Dealing: Contract, Ethics, and Reason*, Ithaca: Cornell University Press.

Guterres, António. 2020. "Tackling the inequality pandemic: a new social contract for a new era," The 18th Nelson Mandela Lecture delivered by the Secretary-General, United Nations.

Hartman, Todd K., et al. 2021. "Different conspiracy theories have different psychological and social determinants: comparison of three theories about the origins of the COVID-19 virus in a representative sample of the UK population," *Frontiers in Political Science*, 3, pp. 1–17: doi: 10.3389/fpos.2021.642510

Hume, David. 1998 [1751]. *An Enquiry Concerning the Principles of Morals*, ed. Tom L. Beauchamp, Oxford: Clarendon Press.

Lantian, Anthony, et al. 2017. "I know things they don't know': The role of need for uniqueness in belief in conspiracy theories," *Social Psychology*, 48, pp. 160–173.

Madgavkar, Anu et al. 2020. "COVID-19 has revived the social contract in advanced economies – for now. What will stick once the crisis abates?" *McKinsey Global Institute*: https://www.mckinsey.com/industries/public-and-social-sector/our-insights/

covid-19-has-revived-the-social-contract-in-advanced-economies-for-now-what-will-stick-once-the-crisis-abates

Olliaro, Piero, Torreele, Els and Vaillant, Michel. 2021. "Comment: COVID-19 vaccine efficacy and effectiveness–the elephant (not) in the room," *The Lancet: Microbe*, 2, pp. 279–280: doi: 10.1016/S2666-5247(21)00069-0

Pigden, Charles. 2007. "Conspiracy theories and the conventional wisdom," *Episteme*, 4, pp. 219–232.

———. 2012. "A 'sensible knave?' Hume, Jane Austen and Mr Elliot," *Intellectual History Review*, 22, pp. 465–480.

Plato. 1989. "The Republic." In eds. Edith Hamilton and Huntington Cairns, *Plato: The Collected Dialogues*, Princeton: Princeton University Press.

Räikkä, Juha and Ritola, Juho. 2020. "Philosophy and conspiracy theories." In eds. Michael Butter and Peter Knight, *Routledge Handbook of Conspiracy Theories*, Abingdon: Routledge, pp. 56–66.

Shaftesbury, 2001 [1711]. 3rd Earl of (Anthony Ashley Cooper) *Characteristics of Men, Manners, Opinions, Times*, Indianapolis: Liberty Fund.

Van Mulukom, V., et al. 2022. "Antecedents and consequences of COVID-19 conspiracy beliefs: A systematic review," *Social Science & Medicine*, 301, pp. 1–14: doi: 10.1016/j.socscimed.2022.114912

Wellcome Global Monitor. 2020. "How COVID-19 affected people's lives and their views about science," Gallup: Wellcome Trust, London.

Wolff, Jonathan. 2022. "The COVID-risk social contract is under negotiation," *The Atlantic*, January 17, 2022: https://www.theatlantic.com/ideas/archive/2022/01/new-risk-social-contract-covid-ethics/621246/

12 Chance, consent, and COVID-19

Ryan Doody

12.1 The case for (and against) mandatory lockdowns

On March 16, 2020, in response to the spread of SARS-CoV-2 (COVID-19), the premier of the Australian state of Victoria declared a state of emergency. Using special powers, he imposed a number of restrictions intended to slow viral transmission. These restrictions – colloquially referred to as a *lockdown* – required residents of impacted areas to remain in their houses and only permitted them to leave under limited circumstances to conduct essential activities. The measures also imposed a mandatory 14-day isolation period on travelers entering the state, and a moratorium on mass gatherings. They required the closure of nonessential businesses and schools. Beginning in August 2020, there was also a nightly curfew. In total, there would be 6 lockdowns in Victoria, over a period of 18 months, lasting for a cumulative total of 262 days.

Victoria was far from the only region impacted by mandatory lockdown measures during the pandemic, but given both the extent and duration of the restrictions, it serves as a particularly stark example. In particular, its example evokes a concern held by many liberally-minded witnesses to lockdown measures: namely, that they appeared to involve a somewhat tragic clash between serious public health interests and considerations of individual rights. Vocal opponents of the lockdown measures, and of the nocturnal curfew, in particular – including Victorian Liberal Party MP Tim Wilson, the plaintiff in a lawsuit contesting the measures (*Loielo v Giles*), and countless protesters – complained that the lockdowns infringed upon important *civil liberties* such as the rights to free movement and assembly. In response, the premier of Victoria, Daniel Andrews, defended the lockdown: "[I]t's not about human rights; it's about human life." The measures, Andrews argued, were necessary to suppress transmission of a lethal virus – they were necessary to protect human life.

Supposing that mandatory lockdown measures are sometimes necessary to prevent serious harm to the public, when is the state justified in using them? It's not implausible to think that, insofar as lockdowns

DOI: 10.4324/9781003310129-15

infringe important civil liberties, a high bar of effectiveness must be met – they must be necessary to prevent *a great deal* of grievous harm – to be justifiable. As a general rule, if a policy infringes on someone's rights, it shouldn't be implemented – unless the considerations in favor of doing so are of significant enough moral weight. After all, the thought goes, rights are no small thing; their infringement shouldn't be taken lightly. And an important role (indeed, on some views, the primary duty) of the state is to protect citizens' rights.

In Victoria, people like Tim Wilson, who opposed mandatory lockdown measures, argued that the very high bar for licensing rights infringements had not been met. They variously questioned how *effective* lockdown measures actually were, whether they were really *necessary* to achieve desired results, and disputed operative assumptions about what the threshold for public good should be in order to justify rights violations. On the other hand, proponents of mandatory lockdown measures, like Dan Andrews, argued that the bar *had* been met: e.g., the social damage averted and the number of lives to be saved were significant enough to override the strong presumption against violating rights – "it's not about human rights; it's about human life."

However, casting the debate in these terms, as representative as it might be of public discourse at the time, arguably concedes too much to those who, like Tim Wilson, opposed mandatory lockdowns. For, the thought goes, despite appearances, lockdown measures *do not* violate important rights. Why? Because no one has a right to impose a significant risk of grievous harm on others (this follows from the right that each of us enjoys against such impositions) – and, in the context of the COVID-19 pandemic, participating in the sorts of activities restricted by the lockdown measures would impose such a risk. Going to a bar and "getting on the beers" (to use the premier's memorable expression) would arguably impose such a risk on others. Classical liberal thought tells us that while you might enjoy a presumptive right to wave your arms around in such-and-such a fashion, if doing so on this particular occasion also amounts to doing me grievous harm, then you don't have such a right (at least, on this occasion) after all. And as for waving arms, so, we might say, for getting on the beers. Further, as mentioned earlier, the state – while perhaps lacking adequate justification to regulate issues of personal morality – plausibly *does* have an interest in regulating behavior that violates important *rights*. And so, if citizens have a right against being subjected to a significant risk of grievous harm, then the state is justified in using coercive force to prevent the imposition of such risk.

On this view, the "right against risk impositions" plays two roles in justifying mandatory lockdown measures. First, it *blocks* the objection that such measures infringe upon important rights. Second, if the state is justified in intervening to prevent rights violations, it also helps to make a *positive* case for implementing mandatory lockdown measures.

The activities that such measures prohibit are ones that we, in the context of a pandemic, do not have a right to engage in, and, insofar as those activities infringe the rights of others, the state is justified in prohibiting them.

This chapter explores whether this defense of mandatory lockdown measures can succeed. It, first, considers whether the following claim is true and, in so doing, asks how the risk to which it refers is best understood:

> *Right Against Risk*: We have a right against others not to be subjected to a significant risk of grievous harm.

Second, it considers the following objection:

> *Waived Rights*: Even if we do have a right against being subjected to a significant risk of grievous harm, those who voluntarily choose to engage in the activities prohibited by mandatory lockdown measures, if fully appraised of the risks involved, effectively waive this right.

Following this objection, if everyone who, e.g., gathers at the bar effectively *waives* their right against the risk of grievous harm that might result from contracting COVID-19, no one at the bar is in danger of infringing the (unwaived) rights of others. And thus mandatory lockdown measures cannot be justified on the grounds that they prevent rights violations – rights that have been waived cannot be violated. And if going to the bar doesn't violate anyone's rights, given the presumptive right to assemble where we please, the state's use of coercive force to prevent us from doing so appears to infringe rights after all.

The chapter argues that this objection fails. What it takes for one to waive such a right is significantly more nuanced than the objection can allow. And, in any realistic case, there will be legitimate third parties whose rights have not been waived.

12.2 A right against risk

It's not implausible to think that we each have a right against being harmed – especially if that harm is significant. Do we each also have a right against being subjected to a *risk* of harm (especially if that harm is significant)? And, if so, how is this right best understood? And would engaging in those activities prohibited by mandatory lockdown measures (e.g., gathering at the bar) constitute a violation of such a right?

These questions, to differing extents, turn on what it is to have a *right*. Opinions, of course, vary greatly. I will not argue for any particular conception of rights here. Instead, let's focus on the following three features that might plausibly characterize the possession of a right.

DUTY: If A has a right against B's φing, then B has (at least) a *pro tanto* duty not to φ.

ENFORCEMENT: If A has a right against B, then it is *pro tanto* justified for A – and, perhaps, certain ordained third parties, like the state – to prevent B from violating this right.

COMPENSATION: If B infringes one of A's rights, then A has a right to be compensated by B in the appropriate way.

A quick word about each. According to DUTY, to have a right is, in part, for others to have a corresponding duty. This duty needn't be absolute; it can be outweighed by other considerations.[1] Also, this duty might best be thought of as a *directed duty* – so that if B were to φ, not only would B do wrong (assuming the duty hasn't been outweighed), B *wrongs* A in particular. Not all directed duties correspond to rights, however – and some philosophers appeal to something like ENFORCEMENT to account for the difference.[2] Even if that's not true in general, ENFORCEMENT is of particular interest given our purposes because the central question of this chapter concerns the sorts of restrictions that the state is justified in imposing. Like the correlative duty in DUTY, the justification one has to prevent B's infringement of A's right is *pro tanto*: it can be overridden by other considerations. Finally, COMPENSATION says that, at the very least, having a right generates a duty of appropriate compensation in the event that that right is infringed. It might be (all things considered) morally permissible for B to φ, and it might be (all things considered) morally impermissible for A (or the state) to *prevent* B from φing, but – if A has a right against B's φing – B owes A some form of compensation for the infringement.[3]

In addition to assuming that we each have a right against being harmed, I will also assume that, during the height of the COVID-19 pandemic, many everyday activities (e.g., gathering at the bar) involved imposing a *risk of harm* on others. This can be true, I contend, even if one isn't actually contagious or incubating the virus at all – all that's required is that one not be *certain* whether they're infectious. That is, we will operate with a *subjective conception* of risk.[4] For that (and other) reasons, it's very hard to say exactly *how much* risk one imposes on another by, e.g., going to the bar. Supposing (for the sake of argument) that one is experiencing no symptoms, the question turns on how likely one is to be an asymptomatic carrier anyway, how likely one is to transmit the virus if one is carrying it, and how likely those who are exposed are to suffer significant harm (e.g., death) from the exposure.

In any case, of particular interest to us are *pure risk impositions*: cases in which someone imposes a risk of an unwanted outcome, but doesn't actually cause an unwanted outcome.[5] For example, suppose that X imposes a risk on Y – by, e.g., exposing them to COVID-19 – that does not eventuate, and that Y never learns of (and, so, is not a source of psychological distress). Cases like these are of particular interest because, if the harm *did* eventuate or if the action caused harm in some other way, Y's (uncontroversial) right against being *actually* harmed would be infringed.[6] And the question before us is whether Y also has a right against the imposition of a *risk* of harm – and, if so, how that right is best understood.

12.2.1 The risk thesis

Perhaps the most straightforward view (defended by McCarthy 1997) is the following:

> *The Risk Thesis*: We each have the right that others not impose risks of harm on us.

Because, during a pandemic, those activities prohibited by mandatory lockdown measures (e.g., gathering at the bar) impose a risk of harm on others, on this view, such activities infringe the rights of others. Consequently, we each then have a *pro tanto* duty not to engage in such activities (from DUTY), and the state is *pro tanto* justified in preventing us from doing so (from ENFORCEMENT). And so, if *The Risk Thesis* is correct, mandatory lockdown measures are *pro tanto* justified.

The Risk Thesis, however, faces a powerful objection: because nearly all actions involve imposing at least *some* risk on somebody, there's little one can do to avoid infringing someone's rights. The best one can do, it seems, is as little as possible. The only morally defensible action – whether during a pandemic or not – is to sit silently and motionlessly at home. But that, of course, is absurd. This is the *Paralysis Problem*.[7] Let's investigate it further.

THE PARALYSIS ARGUMENT

P1	If *The Risk Thesis* is correct, then each person has a right against you imposing a risk of harm on them.
P2	Nearly all of your actions (with, perhaps, the exception of sitting silently and motionlessly at home) impose a risk of harm on someone.
P3	If φing imposes a risk of harm on someone, and they have a right against you doing so, it's morally impermissible for you to φ.
C	If *The Risk Thesis* is correct, there's nearly nothing it's morally permissible to do (with, perhaps, the exception of sitting silently and motionlessly at home).

But surely it's okay for some people to leave the house sometimes. And so, if the argument is sound, *The Risk Thesis* must go. Is the argument sound? The first premise is merely a restatement of *The Risk Thesis* itself, so there's no use denying that. The second premise, although partly an empirical matter, is plausible enough. A risk, no matter how small, is still a risk, and there are hardly any actions certain to carry no risks whatsoever.

That leaves the third premise. If the right against risk impositions were *inalienable* and *absolute*, the third premise would be plausible: imposing a risk on someone who had an inalienable and absolute right against you doing so would be morally impermissible. But defenders of *The Risk Thesis* needn't think the right is inalienable nor absolute.[8]

Plausibly, the right against risk impositions can be *waived* (if, for example, its bearer *consents* to the risk), which potentially renders the imposition morally permissible (see Section 12.3 for more discussion). And, plausibly, the right can be *overridden* – if, for example, the amount of good that would result from the infringement outweighs its badness – thus rendering its infringement morally permissible. And, the thought goes, the smaller the risk, the easier it is to be outweighed. And so, perhaps, paralysis can be avoided after all.

But *The Risk Thesis* is not yet in the clear. Even if my *pro tanto* duty not to impose a risk on you can be outweighed, rendering my infringement of your right morally permissible, I've infringed your rights all the same. And, according to COMPENSATION, if I've infringed one of your rights, I owe you compensation. But – when the risk is vanishingly small and no actual harm eventuates – it's not plausible that I owe you compensation.[9] Furthermore, given that nearly all actions impose some risk on others, if *The Risk Thesis* were correct, we would need to engage in a quixotic attempt to identify and indemnify a potentially enormous number of people in order to leave the house. And that's its own kind of paralysis.[10]

Finally, according to ENFORCEMENT, if *The Risk Thesis* is correct, the state would be *pro tanto* justified in confining each of us to our respective rooms in order to prevent us from imposing a risk (however small) on anyone else. If we take the view seriously, mandatory lockdown measures (in their most extreme form) would be justified, not only in the face of a deadly pandemic but always. And that's too extreme. Some risks are just too small to justify that much.

12.2.2 The high-risk thesis

The shortcomings of the previous view naturally suggest an alternative (defended by Song, 2019):

> *The High-Risk Thesis*: We each have the right that others not impose a *suitably high* risk of harm on us.

According to *The High-Risk Thesis*, some risk impositions violate rights while others don't. Because many everyday activities during a pandemic impose higher risks on others than they would normally, on this view, the pandemic can turn previously permissible activities into ones that infringe rights. And, the thought goes, this affords us the resources to justify mandatory lockdown measures but avoid paralysis.

The High-Risk Thesis, however, faces several well-known problems. First, there's the question of how high is "suitably" high? It's unclear what motivates drawing the line one place rather than another – but, admittedly, we should expect some vagueness here. Even still, it's not obvious that there's a consistent way of drawing the line that will account for our intuitions about cases. Furthermore, as Altham (1983, 18–19) argues, a simple threshold will not do – the seriousness of a risk imposition is, plausibly, a function of *both* the size of the risk and the seriousness of the harm that might result. A "suitably high" risk of death is surely lower than a "suitably high" risk of mild discomfort.

Second: building on the previous problem, given that many of our actions have various potential effects, there's often no such thing as *the* harm that might result, and thus no such thing as *the* size of the risk of harm that an act imposes (Thomson 1990, 245). For example, being exposed to COVID-19 might result in a case of very mild (but unpleasant) symptoms, or of Long COVID, or of sufficient seriousness to warrant hospitalization, or of death. Suppose that, for each of these particular harms, the probability of *it* resulting is fairly low – none of them, let's say, count as "suitably high." But, suppose further, that the probability of suffering some harm or other *is* suitably high. Whether "the" risk of being exposed to COVID-19 is "suitably high" depends on how we individuate potential harms. But it's not obvious why that should matter.

Third, the view issues implausible verdicts when one can either impose a high risk on a few or spread the risk across very many more. Here's an example. It's March 2020, and you've contracted COVID-19. You have two options. You can isolate in your apartment, exposing your roommates to a reasonably high risk of contracting it also. Or you can take a series of short bus trips to a remote cabin, which involves incidental encounters with many more people. Because these encounters are so brief, you impose only a small risk on each. Let's suppose (given social distancing and mask wearing) that the risk you pose is so small that, if *The High-Risk Thesis* is correct, each of your fellow travelers has no right against you imposing it. Because the risk you pose to your roommates is (let us suppose) high enough that they do have a right against you imposing it on them, *The High-Risk Thesis* seems to imply, implausibly, that you should take the bus trip – even if you know you will encounter so many people in your travels that the overall chance of grievously harming *someone* is greater than it would be if you stayed home.[11]

In response, one could argue that the smaller risks you impose on the many travelers *add up* to something worse than staying home – ultimately rendering the bus trip impermissible. But because, for each traveler, your trip would impose only a permissible amount of risk, if it's nevertheless impermissible to impose that risk on all of them, we have a failure of agglomeration: you ought to do this, you ought to do that, and you ought to do the other, but you shouldn't do this, that, and the other. In which case it appears there's no way for you to satisfy all that you ought to do. It's better, then, for proponents of *The High-Risk Thesis* to just accept the conclusion: you ought to impose the risk on the very many rather than impose a higher risk on the very few. On this picture, your moral duties are directed toward each *individual*, not to some aggregate or fusion or class. And, although you can be confident that *somebody* – whoever they are – is likely to be harmed by your action, because that harm is merely a *foreseen* rather than *intended* consequence, it's not clear how worrisome this objection is.[12]

Lastly, *The High-Risk Thesis*, by putting all its emphasis on the size of the risk, fails to capture an important class of intuitively impermissible risk impositions. Let $1/n$ fall well below the "suitably high" threshold – suppose it's, to borrow an example from Thomson (1986a, 177–179), the risk of death that turning on your gas stove would impose on your neighbor. Now imagine that B plays Russian roulette on A using a gun with one bullet and n chambers. B imposes the same degree of risk on A that you impose on your neighbor. Intuitively, what B does to A is impermissible, whereas what you do to your neighbor is not impermissible.[13] What's the difference?

Examples like these put pressure on *The High-Risk Thesis*. Because these examples involve the same degree of risk but inspire different moral reactions, any view that attends only to facts about the size of the risk imposition will, at best, only supply part of the story. There are three ways of responding to this pressure. First, one can resist it: continue to believe *The High-Risk Thesis*, and explain the different moral reactions in some other way. In particular, because it's implausible that you infringe on your neighbor's rights every time you light your stove (on pains of the *Paralysis Problem*), one needs to explain why we think B has wronged A despite causing her no actual harm and without infringing her rights. Second, one can reject *The High-Risk Thesis* in favor of some entirely different account of when a risk imposition infringes a right – one according to which the *size* of the risk isn't of central importance – and hope that that account fares better. Finally, one can take *The High-Risk Thesis* to provide merely a sufficient condition on what rights we have against risk impositions; imposing a "suitably high" risk of harm is part of the story, not the whole story. We'll look at each option in turn.

If B doesn't actually harm A and doesn't infringe A's right against the imposition of a "suitably high" risk of harm, why does it seem like B *wrongs* A by playing Russian roulette on her? According to Holm (2016, 921), "the moral wrongness resides in *the reasons* that the agent has for performing the action," which, in this case, presumably involves the *intention* to impose a risk on A – after all, with Russian roulette, imposing a risk on another is basically the point! On the other hand, the risk you impose on your neighbor is *not* "the point" – the point is to make coffee; the risk is merely a foreseeable side effect. B has perverse motives, while you do not.[14] And according to Holm (2016, 921), "an agent may be blameworthy for performing an otherwise permissible risk-imposing action due to the agent's reasons for acting." So, the difference is B is *blameworthy* for imposing a 1/n risk of death, whereas you are not blameworthy for imposing a 1/n risk of death.

But this explanation is somewhat unsatisfying. While it's true that B's character leaves something to be desired, it also seems like B *wrongs* A. And, presumably, it takes more than a bad motive to wrong someone. But, then, if B hasn't *done* anything wrong, what is B blameworthy for? At the risk of going in circles, perhaps B is blameworthy for their bad motive: their desire for the rush derived from imposing a risk on A. But now consider B*, who is motivationally just like B, but who doesn't act on their desire to play Russian roulette on A. B* fantasizes about doing so but never actually pulls the trigger. Is B* just as blameworthy? Perhaps. Has B* *wronged* A? I think no – or, at least, not to the same extent B has. Something more, or something different, must account for the difference.

12.2.3 *The intention thesis*

Perhaps, then, we ought to reject *The High-Risk Thesis* entirely, and instead accept something like the following view (discussed in McKerlie 1986, 243–245):

> *The Intention Thesis*: We each have the right that others not perform actions that aim to impose a risk of harm on us.

On this view, whether a risk imposition violates someone's rights depends not on the size of the risk but on whether that risk imposition is an intended result of the imposer's aim. We don't have rights against risk impositions when they are merely foreseeable side effects of the imposer's aim. We do have a right against actions that are aimed at imposing a risk of harm on us. So, on this view, A has a right against B's playing Russian roulette on her, but your neighbor doesn't have a right against you using your stove – even though both activities impose the same sized risk of death.

I'll raise three issues for *The Intention Thesis*. First, the view is arguably too lenient. Risk imposition needn't be intentional to be impermissible. Suppose B loves to fire his pistol in the air, and suppose that, when he does so, he imposes a high risk of death on A. Imposing this risk is not

B's *intention*, it's merely a foreseeable side effect of an activity he loves. There are things B could do to make it less likely that A is hit by a stray bullet (e.g., he could ensure A isn't around when he fires his gun), but he elects not to because he's utterly indifferent to what effects his behavior has on A's well-being. B's not malicious, he's grossly negligent. Or, a germane example: suppose B is contagious with COVID-19 and knowingly exposes A to the virus, not because he *intends* to impose this risk on A but because he simply doesn't care enough to do otherwise. In both examples, B acts impermissibly – he *wrongs* A. The best explanation of why (given that, let us suppose, no actual harm eventuates) is that A has a right against being treated in these ways.

The second issue is more theoretical. A compelling thought about having a right is that it grants you sovereignty over certain choices; rights provide you with a foundation on which to build your autonomy. By infringing one of your rights, I damage your autonomy by interfering in a domain of choices that, ultimately, are yours to make. But this picture is in tension with *The Intention Thesis* because an action can undermine one's autonomy without that being its *intended* purpose. As McKerlie (1986, 244–245) elaborates,

> [*The Intention Thesis*] makes the force of the rights of others depend on the structure of my plans. If I have one thing rather than another as my goal, or if something figures in my project as a by-product of my pursuit of my goal rather than as a means to the goal, then those rights have no stopping power against my action. A right becomes a sort of reflector that only has force when a hostile intention plays on it. I think instead that the rights of others have an independent force that constrains our plans and intentions. The rights start in their lives, not in our own, and they derive their force from their place in those other lives. When I discover that the route to my goal would also intrude in another life in one of the proscribed ways I must change my plans.

Why should *your* rights depend on *my* plans? Instead, shouldn't my plans, in part, depend on your rights?

Finally, let's step back and consider *The Intention Thesis* in the context of the pandemic. In particular, if that view is correct, would this bolster or subvert the case for mandatory lockdown measures? The answer is that it would subvert it. Consider an activity prohibited by the lockdown measures: e.g., going to the bar. On this view, so long as your *aim* is something *other* than to impose a risk of catching COVID-19 onto others, going to the bar doesn't infringe anyone's rights. If your motivation for going to the bar is to have a good time, not to spread COVID-19, then you are in the clear – even if your presence at the bar will foreseeably impose a risk on others. Because you (and, presumably, the other bar-goers too) don't infringe anyone's rights by going to the bar, this fore-closes a promising way in which the state might be justified in enforcing a mandatory lockdown. The lesson is that *The Intention Thesis* is implausibly permissive.

12.2.4 A hybrid view

Both *The High-Risk Thesis* and *The Intention Thesis* are too permissive but in different ways. *The High-Risk Thesis* doesn't secure us a right against being made the victim of involuntary Russian roulette so long as the risk of death is low enough. But it seems like we do have a right against others performing actions intended to impose a risk of harm on us – even if that risk is quite low. On the other hand, *The Intention Thesis* doesn't secure us rights against the risks imposed from gross negligence. Given that they each plug a hole found in the other, why not combine them?

> *The HI-brid Thesis*: We each have the right that others not perform actions that aim to impose a risk (however small) of harm on us and that others (whatever their motives) not impose a suitably high risk of harm on us.

The HI-brid Thesis is a hybrid. It grants A a right against B's playing Russian roulette on her (no matter how many chambers of the gun); it grants A a right against B imposing a high risk on her (no matter his intentions), but it doesn't grant your neighbor a right against you lighting your gas stove to make coffee. But while *The HI-brid Thesis* might get the cases right, if it does, it does so in an unsatisfying way; it's gerrymandered and seems to lack any unifying underlying theoretical motivation. Furthermore, it inherits problems from both of the views it hybridizes: e.g., it's not clear what "suitably high" means or why it should matter, it's unclear why *your* rights are sensitive to the structure of *my* plans, and so on.

These flaws aren't fatal – it's certainly possible that a compelling underlying motivation that both better unifies the thesis' two ideas and answers the objections could be provided. And while doing so is outside the scope of this chapter, I'll point to what to me seems to be a potentially promising candidate: that we each have a right to be treated with *respect*.

> *The Respect Thesis*: We each have the right that others not perform actions that fail to express proper respect for us and our projects.

Actions that *aim* to impose a risk on us (e.g., Russian roulette) are disrespectful – even if the size of that risk is small. When B imposes a risk on A *intentionally*, B treats A like a plaything, and that fails to express proper respect for her. Furthermore, actions that impose higher risks of harm, arguably, express greater disrespect.[15] Treating someone with respect requires you to take their interests (including their interest in not being harmed) into account when deciding what to do. That an action *might* cause them harm provides you with a reason against doing it, a reason whose strength is proportionate to how likely that harm is. So, the more risk an action imposes on someone, the stronger the reasons against performing it. And while you may have reasons to perform it, if that risk is suitably high, performing it anyway suggests that you've improperly undervalued the interests of the person your action might harm. And that's disrespectful.

More would need to be said to fully defend the view, of course, but let's assume it is true for now. Then, people have a right against being subjected to a suitably high risk of harm. And this might serve to justify mandatory lockdown measures. If certain activities impose, on some particular people, a suitably high risk of harm, then – unless those particular people have *waived* their right – engaging in those activities violates those people's rights, and thus (from ENFORCEMENT) the state can be justified in restricting those activities by means of tools like lockdowns. It's hard to estimate exactly how much risk a person imposes on others by engaging in activities like bar-going, but it's not implausible to think that – at least, during the height of the COVID-19 pandemic – the risks are "suitably high."

But if everyone subjected to this suitably high risk has *waived* their right against having it imposed on them, imposing it on them isn't a violation – and ENFORCEMENT has no force. This brings us to our final subject of examination: whether those who knowingly and voluntarily choose to engage in activities that are known to be risky effectively waive their right against risk impositions.

12.3 Consent and COVID

Suppose that, by going to the bar, B will impose a suitably high risk of harm on A. Why? Suppose, plausibly enough, it's because A will also be at the bar – and by being in close proximity, there's a suitably high chance of B transmitting the virus to A. Assuming that A has a right against others imposing a suitably high risk of harm on her, does B violate this right of A's by going to the bar? Not if A has waived her right. And, one might argue, by wittingly and voluntarily choosing to go to the bar – an activity known to carry certain risks during a pandemic – A effectively does just that. *Mutatis mutandis* for many of the other activities prohibited by mandatory lockdown measures. And so, the argument goes, ENFORCEMENT doesn't provide adequate justification for such measures.

Let's take a closer look at this argument to see if it holds up. The argument appeals to a plausible idea governing the relationship between *consent* and the *waiving* of a right:

The Consent Thesis: If A validly consents to B φing, then A effectively waives her right against B φing (supposing she has one).

If A has a right against B doing something to her, this right can be waived through an act of valid consent. What is it for an act of consent to be valid? This is a notoriously vexed issue, but there are a number of conditions that seem necessary: the person issuing the consent must be sufficiently *competent*; the consent must be given *voluntarily*; and the person issuing the consent must be *adequately informed* about what she is consenting to.[16] Each of these conditions themselves raises a host of complicated issues, but I will trust that they are clear enough for now.

We are concerned with A's right against others imposing a risk of harm on her. Substituting that into *The Consent Thesis* we get:

(1)   If A validly consents to B imposing a risk of harm on her, then A effectively waives her right against B imposing a risk of harm on her.

This instance of *The Consent Thesis* raises an interesting question about *what it is* to consent to a risk. In particular, if you consent to a risk, do you then have no grounds for complaint if the risk eventuates? Thomson (1986a, 188–191) explores this issue in some detail.[17] She argues that there's no simple answer by contrasting two different cases. She observes, "[O]ne who loses in a nonfradulent lottery, which he entered without duress, has no ground for complaint when he loses" (190). (Call this *Lottery Ticket*.) But that same person surely has grounds for complaint in the following example (call it *Unpleasant Way*):

> Suppose there are two ways in which I can get home from the station at the end of the day. The first is pleasant, passes through a brightly lit middle-class shopping area, is quite safe, but is long. The second way is unpleasant, passes through an ill-lit area of warehouses, is unsafe, but is short. Nobody has ever been mugged while walking along Pleasant Way; people have from time to time been mugged on Unpleasant Way. Here I am, at the station; I am tired; I think "The hell, I'll chance it, I'll go home via Unpleasant Way." I then promptly get mugged.
>
> (Thomson 1986a, 189–190)

It's not clear what accounts for the difference.[18] This, in my opinion, remains "a nice problem" (190). But it needn't be our problem. Whether or not A would have "grounds for complaint" were she to contract COVID-19 from B at the bar, our problem concerns whether A's actions suffice to waive her right against B imposing that *risk* on her.

(2)   By wittingly and voluntarily going to the bar, A validly consents to B imposing a risk of harm on her.

If A wittingly and voluntarily goes to the bar during the pandemic, she thereby accepts the risks that come with it. That she "accepts the risks" is just another way of saying that she consents to them. This wouldn't be true, of course, if A were unaware of the dangers involved or if she was coerced or unduly induced into going. But she's not and she wasn't: she chooses to go to the bar wittingly and voluntarily.

But (2) can be resisted. While it may be that by wittingly and voluntarily going to the bar, A accepts the relevant risks, it doesn't follow that she validly consents to *B in particular* – or anyone else, for that matter – imposing such a risk on her. Consent is inter*personal*: it's something that one person grants to another who they stand in some relation to. One can "accept the risks" of some course of action – like leaving their umbrella at home when it might rain – without there being anyone to whom they give their consent. And, one might think, this can be so even when the risks in question stem not from the weather but from others.

In fact, Thomson (1986a, 190) makes a similar point concerning the difference between *Lottery Ticket* and *Unpleasant Way*: "there is no person or persons such that I consented to his or their imposing a risk of being mugged on me." In buying a lottery ticket, however, there is a person or persons (e.g., whoever is administering the drawing) such that one consents to the risk of losing to. But, upon reflection, it's not clear this difference makes a difference. Consider the following:

> *Poker Table*: You sit down at the poker table at your local casino and settle in for a night of high-stakes play. You've never met anyone else at the table, and players come and go throughout the night. After hours of play, luck is not on your side: you lose everything to the late-arriving man in sunglasses on your left.

You wittingly and voluntarily agree to play poker, accepting the risk that you might lose it all. But just like A's trip to the bar and Thomson's trip down Unpleasant Way, there is no person or persons in particular to whom you've consented to potentially lose it all. When you joined the table, you didn't know who all else might join as the night wore on. But *Poker Table* seems more like *Lottery Ticket*: you've consented and you have no grounds to complain when you lose.

Here's a suggestion. When you join the poker table, in addition to accepting the risk of losing, you also *impose* a similar risk on your fellow players. Similarly, when you buy the lottery ticket, in addition to accepting the risk of losing, you also accept a chance of winning – which imposes a risk on whoever must pay out if you do. Nothing similar is true in *Unpleasant Way* however: by taking that route, you accept the risk of being mugged, but you do not impose a comparable risk on those who impose that risk on you.[19] The difference appears to be one of *reciprocity*: in accepting an imposition of risk from a person or persons, you in turn impose a risk on them.[20] Why might this matter? Here's a thought: wittingly and voluntarily imposing a (suitably high) risk on someone functions to *personalize* the relationship – so that accepting the risks imposed on you suffices for consent. By imposing a risk on B, A opens herself to consenting to the risk that B imposes on her.[21]

(2′)   By wittingly and voluntarily engaging in a reciprocal risk imposition with B, A validly consents to B imposing a risk of harm on her.

In our example, by wittingly and voluntarily going to the bar, A thereby wittingly and voluntarily engages in a reciprocal risk imposition with B (as well as whoever else might be at the bar that day). And so, from (1) and (2′), we can conclude:

By wittingly and voluntarily going to the bar, A effectively waives her right against B imposing a risk of harm on her.

This, of course, also holds for B, and for whoever else goes to the bar as well. So, each person who goes to the bar effectively waives their right against each of the others imposing a risk on them – so long as their going is done wittingly and voluntarily.

(3)   Many of those activities prohibited by mandatory lockdown measures are such that those who would engage in them would do so wittingly and voluntarily.

And so, for a wide class of activities (like going to the bar), so long as the public is made well aware of the risks involved, those who choose to engage in those activities effectively waive their rights against having the risks of COVID-19 imposed on them. And so, because no one who voluntarily engages in those activities is in danger of having their rights violated, the state's justification for instituting mandatory lockdown measures cannot be grounded in preventing rights violations.

12.3.1 Responding to the consent argument

This is a compelling argument. There is something to the thought that, if I am doing basically the same thing to you that you are doing to me, I lose my standing to complain about what you're doing to me. There is, at the least, something *hypocritical* about condemning someone for the very same thing you're doing to them. Of course, it doesn't follow from the fact that no one can non-hypocritically complain about what you've done, that you've done nothing wrong.[22] But even if it did, I think the argument is ultimately unsuccessful anyway – for somewhat prosaic reasons.

Let's grant (1) and (2') for the sake of argument. I will raise a problem for (3). It's simply not true that those who would engage in the activities prohibited by mandatory lockdown measures would do so knowingly and voluntarily. Perhaps some would, but it's unrealistic to imagine that all would. Here are two examples.

First, consider someone – call her "Missy" – who has formed many radically false beliefs about the pandemic (perhaps owing to the large amount of misinformation especially prevalent at the beginning), which leads her to systematically underappreciate the risks that she imposes on others and that they present to her. If Missy decides to spend the day at the bar, does she engage in that activity *wittingly*? We can assume, of course, that she knows what a bar is, and so there's a sense in which she knows what she is doing by going to the bar. But given her many and varied false beliefs about the dangers of COVID-19, she fails to appreciate that to spend the day at the bar is to do something that exposes her and others to an elevated level of risk. There's a sense, then, in which she doesn't know what she's doing; she doesn't go to the bar wittingly. And so it's not obvious that her right against being subjected to a suitably high risk isn't violated.

Second, consider someone – call her "Essie" – who is an essential worker, working in food service. Essie spends the day at the bar, let's suppose, because she gets paid to work there. And while it's true that Essie isn't forced to work at the bar, she definitely wouldn't spend her time there if not for the promise of remuneration and the threat of unemployment. Does Essie go to the bar voluntarily? In a sense, yes. She appreciates the risks involved, and given the size of her paycheck and the other options available to her, she figures it's worth it. But her presence at the bar seems importantly less voluntarily than that of her clientele. And so it's not obvious that her right against being subjected to a suitably high risk isn't violated.

One final point. The argument, if successful, establishes that no one who voluntarily engages in activities that would be prohibited under the lockdown is in danger of having their rights violated. We've just questioned whether that argument is successful. But there is a further worry. Even if it is, it doesn't follow that the state isn't justified in instituting mandatory lockdown measures on the grounds of preventing the rights violations of *others* – in particular, the rights of health-care workers and all of us who have a stake in a well-functioning health-care system. Here's the thought. Even if you, as well as everyone else at the bar, have elected to waive your right against the risks of COVID-19, you have all collectively made it more likely that some number of you will require additional health care, including hospitalization. And while that might be a risk that you and the other bar-goers are happy to bear, it's not a risk that you bear alone – we all have an interest in a well-functioning health-care system that isn't overrun and depleted by victims of COVID-19. This might provide the state with ample justification to institute restrictions when doing so is necessary to sustain the health-care system.

12.4 Conclusion

This chapter did several things. First, it explored whether we each – in addition to having a right against being harmed – have a right against being subjected to a *risk* of harm. We surveyed several of the extant positions and cautiously sketched a novel one. Second, it considered an argument against mandatory lockdown measures on the grounds that those whose rights the measures are meant to protect have, in virtue of engaging in the activities in question, effectively waived those rights. We then looked at several objections to this argument and closed by noting that even if the argument is successful, pandemic bar-goers shouldn't rush to get on the beers. The integrity of the health-care system, and the rights of its workers and clientele, may yet supply the state with a plausible rights-based ground to justify mandatory lockdowns.

Notes

1 Gewirth (1981, 16) argues that there is at least one absolute right: the "right not to be made the intended victims of a homicidal project." If he's correct, then B will have more than a *pro tanto* duty – hence, the clause "at least" in DUTY.

2 See, for example, Wenar (2013, 209, 214), and "in my view enforceability (…) distinguishes directed duties we call rights from those we do not" (Cruft 2013, 209). Thomson (1986b, 161) also regards something like ENFORCE-MENT as "a plausible idea."

3 Consider the discussion in Thomson (1980) of the beleaguered backpacker, who, imperiled by a blizzard, breaks into someone's boarded-up cabin to escape the elements. Because the backpacker would otherwise die, it's morally permissible for them to do so; it would be morally impermissible for us to prevent them from doing so; but they nevertheless infringe the cabin owner's property rights – and, correspondingly, owe them compensation.

4 Among subjective conceptions of risk, we can distinguish belief-relative from evidence-relative conceptions. The former concern the actual beliefs of the agent, the latter concerns the beliefs the agent *should* have given their evidence. Nothing in the ensuing discussion will turn on this distinction. These two notions can, in turn, be distinguished from a fact-relative conception of risk, which understands risk in terms of facts that are independent of agent's beliefs and evidence (e.g., objective chances) – but, for reasons outside the scope of this chapter, I confess to finding this notion obscure.

5 The distinction between pure and impure risk impositions is introduced and discussed in Thomson (1986a).

6 According to some, an imposition of a risk of harm – whether or not it eventuates – is itself a harm (Finkelstein 2003; Oberdiek 2017; Placani 2017). On these views, there is a sense in which pure risk impositions don't exist. For reasons outside the scope of this chapter, I don't find these views particularly plausible (for some indication of why, see Maheshwari 2021; Rowe 2021), and so I shall set them aside.

7 The name for the objection comes from Hayenhjelm and Wolff (2012, e37), who regard it as "the central philosophical problem" concerning the morality of risk-impositions. It's been discussed by many, including Fried (1970, 192–193), Kagan (1989, 87–88), McCarthy (1997), Nozick (1974, 73–78), Thomson

(1986b), and Holm (2016). Thomson (1990, 244–245) raises a similar, but distinct issue (which Holm, 2016, refers to as the "Proliferation Problem").

8 McCarthy (1997, 215) is one such defender. He thinks that an imposition of risk can be rendered morally permissible (despite infringing a right) if the imposition is consented to or "if the good that would come of bringing about [the imposition] would sufficiently outweigh the burden to the bearer of the right." He calls the former point the Consent Idea, and calls the latter the Trade-off Idea. See Holm (2016) for more discussion.

9 Thomson (1986b, 165) makes a similar argument: because I do not owe you compensation for imposing a risk on you, we have "a ground for thinking that I do not infringe a right of yours when I do so."

10 McCarthy (1997) argues that this problem can be overcome because he thinks, in cases like this, the only compensation owed is the promise to make amends in the event that the risk of harm eventuates. Although, of course, we should make amends if the harm eventuates; it's unclear why this is all that should be required if it's true that we have a right against *pure* risk impositions (see Holm 2016, for further discussion).

11 McKerlie (1986) and Railton (1985) are, to my knowledge, the first to raise this issue. McCarthy (1997, 213–214) discusses the problem, arguing that it provides a point in favor of *The Risk Thesis*. Holm (2016, 922–923) argues that the objection is inconclusive because proponents of *The High-Risk Thesis* needn't find this implication of their view objectionable. Song (2019, 776) argues that proponents can appeal to moral considerations other than rights violations (e.g., expected harm) to rescue the verdict that it's worse to impose risk on the many rather than the few.

12 Aboodi et al. (2008, 266–268) make the same point in response to a different but closely related objection to the "threshold version" of a deontological moral theory under uncertainty. Although not presented as such, *The High-Risk Thesis* is essentially just that.

13 This puzzle, as well as the diagnosis below, appears in Thomson (1986b, 167) and (McKerlie 1986, 241). (Nozick (1974, 74, 81–82) raises the puzzle, too, but floats a different solution.) It's raised as an objection to *The High-Risk Thesis*, in particular, in McCarthy (1997, 213), who takes it to be a reason to reject the view; and in Holm (2016, 920–922) and Song (2019, 775–776), who both think the objection can be answered.

14 Appealing to the distinction between *intended* effects and *foreseeable* side-effects to account for the difference is popular (Holm 2016; McCarthy 1997; McKerlie 1986; Song 2019; Thomson 1986b), but not universal. Nozick (1974, 74), in discussing a similar example concerning driving and Russian roulette, offers two other explanations: first, that Russian roulette, unlike driving, has insufficient social value; and second, that it's "not a normal part of almost everyone's life," (Nozick 1974, 82). Nozick's first explanation (about social value) fails when applied to our example: so long as B enjoys the activity (finds it energizing, etc.), it's not obvious that it has less social value than your home-brewed coffee habit. His second explanation fares better: making coffee is a normal part of almost everyone's life. But as Nozick himself points out, this approach places a lot of weight on the scheme used to classify actions.

15 Lazar (2019, 25) develops a similar idea, arguing that "killing someone more riskily shows greater disrespect for him by more grievously undervaluing his standing and interests".

16 See Eyal (2019) for a general survey of issues concerning *informed consent*. See Dougherty (2021) for a discussion of how ignorance can affect the content of what one counts as having consented to.

17 Davis (2022, 475) explores this issue, too – specifically in the context of COVID-19: "your having accepted the risks that I might unintentionally transmit a deadly virus to you means that, if indeed I do unintentionally transmit the virus to you and you later die from it, I do not thereby wrong you. You knew the risks and you accepted them." He ultimately rejects this argument.

18 One possibility is that you "know the probabilities" in *Lottery Ticket* but not in *Unpleasant Way*. But that won't do. Consider, instead of playing the lottery, playing a slot machine. You don't "know the probabilities" of winning, but if you walk away from the machine a loser, you don't have grounds for complaint.

19 Suppose, instead, that you take Unpleasant Way, not because it's a shorter route home, but because you're interested in finding someone to mug. In this version, you *do* impose a risk of mugging on the others – and so the risks involved are reciprocal. But now this case seems more like *Poker Table*. If one of the other muggers gets the drop on you, that's just fair play.

20 Many have highlighted the potential importance of reciprocal risk-impositions. See, for example, Fried (1970); Song (2019). For discussions of it in the context of the COVID-19 pandemic, see Davis (2022); Lang (2020); Lazar and Barry (2020).

21 This – admittedly underdeveloped – suggestion finds some indirect support from thew ways in which reciprocal risk impositions *don't* seem to matter. Imagine, for example, that I (unbeknown to you) subject you to an involuntary game of Russian roulette. I impose a risk on you. But also suppose that I know the gun is just as likely to backfire, killing me, as it is to kill you. From my point of view, the risks of the activity are mutual. But this goes no way at all toward justifying my actions. Imagine instead that, while I'm playing Russian roulette on you, you are (unbeknownst to me) playing Russian roulette on me – perhaps with the aid of stealth drones. The risks are reciprocal (albeit unbeknownst to us), but again this fails to justify our actions. Lastly, imagine that I know the person I'm imposing a risk on is, in turn, imposing a risk on me – and that I know that they know this too. This case is different from the previous two, which suggests that it's not the reciprocity of the risks *itself* that matters, but what we know about the relationship that obtains between us.

22 Davis (2022, 481) (drawing on Cohen 2006) makes the same point: "the fact that we behaved the same way does not make the wrongdoer's actions any less wrong, but it does make us poorly positioned to criticize them." On the other hand, Lang (2020) appears to disagree (at least about this case): "If I am wronging you and am also being wronged by you, and you are wronging me and are also being wronged by me, then it will turn out…that neither of us is wronging the other." I'm inclined to agree with Davis here, but the objection in the text lands either way.

References

Aboodi, Ron, Adi Borer, and David Enoch. 2008. Deontology, individualism, and uncertainty: A reply to Jackson and Smith. *Journal of Philosophy*, 105(5): 259–272.

Altham, J.E.J. 1983. Ethics of risk. *Proceedings of the Aristotelian Society*, 84: 15–29. DOI: 10.1093/aristotelian/84.1.15

Cohen, G.A. 2006. Casting the first stone: Who can, and who can't, condemn the terrorists? *Royal Institute of Philosophy Supplement*, 58: 113–136. DOI: 10.1017/S1358246100009334

Cruft, Rowan. 2013. Why is it disrespectful to violate rights? *Proceedings of the Aristotelian Society*, 113: 201–224. DOI: 10.1111/j.1467-9264.2013. 00352.x

Davis, Jeremy. 2022. The ethics of killing in a pandemic: Unintentional virus transmission, reciprocal risk imposition, and standards of blame. *Journal of Applied Philosophy*, 39(3): 471–486. DOI: 10.1111/japp.12574

Dougherty, Tom. 2021. *The Scope of Consent* (Oxford: Oxford University Press).

Eyal, Nir. 2019. Informed Consent. *The Stanford Encyclopedia of Philosophy*, Edward N. Zalta (ed.). URL: https://plato.stanford.edu/archives/spr2019/entries/informed-consent/

Finkelstein, Claire Oakes. 2003. Is risk a harm? *University of Pennsylvania Law Review*, 151(3): 963–1001

Fried, Charles. 1970. *Anatomy of Value* (Cambridge, MA: Harvard University Press).

Gewirth, Alan. 1981. Are there any absolute rights? *The Philosophical Quarterly*, 31(122): 1–16. DOI: 10.2307/2218674

Hayenhjelm, Madeleine and Jonathan Wolff. 2012. The moral problem of risk impositions: A survey of the literature. *The European Journal of Philosophy*, 20(S1): 26–51. DOI: 10.1111/j.1468-0378.2011.00482.x

Holm, Sune. 2016. A Right against Risk-Imposition and the Problem of Paralysis. *Ethical Theory and Moral Practice*, 19: 917–930. DOI: 10.1007/s10677-016-9697-6

Kagan, Shelly. 1989. *The Limits of Morality* (Oxford: Oxford University Press).

Lang, Gerald. 2020. Costs and risk impositions in a pandemic. *Public Ethics*. URL: https://www.publicethics.org/post/costs-and-risk-imposition-in-a-pandemic

Lazar, Seth. 2019. Risky killing: How risks worsen violations of objective rights. *Journal of Moral Philosophy*, 16(1): 1–26.

Lazar, Seth and Christian Barry. 2020. Justifying lockdown. *Ethics and International Affairs*. URL: https://www.ethicsandinternationalaffairs. org/2020/justifying-lockdown/

Maheshwari, Kritika. 2021. On the harm of imposing risk of harm. *Ethical Theory and Moral Practice*, 24: 965–980. DOI: 10.1007/s10677-021-10227-y

McCarthy, David. 1997. Rights, explanation, and risk. *Ethics*, 107(2): 205–225.

McKerlie, Dennis. 1986. Rights and risk. *Canadian Journal of Philosophy*, 16(2): 239–251.

Nozick, Robert. 1974. *Anarchy, State, and Utopia* (New York, NY: Basic Books).

Oberdiek, J. 2017. *Imposing Risks: A Normative Framework* (Oxford: Oxford University Press).

Placani, A. 2017. When the risk of harm harms. *Law and Philosophy*, 36(1): 77–100.

Railton, Peter. 1985. Locke, stock, and peril: Natural property rights, pollution, and risk. In *To Breathe Freely*, edited by Mary Gibson (Rowman & Littlefield Publishers), pp. 89–123.

Rowe, Thomas. 2021. Can a risk of harm itself be a harm? *Analysis*, 81(4): 694–701. DOI: 10.1093/analys/anab033

Song, Fei. 2019. Rights against high-level risk impositions. *Ethical Theory and Moral Practice*, 22: 763–778. DOI: 10.1007/s10677-019-09994-6

Thomson, Judith Jarvis. 1980. Rights and compensation. *Nous*, 14(1): 3–15.

224   *Ryan Doody*

———. 1986a. Imposing Risks. In *Rights, Restitution, and Risk*, edited by William Parent, chap. 11 (Cambridge, MA: Harvard University Press), pp. 173–191.

———. 1986b. Some questions about government regulation of behavior. In *Rights, Restitution, and Risk*, edited by William Parent (Cambridge, MA: Harvard University Press), pp. 154–172.

———. 1990. *Realm of Rights* (Harvard University Press).

Wenar, Leif. 2013. The nature of claim-rights. *Ethics*, 123: 202–229.

13 Allocation of scarce intensive care units in COVID-19 and ageism

Alcino Eduardo Bonella

13.1 Introduction

In the scenario of extreme scarcity of hospital resources for the high volume of patients in the COVID-19 pandemic, some protocols proposed or adopted, and some specialized papers, incorporated cycle life or age criterion as a relevant factor for the allocation of intensive care unit (ICU) beds and ventilators. In general, what is questioned are which factors could be used, such as the severity of the patient's situation, the order of arrival to the hospital, the higher or lower chances of recovering from the disease, the age, a draw. It is a common observation that the age factor should never be used alone, but without totally condemning its use incorporated with other criteria. What can we think, from an ethical point of view, about the use of age? At first sight, our intuitions seem to conflict: one of the forms of discrimination, in the negative and condemnable sense of the expression, consists in arbitrarily disfavoring someone just because they are older; we have the intuition to condemn what can then be called ageism. However, with a little more information, and observing the most immediate attitude of medical teams at the beginning of the pandemic (as in the Italian or Spanish case, in which they even published guidelines indicating the use of age to prioritize the youngest since they had a better chance of success with the intervention), we are left in doubt whether the use of the age factor, prioritizing, for example, in the case of COVID-19, the youngest, corresponds to something reprehensible or if the problem would not be exactly not using life cycles or age. With further reflection, the ethical challenge is that there is probably more harm in losing a younger life than an older one. When our intuitions conflict, we need critical ethical thinking, which does not rely solely or even heavily on them, because one's own intuitions or past experiences, however wise, should appeal to practical reasoning and the facts of the situation. I will try to present the outline of this in the issue of the use of age in the allocation of ICUs during the COVID-19 pandemic. Although an outline, there is apparently soundness in favor of using age and giving priority to younger people. The thesis to be defended is that this is the right thing to do. Let's see.

DOI: 10.4324/9781003310129-16

13.2 The use of age in allocation guidelines under scarcity

Usually, we start investigating ICU allocation by verifying what is said at the medical councils (such as the Federal Council of Medicine of Brazil) and the associations of intensive care medicine (such as the Brazilian Association of Intensive Care Medicine); we also look at principles and arguments in available ethical theories, as well as proposals for guidelines and protocols made by specialized groups of academics and officially made by affected countries. All things considered, we can think about ethical allocation guidelines without mediation, by ourselves, and also about more specific aspects, such as the relevance of using the "age" factor for allocation in the COVID-19 context.

Something that stands out in this research for the more general theme of allocation in scarcity, the most fundamental ethical perspective for a scenario of extreme scarcity, is the equitable maximization of the benefits of intensive care, in other words, trying to save the greatest possible number of human lives. In a hospital calamity, when so many human lives are at stake in a short period of time, and in the face of extremely scarce resources, we have an acute public health and medical ethics problem. Such as occurs in huge natural disasters, the priority should be saving as many people as possible. Thus, for a correct allocation in the ICU, what appears to be more decisive is the higher patient recovery probability: it is not the severity of the patient's condition, much less the order of arrival at the hospital (Emanuel et al. 2020). Patients with a higher chance of recovering from the disease tend to spend less time in the ICU, have a higher chance of being saved, and, if treated as a priority, it can lead to more people being saved, which is the goal in cases like this. Besides, for the maximization to be equitable or to maintain the equal consideration of citizens, another fundamental aspect from an ethical perspective is that the resource allocation should be provided impartially to all patients, in a way that all demands receive due consideration and no patient is completely left out, without their demand being compared to other people's need for an ICU. (Beauchamp and Childress 2019). According to the factual knowledge available, however, many more deaths will occur without suitable prioritization.

An adequate order of priority care would avoid *a priori* patient exclusions, so that the calamity itself and the availability of resources are what will, in fact, determine who receives treatment and at what time. It seems that it is possible to find equitable directives and allocation guidelines, which figure among principles of maximization and impartiality (Center for Law, Medicine and Life Sciences 2020; White 2020; Azevedo et al. 2020; Azevedo et al. 2021. First of all, however, it is important that the competent authorities establish the guidelines publicly and declare the duration of the calamity period during which such measures must be observed and that it is made clear that the guidelines will apply (i) to the extraordinary situation that is happening (and not the normal routine of hospitals and emergency rooms), (ii) in all locations in the country or state where the situation is exceptional, and (iii) that they are directed equally to all patients who need an ICU and not just to patients diagnosed with the pandemic disease, in this case, COVID-19. (Emanuel et al. 2020; White and Lo 2020). Being affected by COVID-19 should not, on its own, give any patient either higher or lower priority over other patients. All people must be allocated by the same special guidelines. Another preliminary aspect is that medical triage teams should be created and established in each institution with ICUs, separate from the intensive care teams, for the admission of critically ill patients, according to these special guidelines. Such measures aim to mitigate the medical dilemma of selecting priority patients and to diminish the tension between the intensive care of the individual patient (clinical ethics) and the attention to the collective of patients waiting for treatment, aiming to save the greatest number of people (ethics of public health). It will be up to the triage team, preferably formed by specialized professionals, to classify patients according to a certain priority, in this case, the degree of higher chance of recovery. It would be better, if possible, for triage to use quantitative clinical assessment scores, which is justified by the concern to mitigate selection bias and increase protection from the risks of excessively subjective assessments, for both patients and professionals. Clinical scores, especially those related to infectious conditions, such as the SOFA (Sequential Organ Failure Assessment), will provide greater objectivity to decisions, mainly in situations in which professionals need to justify these decisions to patients and family members. Furthermore, such scores will allow priorities to be expressed objectively (Ferreira et al. 2001; White 2020).

Using total scores, like SOFA, we can obtain a patient classification in order of priority care, from the lowest score to the highest. Note that such an assessment does not fail to give equal consideration to all patients: all are eligible for admission to the ICU, and the classification criteria are impartial including all those in need. As resources become less scarce, more patients will be served, but still according to the priorities established in the special guidelines.

Unfortunately, during the COVID-19 pandemic, in order to save more lives, patients who are more critical, but with a worse prognosis for recovery, will be at a lower priority level than patients in a less critical condition, but with a higher chance of recovery (Beauchamp and Childress 2019; White and Lo 2020). Perhaps there could be a combination of some different scores, to obtain a final score that is more suitable to the situation, and that depends on the experts telling us how this would be the case (Emanuel et al. 2020; White 2020). For example, combining severity, morbidity, and reversibility scores. It must be remembered that a combination of scores must be adjusted to the aim of saving the greatest number of lives (for the higher chance of recovery, in cases such as

COVID-19) but also be reasonably realistic so that it can be applied quickly by the triage team, taking into consideration the technology available in each location.

Moreover, there is always the possibility of rare situations that should classify patients regardless of total scores. One, for example, would be to give priority to health professionals who work on the front line of ICUs, and who should be ahead of everyone, or in the high priority group. In this case, reasons that could justify this priority are save such professionals who were and could be essential for the intensive care of patients; to maintain the morale of the teams (something called in the literature *the instrumental value of the guideline*), which is also part of the effort to save more lives; and a way of fulfilling a moral duty of reciprocity toward such professionals. Another situation, which would place patients inversely, last, or in the low priority group, is that of people whose clinical conditions do not recommend intensive care, such as terminally ill patients or with incurable diseases in an advanced stage, or in critical and irreversible situations. These are candidates for other types of care outside the ICU, such as palliative care, which must be available alongside intensive care. In order not to exclude such patients, if they or their families insist on intensive treatment, they should be equally included in the priority queue, but, in this case, with the lowest priority, and then be immediately allocated among the last. Such criteria are normally used even in ordinary situations, outside of calamities, and with the guideline of maximizing the saving of more lives, it is highlighted in importance. Now we can already consider the problem of using age or cycles of life among the factors. They would be contemplated in objective scores that assess the probability of recovery, but if age is a factor that worsens such scores, or if the scores integrate morbidity and functionality of patients, or if there is an explicit weight, in the scores, for the cycles of life, so we will be using the age factor. One way to avoid classification directly by age or life cycle is to leave this factor for when there is a tie in age-independent clinical scores, within a certain group of patients classified in the order of the guidelines. Considering the indicated literature and in the event of scores of the same value, the tiebreaker should take the idea of the patient's cycle of life into account. In the case of COVID-19, an idea is that people aged up to 40 years old (initial cycle) have higher priority than those between 41 and 75 (intermediate cycle), and both have priority over people above that age (final cycle). This criterion allows, at the same time, in pandemics with the characteristics of COVID-19, to achieve the aim of saving more lives, since a higher age, in general, is related to a worse prognosis in the ICU (again, in COVID-19), and protecting society against the greatest loss of lives and of aggregated life years, which is normally one of the goals of health care in general. In addition, the cycle-of-life criterion expresses – this is the thesis of this chapter – impartiality in dealing with patients who have not yet gone through the expected cycles of a complete human life and suffer greater losses in terms of years to live (Emanuel et al. 2020; White 2020).

Premature death is one of the great harms of death in general. And the damage is greater than death in the final life cycle, both for the individuals affected and for society as a whole. An important observation is that the cycle-of-life criterion does not mobilize age purely and simply, as when prioritizing someone who is 54 over someone who is 57, but the age group is distributed in broad groups. Within "priority groups," there are no scores by age. Another aspect to be emphasized is the need for palliative care teams and other adequate care for patients outside the ICU. It is also imperative to have the existence of a commission for evaluation and permanent monitoring of guidelines and their application, especially if the age factor was used.

13.3 Discussing the ethics of the life cycle factor: Would it be ageism?

An immediate objection to the use of the age factor is whether the choice of "life cycles" would not be a form of age-based (wrong) discrimination. But what moral beliefs could they be based on, given our current critical awareness of the error of negatively discriminating on the basis of age? To what extent could the time of life be a value and one that substantiates the rights of the youngest over the oldest, in addition to a value that we would be justified in wanting to distribute equally? Is it possible to accept, using the equal consideration of interests, guidelines in which there would be an equal right to experience the various life cycles overriding the right to continue living of those who have already reached a certain age? The main objection seems to be that despite an overlay of good philosophy and good ethics, the use of the age factor seems to imply that the lives of all patients are not of equal value (Gonçalves and Dias 2020).

13.3.1 Equal value without factual equality?

In response to the challenges noted earlier, and starting with the last point, it can be said that equality of consideration in situations of extreme scarcity does not necessarily imply strict equality of resources, nor does it necessarily exclude prioritization based on various factors (even age) in situations of extreme scarcity. For example, young people also have the same value as the elderly, but they should be the last to receive vaccines for COVID-19, as vaccines are a preventive treatment; in this situation, it is the elderly who are most exposed to the risks and harms if they contract the disease. On the other hand, the elderly have the same value as the youngest, but it is the youngest who should receive priority in ICUs, which are curative treatment; in this situation, as we know in the case of COVID-19, it is the youngest who are most exposed to the harm of premature death (Emanuel et al. 2020; Persad 2009; Singer 2020).

There is nothing inconsistent between such prioritizations in scarcity, on the one hand, and equal consideration of interests, on the other. Remember that in an earthquake or in a nuclear accident, everyone deserves equal consideration and everyone has the same value as people, and yet, an exactly equal distribution of paramedic attention, in an emergency, is, besides imprudent (as it can leave everyone who receives the same treatment in a worse situation), irresponsible, as it risks failing to promote the benefit to a greater number of patients, or even to save a smaller portion of them (that is, the opportunity to save more people is lost). Also in war medicine, priority is given to the care of those who have a greater expectation of surviving and are younger, and it is from field war hospitals that the term *triage* comes. Well, the same scenario occurs in a potential hospital burnout in a pandemic like COVID-19.

If the greatest value is to save more lives and a basic criterion for this is the greater probability of recovery, then it makes sense that the person's social or economic condition should not matter and that social factors external to medicine need to be avoided in order to provide not only the most beneficent treatment but also to be equitable in doing so, in terms of medical ethics. Perhaps age is seen by people outside the health area as a social criterion or external to medicine, but age as a generic factor is not the criterion for considering the years of life saved in a decision related to health care: the years of lives saved are commonly considered in ethical evaluations of public health and debates in philosophy of medicine and bioethics. It should be noted that the guidelines can integrate life cycles and not gross age, partially agreeing with the mistrust and the type of criticism that is leveled at the use of the age factor; besides, it's possible to suggest that age should not be used alone, nor use such factor as something preponderant; age could only be mobilized as a tiebreaker, for instance.

13.3.2 Under what beliefs and values is this argument based?

The cycle-of-life criterion can be justified in medical terms (clinical and epidemiological), either by the specificities of a pandemic such as COVID-19 or the use of ICUs in general (again, the more cycles one has lived, in general, the expectation of surviving is lower and surviving with less treatment time, which increases the probability of dying and decreases the probability of saving more people) or because of the medical aim of extending the years of life in good health. Those who defend the consideration of cycles or even age *per se* (Beauchamp and Childress 2019; Daniels 2008; Emanuel et al. 2020; Savulescu et al. 2020; Singer 2020; White 2020) usually do this assuming that one of the goals of medicine and public health is to promote the greatest number of years of life aggregated in a given population. Even in clinical practice (individual medicine), in addition to rescue or cure, the aim is longevity with health for the person under care. This is normally accepted as a common aspect of medical practices, especially public health systems, unlike social or political criteria external to medicine, or even new criteria based on new philosophical standards or social or reparative justice; these approaches need more study and care, for being new and little experienced in medicine. Consequently, the use of life cycles is not discriminatory; therefore, it is not ageism, because years of life are not an arbitrary criterion in the case of medical treatments or health policies since the more premature the death, the greater the loss, and also the "less favored" in the case in question are those who will live less, compared to those who have already enjoyed the expected cycles in a lifetime. Equal consideration not only does not exclude prioritizing in a scenario of scarcity, but it seems to indicate, in circumstances such as COVID-19, that priority in ICUs should be given to younger people.

The age factor is not really the most appropriate factor because the most important guideline is to save more lives, and the determining criterion is the greater expectation of recovery, which is already the criterion generally adopted for intensive care medicine. People with a low probability of recovery are given lower priority in many protocols, and so far there has been no rejection or controversy around this. Both for the protocols that already existed before COVID-19, and for special guidelines in pandemics, a person that is 69 years old, but with a high probability of recovery, based on his clinical status, should still have priority over a person who is 25 years old, but with a very low probability of recovery, given his clinical status (as measured by SOFA). Age is not the most important thing. Furthermore, as we said earlier, people who are, for example, 69 years old will not automatically be given priority over people who are 61 or 56; the guideline may refer to cycles, or be used just for tiebreaking purposes, when the most important criteria are not sufficient for the triage team to make a decision.

13.3.3 Is "lifetime" an asset to want to distribute? Can a longer life become valuable in itself?

The answer is "yes" due to the previous points, but if it were not taken as part of medical criteria already used in evaluations or in medical practice, one can easily justify the perspective of priority of the youngest over the oldest for allocation of scarce resources related to saving lives. Saving lives really means extending years of lives since we're all going to die anyway. Many things happen throughout a lifetime: games, school, college, or already working; some people get married, have children, separate, remarry, get jobs or start businesses, study again, try spiritual practices, become grandparents, retire, etc. These are all valuable stages in a person's life. The cycle-of-life criterion does not discriminate against the elderly; on the contrary, it recognizes advanced age as a valuable phase of a complete human life: so valuable that the purpose of the criteria is to ensure that people have the opportunity to reach this phase as well as possible. In addition, this age factor is proposed in a protocol for an abnormal and exceptional situation of a public calamity, such as pandemics, like COVID-19.

Let's imagine that, as a society, we decide that this is not a valid criterion in general or in ordinary situations: the problem will continue to exist, at least in emergencies. That is, when the number of patients becomes significantly higher than the resources available in ICUs, health professionals will continue to have to make decisions about who to treat first. It is not an exotic intuition that premature death, in general, is more harmful or maleficent to those who die, precisely because of the years of life that death abruptly takes away from them, compared to death in seniority. And, again, seniority has already enjoyed these years (more of them), compared to those who will die prematurely. It should be noted again that in the case of the distribution of scarce vaccines, the younger life cycles should receive less priority since the older they are, the greater the importance and need for prevention. Age is simply one of the ethically important medical facts to endorse the greatest benefit if not everyone can benefit immediately.

13.3.4 *Can the right to live more years for some people legitimately overcome the right to continue living for others?*

Despite the various reasons listed in favor of the reasonableness of the cycle-of-life criterion, we recognize that it is an issue legitimately controversial. It was even criticized and, in some places, withdrawn from the initially proposed criteria (AMIB and ABRAMEDE 2020), justifying this in part to make the protocol more representative of current moral values (AMIB 2020). However, not once was it stated that young people have *more rights* to live longer than elderly people to continue living, or that, merely because they are younger, they have the right to reach the life cycles that would be cut off by the disease. This is not an argument about who has more rights to something; it is an argument about what is best to do in extraordinary circumstances. That is, if we have to choose between someone younger and someone older, both having the same prognosis, which medical outcome would be worse, saving the younger one or saving the older one? Failing to give some priority to saving those who would live longer (if attended sooner) has as a possible consequence (and, unfortunately, more likely in cases such as COVID-19) the death of the youngest in favor of the shorter survival of the oldest. The decision concerns considerations about how to get the best results with the available resources, given the impossibility of achieving the best outcome – saving or offering the best probability of saving equally to both or even saving everyone (Savalescu and Wilkinson 2020).

Some people suggested that the age factor was "contaminated" by a capitalist bias, such as the concern with mere productivity in the market, and that it was being assumed uncritically. As I said earlier, we must completely agree that one should not consider the higher or lower "social value of an individual" when dealing with medical rationing and that their socioeconomic status should not be an allocation criterion. This is also true for a socialist or strongly social-democratic society. In this sense, the introduction of values external to *medical utility* is difficult to justify and opens the door to all kinds of arbitrariness. Nevertheless, as we have seen, cycle of life fits rationally both in scenarios such as those of COVID-19 (higher mortality due to older age) and in the already conventional standards of health assessment and public health systems (weighting of aggregated life years). This is a central part of the explanations for the several protocols suggested or already in force, even in countries that are champions of concern for the elderly and vulnerable and with solid universalized public systems, such as Italy, Spain, England, Germany, and others, which mobilize the criterion of age. Hence, living longer is a good criterion for assessing the medical benefit, and if we were to think in terms of rights, the right to live the life cycles not yet lived by some can legitimately overlap, in conflict of interests given scarcity, the right to continue living for those who have already enjoyed the same cycles, those *who have lived longer* (Singer 2020).

An important remark concerns the observation that the acceptance of the age factor, especially the cycle-of-life criterion, is not the result of broad social consensus. An example would be the fact that the Brazilian AMIB and ABRAMED, after a debate with many medical associations and jurists, gave up the criterion of life cycles (and draw) in the second version of their recommendations. However, one can still propose the discussion of the age factor as a contribution to the debate, which may or may not result in a consensus, and is also a contribution to government and health authorities competent to establish emergency protocols. This competence is also part of democratic institutions and the democratic-constitutional regime such as the current ones and, as there is in many places, the competence of national or regional medical councils. Councils in developed and some developing countries (such as Brazil) normally already use survival and weighting of aggregated life years as central allocation components, which shows that it is not the case that no one has agreed to the use of the age factor. Everyone also generally agrees with the guideline of maximizing the life-saving benefit. According to what was established by a Brazilian state medical council (by Resolution CREMERS 2020), by the principle of benefit,

> urgency and utility are weighed, *considering the survival of the population of people with indication of receiving the resource* (including the cases that will receive it and those that will not), *with the aim of*

producing the greatest impact on the survival of that population as a whole and not of particular individuals. Thus, according to this logic, *priority is given to cases with the greatest difference between life expectancies if they receive or if they do not receive the resource.*

We must endorse this without fear of ageism.

Acknowledgments

The author greatly appreciates the contributions of Darlei Dall`Agnol, Marco Azevedo, and Marcelo Araújo in the discussion group Dilemmas COVID-19, from which originated the research initiative Bioethics, Distributive Justice, and Pandemics, funded by CNPq (Grant Nr. 409953/2022-9).

References

AMIB: Associação de Medicina Intensiva Brasileira. 2020. *Protocolo AMIB de alocação de recursos em esgotamento durante a pandemia por COVID-19.* URL https://www.amib.org.br/fileadmin/user_upload/amib/2020/abril/24/ Protocolo_AMIB_de_alocacao_de_recursos_em_esgotamento_durante_a_ pandemia_por_COVID-19.pdf.

AMIB: Associação de Medicina Intensiva Brasileira and ABRAMED, Associação Brasileira de Medicina de Emergência. 2020. *Recomendações de alocação de recursos em esgotamento durante a pandemia de COVID-19.* URL https:// crmsc.org.br/wp-content/uploads/2020/08/Versa%CC%83o-2-0106- Protocolo-AMIB-de-alocac%CC%A7a%CC%83o-de-recursos-em- esgotamento-durante-a-pandemia-por-COVID.pdf

Azevedo, M. A., Bonella, A. E., Dall'Agnol, D., Araújo, M. 2020. Diretrizes para alocação de tratamento em UTI durante a pandemia por Covid-19. *Crítica na Rede.* URL https://criticanarede.com/covid-uti.html

——— 2021. Repensando a ética da alocação de recursos hospitalares escassos durante a pandemia da covid-19. In: Rosario, M. C., Azevedo, M. A. *Anais dos XXXIII Colóquio Internacional de Filosofia Unisinos e IV Simpósio de Filosofia da Medicina.* (São Leopoldo, Editora da Unisinos), pp. 04–32.

Beauchamp, Tom and Childress, James. 2019. *Principles of Biomedical Ethics* (New York: Oxford University Press).

Center for Law, Medicine and Life Sciences. 2020. *COVID-19: Literature on the Legal and Ethical Issues Facing Front-Line* (Cambridge: University of Cambridge Healthcare Professionals)

CREMERS: Conselho Regional de Medicina do Estado do Rio Grande do Sul. 2020. *Resolução CREMERS n° 13/2020.* URL https://cremers.org.br/wp- content/uploads/2021/04/Resolucao-no-13-2020-1.pdf

Daniels, N. 2008. *Just Health: Meeting Health Needs Fairly* (Cambridge: Cambridge University Press).

Emanuel, E. J., Persad, G., Upshup, R., et al. 2020. "Fair allocation of scarce medical resources in the time of COVID-19." *New England Journal of Medicine*, 382: 2049–2055, DOI: 10.1056/NEJMsb2005114

Ferreira, F. L.; Bota, D. P.; Bross, A.; Mélot, C.; Vincent, J. 2001. "Serial evaluation of the SOFA score to predict outcome in critically ill patients". *JAMA: The Journal of the American Medical Association*, 286(14): 1754–1758, DOI: 10.1001/jama.286.14.1754.

Gonçalves, Letícia; Dias, M. C. 2020. "Discussões bioéticas sobre a alocação de recursos durante a pandemia da COVID-19 no Brasil." *Revista Diversitates International Journal, DIVERSITATES, v. 12, 18.*

Persad, G. 2009. "Evaluating the legality of age-based criteria in health care: From non-discrimination and discretion to distributive justice." *Boston College Law Review*, 60(3): 889–949.

Savulescu, Julian; Cameron, James; Wilkinson. 2020. "Equality or utility? Ethics and law of rationing ventilators". *British Journal Anaesthesia*, 125(1): 10–15, DOI: 10.1016/j.bja.2020.04.011.

Savalescu, Julian; Wilkinson, Douglas. 2020. *Who Gets the Ventilator in the Coronavirus Pandemic? These Are the Ethical Approaches to Allocating Medical Care.* Australian Corporation News. URL: https://www.abc.net.au/news/2020-03-18/ethics-of-medical-care-ventilator-in-the-coronavirus-pandemic/12063536

Singer, Peter. 2020. *Is Age Discrimination Acceptable?* Project-Syndicate. URL: https://www.project-syndicate.org/commentary/when-is-age-discrimination-acceptable-by-peter-singer-2020-06?barrier=accesspaylog

White, Douglas B. 2020. *A Model Hospital Policy for Allocating Scarce Critical Care Resources.* University of Pittsburgh School of Medicine. University of Pittsburgh, Department of care medicine. URL: https://ccm.pitt.edu/sites/default/files/UnivPittsburgh_ModelHospitalResourcePolicy_2020_04_15.pdf. Acesso em 16/04/2020.

White, Douglas B., Lo, Bernard. 2020. "A framework for rationing ventilators and critical care beds during the COVID-19 pandemic." *JAMA: The Journal of the American Medical Association*, 323(18): 1773–1774, DOI: 10.1001/jama.2020.5046.

Part IV

After COVID-19 life: Some moral issues

14 Faces of responsibility and moral agency in a pandemic age

Evandro Barbosa and Thaís Alves Costa

14.1 The burden of responsibility in a pandemic

Pandemics are not a new phenomenon in human history; therefore, it should come as no surprise that the same infectious agent has more than once generated some pandemic or minor health crisis. As an illustration, the pathogen Yersinia pestis caused three pandemics throughout history: Justinian's Plague, the Black Death, and the Third Plague (Piret and Boivin 2021, Table 1). Only cholera, caused by the pathogen Vibrio cholerae, was the scene of several outbreaks; influenza (with its variants) was responsible for six pandemics, and SARS-CoV variant 2 was responsible for the COVID-19.

This scenario brings the light how many pests remain dormant and, at some point, explode and reach different levels of public health emergencies. Fortunately, scientific progress allows us to address and prevent pandemics more effectively. Consider for a moment pandemics in different historical periods. Take the plague of Justinian (541–544) or the Black Death (1334–1353). During these times, epidemiological knowledge and sanitary measures were lacking compared to the present day. The term "virus" did not even exist then, and it is hard to see how we can hold the people of those times accountable for circumstances that were out of their control (Gage and Kosoy 2005).

By the time of the 1918 influenza our health practices and our understanding of diseases were better; for example, measures for controlling the spread of disease had become better known (Reid et al. 1999; Johnson and Mueller 2002). Political and health authorities in particular had more robust epidemiological science at their disposal, which allowed for more efficient efforts to fight the epidemic.

Now fast-forward a century and consider COVID-19. It is undeniable that we now have much greater knowledge about sanitation and about the causes and effects of pandemics. The rapid identification of the virus and its modes of transmission and the rapid pace at which a vaccine was created demonstrate current scientists' extensive expertise. We now are, or should be, even better able to control epidemics (see Rosen 1993; Porter 1997).

DOI: 10.4324/9781003310129-18

The fact is that challenging contexts like the pandemic make room for inevitable moral debate about the scope of our responsibility in avoiding or reducing them. Since we have more knowledge about how epidemiological crises work and because COVID-19 is a collective phenomenon, the burden of responsibility must be shared among all pandemic agents. The point is how it should be done.

The main purpose of this chapter is to develop an approach that will help us determine the degree of moral responsibility an individual moral agent has to mitigate the effects of a pandemic. We will begin with an overview of how moral agency and responsibility function during pandemics, locating the pandemic itself, the agents involved, and the types of responsibility they may have in a systematic framework that can serve as a foundation for the remainder of the chapter. In Section 14.2, we present the types of pandemic agents and their duties of prevention and mitigation as preparedness and as response. Section 14.3 sheds light on the moral and nonmoral considerations necessary to establish a metric for individual moral responsibility: (a) the external conditions in which the agents find themselves, including the pandemic's severity level; (b) types of institutional incentive, from the top to the bottom; and (c) moral consideration for the harm principle. By considering all these elements together, we aim to establish an acceptable metric for assigning individual moral responsibility during pandemics in Section 14.4.

14.2 The big picture: Agents and responsibilities

Let us now consider how agents and their responsibilities fit into the big picture. As we mentioned, a pandemic is a collective problem with different agents acting at different levels. We suggest dividing these agents into three categories according to their functions in playing the *pandemic game*.

1   **Institutional agents,** including global actors (like the United Nations and World Health Organization), sovereign states, leaders, political agents,[1] and the scientific community
2   **Social agents,** which include corporations,[2] the media, religious organizations, civic associations, social leaders, and social influencers[3]
3   **Personal agents,** which include individuals in general.[4] They can be usefully distinguished by two factors:
    a   The levels of information they possess: well-informed, informed, ill-informed, or biasedly informed (for example, by "fake news")
    b   Their environments: their levels of social, biological, psychological, and economic vulnerability

Just as the pandemic is part of our moral landscape, so are all of the agents involved. It is crucial to establish their duties.[5]

1   The **Duty of Prevention** (*DP*): responsibility for developing and taking a set of measures to avoid damage or harm. In the case of a pandemic, it is about acting to prevent future pandemics.

2   The **Duty of Mitigation as Preparedness** (*DMP*): responsibility for a set of actions that aim to prepare the state and its citizens to face future pandemics. In such cases, good preparation can mitigate the worst consequences of any future pandemic.

3   The **Duty of Mitigation as Response** (*DMR*): responsibility for creating conditions to reduce the intensity or severity of an ongoing phenomenon such as a pandemic, making it less painful by mitigating the harms of the situation.

The combination of agents and duties generates different types of responsibilities regarding the pandemic as a moral phenomenon in itself or as a generator of such phenomena (see Chapter 01). In a broad sense, the duties of prevention and of mitigation as preparedness are directly related to the pandemic itself as a moral phenomenon. In turn, the DMR concerns phenomena or circumstances connected to a pandemic, rather than the pandemic itself. Although our primary purpose is to establish a metric for individual moral responsibility in the face of the last duty, let us first consider the connection between agents and all their respective responsibilities.

We generally expect all actors to take some responsibility for making efforts to prevent or mitigate the effects of a pandemic; however, each position has different demands. Think about institutional agents and the DMR in relation to the COVID-19 situation. The first concrete decision of the WHO in this case was to declare SARS-CoV-2 type of global emergency.[6] The WHO's responsibility consisted of informing the global community that we were officially in a pandemic and recommending the first measures governments should make to contain the virus and mitigate the damage occurring. Institutional agents such as the WHO are at the top level of the chain of agents. Since DMR concerns "creating conditions to reduce the intensity or severity of an ongoing phenomenon," it is expected institutional agents assume a general responsibility for expanding efforts to deal with the pandemic's effects.

As COVID-19 is a worldwide viral spread, there is a global interest in preventing the virus from spreading further. Control measures, often varying based on the regions in which they occur, have ranged from restricting travel between countries, regions, and cities to the most robust (and perhaps effective) measure: total social isolation from other individuals. Additional measures for production and control of the supply of health resources such as masks, gloves, and medicines have also been taken in response to the DMR. In a nutshell, this duty requires institutional commitment because each measure taken at this high level produces a ripple effect.

Institutional agents have also the DP and mitigation as preparedness concerning the pandemic itself. According to Naomi Zack's (2009) account of disaster-preparation planning (in which pandemics count as disasters), fulfilling the moral duty of preparedness is similar to preparing for a "mystery marathon." The competitor cannot accurately predict all the conditions for the day of the race, but still, he or she can understand the general conditions for it, like the distance of the race, the probable weather, and the type of terrain. Such information is critical for good preparation. Madhav et al. (2017) warns that while each global health emergency requires its own response, this does not prevent us from thinking about strategies that could apply during multiple pandemics, which they call "common prerequisites for effective response."

Despite having information about past pandemics and several recent epidemics, especially the most recent avian influenza, we cannot say we are fully prepared for SARS-CoV-2 with good mitigation strategies. Although the scientific community did its part and warned about the danger of future outbreaks, there was no significant response from institutional agents in terms of preparedness to mitigate possible consequences. COVID would have been difficult to deal with under any circumstances, but the lack of institutional preparation for the first pandemic of the 21st century made its effects far more devastating than they had to be. As a result, the severe impact of institutional agents' unpreparedness demonstrates how much responsibility they had, and have, for mitigation.

The DP concerns the responsibility – associated with their ability – that institutional agents have to identify the potential viral spread risk of a pathogen about its effects and transmission capacity. One particular strategy used by One Health approach (OHC 2020; Rabozzi et al. 2012; Okello et al. 2011) is a good option example: it considers the ability to count as what Madhav et al. (2017) call a pandemic spark by jointly considering human health, animal health, and the environment:

> One Health's activities include the surveillance of zoonotic pathogens of pandemic potential at the human-animal interface, dynamic evolution modeling, risk assessments of zoonotic pathogens, and other methods of understanding the interaction between environmental changes and pathogen emergence.
>
> (Madhav et al. 2017, 327)[7]

Even preventive measures were not on global agents' menu for the emergence of COVID-19 once duties of prevention and mitigation as preparedness did not occur systematically despite warnings from the scientific community about a possible plague/epidemic on a global scale. De Araujo (2021) presents five different scenario modelings of epidemics and pandemics (Exercise Cygnus in 2016, Clade X in 2018–2019, Crimson Contagion in 2019, and Event 201: A Global Pandemic Exercise in 2019). The conclusions from these tests indicated the discharge probability of a pandemic and that, in short, we were not adequately prepared to face it.

One of the conclusions of the Independent Panel report (2020, 15) indicated this: "It is clear to the Panel that the world was not prepared and had ignored warnings which resulted in a massive failure: an outbreak of SARS-CoV-2 became a devastating pandemic."[8]

The role of science is pivotal in combating a infectious disease. On one side, the scientific community can be understood as an institutional agent because of its direct connection from an organizational and financial point of view with the state (see Ball 2021). On the other, many institutions and members of this community seem to be well accommodated as social agents. The key is to understand your role in dealing with an outbreak hazard. They possess and produce knowledge about possible future pandemics. However, they are indirectly or conditioned accountable because institutional agents must provide means to build such expertise and warn of potential future pandemic risks. In essence they are not responsible for adopting prevention or mitigation measures in preparation or response. It is the role of institutional actors to do that, and it is up to science to alert and instruct on the best path (see Lavazza and Farina 2020).

The bottom line is that the scientific community plays a critical role in understanding, managing, and ultimately mitigating the effects of infectious diseases possibilities like COVID-19. When a new virus or disease emerges, scientists are often among the first to identify it, study its characteristics, and develop strategies to contain its spread. For that, scientists around the world have collaborated and shared data to accelerate the development of vaccines – with some vaccines being developed in record time. As a result, Organisation for Economic Co-operation and Development (OECD, n.d.) data indicate that between January and November 2020, approximately 75,000 scientific publications related to COVID-19 were published (see Malekpour et al. 2021). Likewise, during the SARS-CoV-2 outbreak the scientific community has been at the forefront of efforts to develop effective vaccines, treatments, and testing protocols. In addition to developing medical interventions, scientists have also played a crucial role in communicating pivotal information about the virus and how to prevent its spread. Among another things, they have provided guidance on social distancing measures, mask wearing, and other preventive measures while combating misinformation and rumors about the virus. This highlights the importance of developing our scientific culture as "the soil in which science and technology grow" (Han 2020, 226).

Another relevant fact is the imbalance in what Madhav et al. call the global distribution of epidemic preparedness (2017, Map. 17.1): the richer the state, the better prepared it is; on the other hand, less economic power indicates less preparation. When consulting the investments made by governments on topics such as the pandemic, we realized that some countries could have spent more energy on preparation or even preventive measures for these cases (see Chan et al. 2010). One of the problems is that contexts of alert and greater risk are in developing countries, so global help for this control would be advantageous. The duty of preparation binds agents to take measures to avoid future pandemics and their associated phenomena. Therefore, agents' level of responsibility can be determined according to their commitment to this duty. Given that, we can say that institutional agents failed in preventing the pandemic we are facing now. If its effects are more significant today than they might have been, it is these agents' responsibility. Also, as the DMP was not effectively fulfilled, mitigation as response needed to be more aggressive.

Above all things, COVID-19 has highlighted the limited and neglectful way states and nations have dealt with pandemic preparedness. As we can see, there are some gaps there. Although global agents have the role of coordinating international efforts to address an infectious outbreak possibility, it is states that have the duty to put those global recommendations into practice. Institutional agents like WHO and the scientific community can provide data on how best to deal with a public health crisis; the World Bank can provide the necessary financial resources to implement these determinations. But responsibility then passes to the state, which must inform itself and take the actions necessary to protect its citizens from the most severe consequences of the pandemic. The state is the intermediary between the global effort and the attitudes of social and individual agents within (and perhaps outside) its territory. States have the most relevant political and legal authority to act that other agents do not have. To sum up, it is up to them in their role as institutional actors to offer some basic mitigation measures, both in preparation and in response to pandemics.

For instance, the guidelines prepared by the WHO (2020) are widely acknowledged as proving the importance of institutional agents assuming their roles in the face of a pandemic. This responsibility comprises many elements. First, we need an efficient supply chain for essential goods. Second, robust health systems (mainly primary care) are needed to intervene at crucial points (detection of disease outbreaks, essential care, support for vaccine distribution, and medical countermeasures). Third, it is vital an efficient surveillance system to detect potential risk factors related to zoonotic pathogens at the human-animal interface. Fourth, there must be an efficient mechanism for coordination among relevant groups: states, the scientific community, health systems, economies, and other social entities. Fifth, it is essential to maintain a good information network, making individuals aware of the dangers pandemics represent (this role is amplified by the joint action of social actors, especially the media). Finally, states should consider using available economic means to mitigate direct and indirect consequences for their citizens, especially those citizens in the most vulnerable conditions – one example is the financial aid that some countries have adopted to facilitate more effective social isolation measures. As we will discuss later, such measures have made it easier for agents to fulfill their individual duties. Campaigns to contain contagion demand an extended or coextensive responsibility, and it is up to the state to offer the minimum conditions necessary for individuals to engage in containing the virus. This brief report paints a rather gloomy picture of the role and responsibility of institutional actors.

Next, let us consider the duties of social agents, a varied group that plays different social roles with different degrees of responsibility. Overall, they aim to sustain the work that began with institutional agents since they are one of the most efficient informational channels between institutions and individual agents. The scope of their action is broad, but we will focus on social agents that directly interfere with the informational level and vulnerability of individual agents: (a) mass media, (b) religion, (c) large corporations, and (d) social leaders. And although other agents exert influence, these are the four main social agents that move the chains towards an essential gear in the dissemination of information based on institutional policies. We can determine social agents' relevance to pandemic duties by analyzing their level of impact on personal agents.

(a) Mass media has a decisive role in accessing and sharing good information and avoiding distortions and the dangers of fake news; after all, they work to connect institutional and individual agents with the scientific community. During COVID-19, misinformation and fake news campaigns led by anti-vaccine movements and COVID denialist groups have been a pervasive negative force in the informational landscape.

(b) Religion has also served as an important social agent, mainly by offering spiritual comfort. Research also indicates the informational importance that religion can play throughout a pandemic. Its influence has a positive – endorsing vaccination campaigns against the coronavirus as Pope Francis did – or negative impact by supporting anti-scientific positions in some minority cases (see McElwee 2021; Galang 2021; Gopez 2021; and Hegarty 2022). Religions are social agents with a crucial role in many individuals' lives, and their roles are not scientific regarding a pandemic responsibility. Despite of its social function is another, it does not mean they have no duty to provide and communicate truthful information about the pandemic and avoid distortions or misinformation.

We can also consider (c) large corporations. Given their economic power, they have a responsibility to act in line with institutional recommendations that are supported supported by science. The duty of mitigation as a response is a sensitive point in this equation. We expect accountability from institutional actors, but it is challenging to balance conflicting interests. Counteracting the spread of COVID-19, a respiratory syndrome whose aerial transmission rate is high, has required social distancing and isolation by lockdown during the most acute phase. But lockdowns have had a very negative impact on the economy. This tension generated endless debates between the economic and scientific fields, as everyone sought to establish a metric for adequately containing the virus without seriously harming the economy. Political actors inflamed things further when they encouraged this type of dispute and, in some cases, neglected warnings from infectious disease experts, epidemiologists, and other scientists.

This is important for one simple reason. According to World Bank (2023), around 3.32 billion workers worldwide, meaning about half of the population, exercise a trade formally or informally. In many cases, jobs require leaving home and interacting with other people rather than virtually. Therefore, any adjustment in this large body of work directly affects the conditions for preventing and controlling the pandemic. Alternatives such as a home office and a good sanitary environment for workers were some of the options adopted. Even maintaining workers' wages was an incentive to stay at home and protect themselves.

As large corporations employ a large number of individuals and coordinate the economic dimension of society, the attitude they take in the face of a challenging pandemic directly interferes with the lives of many individual agents. In this sense, no exemption or omission on their part is possible when a large portion of the population is vulnerable. Therefore, the labor market – led by large corporations – has pandemic duties too.

(d) In addition to the mass media and large corporations, relevant social agents include individuals who can assemble and influence large portions of the population, such as social and religious leaders and even figures with great popular appeal. As their power of persuasion is high, they can decisively interfere in social behavior during a pandemic, positively or negatively.[9] The Kardashians clan, who have more than one billion followers worldwide, can represent this power of influence. On average, one in seven inhabitants of the planet reads or views their social media posts. A single tweet by Kylie Jenner, one of the Kardashian sisters, complaining about Snapchat caused Snap Inc., the parent company of Snapchat, to lose $1.3 billion in market value (Hern 2018). Jenner was not the only reason for this loss, but it is hard to imagine that such power would influence other areas of life, including public attitudes and behaviors during a pandemic.

Regarding the coronavirus, we had a significant number of public figures encouraging vaccination and protective measures, suggesting that their followers observe the duties of prevention, especially the duty of mitigation in response. On the other hand, COVID denialist and anti-vaccine groups proliferated and rallied a portion of the population to obscurantism throughout the pandemic, often through socially known figures. These groups pose a considerable risk to the social order.

This social domain opens the floor for several figures with a social appeal. Bolsonaro, president of Brazil during the pandemic, is a paradigmatic case with over 58 million social media followers. This number represents about one-fourth of the Brazilian population. His denialist tones had a crucial impact on how Brazilians deal with the pandemic. According to De Arruda et al.'s (2021) research, the Brazilian president's denialist rhetoric inhibited greater adherence by the population to control measures. As a result, they estimate that 318,805.03 cases of infection could have been avoided, and around 10,000 lives could have been saved. This is the power and responsibility of those who exercise this social and political leadership.

Therefore, it is undeniable that some responsibility falls on these social agents, even if we do not precisely know the degree. It can be a positive attitude by alerting to the pandemic or a negative one by denying its importance. Even place neutrality carries the weight of an omission in the face of prevention and mitigation duties. In short, social agents play a decisive role, but their duties differ from those of institutional agents. They are not typically responsible for the coordination of efforts to prepare for or respond to pandemics. But still, these agents' social role does require them to take certain actions or avoid certain attitudes when they are duly called upon to do so by legal, political, or social institutional agents.[10]

Finally, the individual agents are at the base of the pyramid and have broad responsibility for prevention and mitigation. Although in many moments they are responsive to the guidance and information that came from institutional and social agents, it does not mean putting aside responsibility at the individual level, just that the pandemic scenario conditions it.

Think about agent responsibilities in the pandemic context. For example, the duty of prevention requires individuals to follow certain sanitary measures established by the state and other global institutions. Similarly, adequate preparedness requires sanitary measures that will drive agents' behavior to mitigate future effects. Or, in an ongoing pandemic, mitigation as a response requires individuals to comply with efforts to reduce the negative impact immediately.

An accurate analysis looming over that point indicates that taking action is individual, but the choice cannot be based on subjective criteria. In this sense, the pandemic context matters to determine the level of vulnerability and access to information that individual agents have at that time. The information they receive affects how respective agents will engage with their duties; hence, misinformation or the lack of information tends to lower individuals' level of commitment. Individual exposure or riskiness also matters since a person with high vulnerability conditions may face more significant challenges in fulfilling a specific prevention or mitigation role, making it difficult for us to create a fair metric of duties.

As we will see in the next section, the degree of responsibility in such situations is conditional upon how institutional and other collective agents fulfill their duties. The more effectively institutional agents perform their role, the more strongly individuals are bound to their duties.

Still, even when institutions and social agents do their part, there are no guarantees that individuals will fulfill their roles because individuals' level of responsibility does not rely merely on external conditions. The burden of responsibility persists under more or less favorable conditions; what changes is the weight of that responsibility.

For now, consider a systematizing framework:

Level	Agents	Responsibility (Pandemic Itself)	Responsibility (Inside)
Institutional Agents (Main Global Agents)	WHO UN Wealthier nations	DP* DMP* DMR*	DMR
Institutional (State or Nation)	Political leaders and agents Scientific community	DP DMP DMR	DMR
Social Agents	Religion Associations Employers (big corporations)	DP DMP DMR	DMR
	Press Leaders Social influencers (different kinds)	Conditional Duty**	Conditional Duty
Individual Agents	Well-informed Informed Poorly informed Misinformed by fake news	DP DMP DMR	DMR
	In conditions of vulnerability (social/biological/psychological/economic/etc.)	Conditional Duty	Conditional Duty

* DP: Duty of Prevention
  DMP: Duty of Mitigation as Preparedness
  DMR: Duty of Mitigation as Response
** It is a conditional duty because the responsibility of these agents depends on institutional agents and some setups.

14.3 A metric for individual responsibility

The large picture presented allowed putting the pieces in their proper place, stating the types of agents and their respective duties in a pandemic. Let's focus on offering criteria for determining individual agents' level of responsibility in relation to the duty of mitigation as a response. For that, we suggest considering the pandemic as a nonideal circumstance. Nonideal circumstances concern individuals' constraints when carrying out their responsibilities based on the pandemic severity and the kind of incentives they receive from the top agents. After that, we will also use the harm principle to determine the personal responsibility level of actions taken in these circumstances.

14.3.1 Level of severity in a pandemic context

Several studies indicate that individuals' context affects both the rational and the emotional elements of their decision-making (Barbosa 2022; Huijsmans et al. 2019; Kim and Grady 2020; Mani et al. 2013; Marshall 2020; Morton 2017). As the influence of a pandemic is negative, it creates nonideal circumstances that impair individuals' agency.

One way to analyze the challenge pandemic context is by its severity at a given moment. It allows us to categorize different phases of it as harder or softer based on some guide marks:

(T) Virus's transmissibility rate
(C) Capacity of the health system to handle the infected
(L) Level of disease lethality

Let us call these the *TCL* criteria. For the first one, a common strategy to identify the transmissibility rate (T) of a disease under certain conditions is to use the reproduction number. It serves to identify the potential for spreading the virus. If the reproduction number is greater than 1, each infected person transmits the disease to at least one more person. In this case, there is an increase in the spread of the virus. But if the reproduction number is less than 1, then the number of infected is decreasing, indicating that transmission is under control, reducing the pressure on the health system and flattening the curve (Achaiah and Subbarajasetty 2020). In turn, to identify the health system's capacity (C), we can use the Structure Efficiency Index as a reference or the elements of outbreak capacity like staff, materials, structures, and systems (see WHO 2020; Izmirlieva 2020; Silva et al. 2020). Finally, the Case Fatality Rate is an efficient metric to identify the lethality level of diseases (L) like the coronavirus, although there is room for improvement (Abou Ghayda et al. 2022; Rinaldi and Paradisi 2020; Wilson et al. 2020).

These criteria can vary but understanding their importance for agents' choices under nonideal circumstances matters. For example, determining the severity level is an efficient way to help institutional agents estimate the risks of spreading and take control of measures, such as social distancing, wearing a mask, or lockdown. When the transmission rate is low, the health system is more likely to be able to support the number of infected patients. This does not necessarily mean that a high transmission rate indicates a collapse of the health-care system because the capacity of health systems depends on the structure and resources of each region or country. However, a high transmission rate combined with overload of the health system indicates that we have entered a harder phase of the pandemic. In such a situation, the health-care system could collapse, and the fatality level could rise considerably. Then, agents are called upon to act to prevent this from happening.

Once agents' actions are influenced by context, individual agents' responsibility flows steadily according to the corresponding pandemic's severity level. If *TCL* criteria determine a harder phase, then individual responsibility increases and control measures are mandatory. Most regions have experienced such conditions at least once during the COVID outbreak and have required measures such as mask wearing, social distancing, and lockdowns. During these harder phases, the most effective mitigation measures should be presented as something more than mere recommendations. Since the duty of mitigation as a response requires conditions to reduce the severity of an ongoing phenomenon, individual agents must follow the health protocols precisely in order to fulfill this duty. Therefore, responsibility cannot be diminished and there is little or no room for maneuvering for individuals not to follow their pandemic duty.[11]

All in all, *TCL* criteria to measure the severity of the pandemic are crucial to determining a good metric for individual responsibility. However, its accuracy is not at stake here. What matters for our purposes is to demonstrate that context matters for taking action. Once we assume that the pandemic environment puts decisive pressure on individual agents, then we can state that external conditions determine – even if indirectly – the internal conditions of agents and the consequent decision-making (Barbosa 2022). As a consequence, we can say that agents' responsibility toward the duty of mitigation as a response to COVID-19 or any other pandemic is conditioned.

14.3.2 Incentives: From the top to the bottom

As we said, individual agents in a pandemic make choices that take into account their context, so neglecting such circumstances blurs our understanding of it as a kind of context challenger. One way to get around this issue is to offer some incentives from the aforementioned for individuals to fulfill their pandemic duties. At this moment, institutional agents come into play, mainly the states; after all, they have an institutional responsibility to provide incentives for individuals to mitigate the effects of a pandemic.

For that, it is essential to understand that individual agents are at different levels of information and vulnerability. In the previous section, we mentioned the role of institutional agents in promoting an appropriate informational level for agents – going directly through the type of information that social agents bring to them. We know that certain incentive campaigns are important as an attempt to promote new health and care habits among agents (Snitow and Brennan 2011).

Whatever incentives or punishments are chosen, it is important to offer informational incentives that can positively affect the choice of individual agents.[12] This encouragement comes in the form of knowledge and scientific advice. A large-scale publicity campaign explaining the effects of the pandemic is crucial for individuals to understand the big picture. Furthermore, if they are encouraged to fulfill their mitigation duty in response via vaccination and social distancing, then the challenging context will be less threatening. One of the tasks of these incentives is to promote a call for pandemic duty and a wave of responsibility. In this sense, when institutional and social agents foster a sense of commitment through incentives, the chances of promoting this wave are much more significant. In addition, incentives of this nature via access to knowledge also serve as a shield for anti-science and anti-vaccination groups, which promote disincentives on the role of individuals in belittling or reducing the impact of a pandemic on society. As a result, the bond of responsibility is broken, which means less sense of duty.

And moving forward, it turns out that individuals in vulnerable conditions are in a more challenging position to fulfill their duties in facing what many have called the "pandemic of inequality" (Nassif-Pires et al. 2020a). The World Bank identified that the poorest people (with the lowest incomes) had the most significant economic losses throughout it and are also the ones that take the longest to recover their financial condition. This inequality is also manifested in the deaths caused by the virus. A study (Sidik 2022) carried out in the United States shows that the mortality rate between groups is also unequal – the fatality rate of American Indians is about 108% higher than that of whites and nearly 180% higher than that of Asian descendants.

Another factor that aggravates the situation is associated with the severity of multiple deprivations that certain groups or people face – similar to the Index of Multiple Deprivation tracks.[13] Areas or neighborhoods with a low average salary of workers, low educational level, and high crime rate tend to suffer more aggressively from the consequences of the virus – "due, for instance, to lack of paid sick leave, dependency on public transportation, inability to afford quarantine, and residency in smaller dwellings sharing space with more people" (Nassif-Pires et al. 2020b, 3). These consequences include considerable financial loss and increased rates of transmissibility and mortality.

All these elements demonstrates that correct sanitary measures cannot be applied alone. The state must offer incentives and create conditions for individual agents to fulfill their pandemic duties – in this case, the duty of mitigation as a response. Virtually all countries have adopted direct or indirect financial support measures for their citizens. So, suppose the state executes its institutional responsibility correctly by, for instance, offering financial assistance for individuals to stay home and avoid contaminating or being contaminated by social contact. If the state has provided the necessary conditions to make good decisions, individuals have far less justification for making excuses or requesting exceptions to avoid participating in the lockdown.

On the other hand, when institutional agents do not fulfill the duty to protect their citizens, the duties of individuals become much more difficult to carry out. As we live in a money-based society, we should draw attention to the fact that, according to the International Monetary Fund, a cumulative loss of $13.8 trillion is estimated by 2024. (see WHO 2020). Also, there are countries with a high rate of inequality and low working and salary conditions, which are more hostile environments – individuals are surrounded by nonideal circumstances. Now, consider lockdown in these situations. In the struggle between health and the economy, many examples demonstrated how the scales tipped toward the economic side for the most vulnerable groups who found themselves facing a dilemma: break the lockdown to go to work or properly respect sanitary measures. That explains why vulnerable individuals have a lower tolerance for the effects of lockdown. Consequently, they are less disposed to more extended periods of isolation, as the economic losses suffered are considerable for their way of life and survival. While everyone was asked to stay at home without the proper incentive, individual responsibility before the duty of mitigation cannot be the same for everyone without distinction.

We need to understand how there is a correlation between the state's duty to promote "good pandemic policies" for mitigation and the role of individuals in this process. This explains how important context and external conditions are in determining the question of moral responsibility during pandemics. There is a difficult metric to establish here. The greater the vulnerability conditions, the greater the degree of difficulty in following public health guidelines may be.

Pandemic duties work to guide individual agent actions in a pandemic. However, while institutional agents are independent of other agents in their choices, the same does not happen with individual agents. It is up to institutional agents – especially the state – to provide information and appropriate conditions that allow decision-making by individual agents in a consistent manner. By failing to offer these incentives, individuals leave what would be the best position for the moment. At that point, their choices are limited, and their liability appears to be limited or lessened considerably.

14.3.3 The harm principle

Amid the ongoing pandemic, we have observed how nonideal circumstances can impede our actions. However, we have also come to understand the significance of incentives provided by both institutional and social agents in motivating individuals to take individual responsibility. The severity of the pandemic and the incentives presented for its mitigation highlight the challenge that individual agents face in fulfilling their duty to curb its effects. This challenge arises from the fact that the pandemic is a collective phenomenon where individual actions directly impact the lives of others.

So, how can we justify the moral significance of individuals fulfilling their pandemic duties? One approach to comprehending and justifying this moral relevance involves evaluating the harm that our actions may inflict on others utilizing Mill's harm principle. According to this principle, "the only legitimate reason for exerting power over any member of a civilized society against their will is to prevent harm to others" (Mill 1859, I).

Overall, observing the duty of mitigation as a response is a way of fulfilling the harm principle. By taking preventive measures, such as wearing a mask, practicing physical distancing, and getting vaccinated, individuals can help reduce the spread of the virus and protect vulnerable populations from harm. Moreover, failing to observe the duty of mitigation as a response can result in harm to others, especially those who are more vulnerable, such as the elderly, immunocompromised individuals, and essential workers. Therefore, individuals have a moral obligation to take action to mitigate the effects of the pandemic, as their actions can have a significant impact on the well-being of others.

Note, however, that the harm principle cannot operate independently but rather in conjunction with nonmoral factors such as the severity indicators of the pandemic and the incentives. At different times of the COVID-19, factors such as the contagion rate and ICU bed occupancy, and their values vary at different stages of the pandemic. Hence, the strength of individual responsibility in adhering to the mitigation rules is highest during the most severe stages of the pandemic when the risk of harm to others is the greatest. During a shortage of hospital beds, failing to follow mitigation measures increases the risk of causing harm to others, making the agent responsible for any harm caused. Therefore, an agent's responsibility for any harm caused to others increases during the most challenging phases of the pandemic.

During phases of the pandemic where there are lower levels of contagion and health systems are better equipped to handle demand, resulting in reduced mortality rates, institutional authorities may ease disease containment measures. In these softer phases, the harm principle suggests that individual liability is reduced, in part due to lower risk levels. The possibility of causing extreme damage is also lower, and any damage that does occur can be more effectively mitigated than during the hard phase. In this way, the principle of harm, combined with the conditions and incentives present in a pandemic context, helps to determine the extent of agents' responsibility in fulfilling their duty of mitigation.

In summary, we can conceive it as a moral suspicion or intuition that individual agents have certain responsibilities in a pandemic. However, this is a vague outline of the degree of individual responsibility because it disregards the context of the pandemic. Now, the combination of severity level factors, incentives for fulfilling duties, and moral consideration of the damage caused may be a metric to determine that degree. And once it is not a static metric, we can consider degrees of responsibility throughout the pandemic. Most important, the metric is not a case-by-case response but a consideration that the context – with its severity and incentives – is relevant to determine individual agents' responsibility.

14.4 Conclusion: A metric for individual accountability

The previous sections of this chapter presented a systematic approach to address the issue of responsibility and moral agency during a pandemic. In Section 14.1, we argue that all agents involved in this context have a burden of responsibility. In turn, section 14.2 identifies three categories of agents – institutional, social, and personal – and discusses their respective roles and responsibilities in preventing and mitigating the impact of a pandemic.

Section 14.3 came up with a metric to determine the individual degree of responsibility in front of the duty of mitigation as a response. For that, we propose three conditions to determine the individual's degree of responsibility in response to the duty of mitigation: (a) severity of the situation, (b) incentives for correct action based on the agent's level of information and vulnerability, and (c) the possibility of harm from the agent's actions. Overall, the burden of responsibility must be shared among all pandemic agents, but the chain of responsibilities is constrained and flows from the top to the bottom. When institutional action needs to be better executed, there is a slippery slope effect by which the duty assigned to individual agents is diminished. Our defense is that external conditions matter for moral agents' decision-making.

It is important to reinforce that the relationship between the different types of agents and the level of responsibility is not a closed metric, as different factors come into play for different agents. Also, a comprehensive account must go beyond enumerating pandemic duties and their consequent responsibility attribution to each agent. Even aware of this difficult task, this chapter tried to provide a potential metric for holding individual agents accountable during a pandemic.

Acknowledgments

We gratefully acknowledge the financial support provided by the National Council for Scientific and Technological Development CNPq, Brazil. Many thanks to the audience at the *Ethic Work Group* and the workshop at XIX Associação Nacional de Pós-Graduação em Filosofia, Brasil, meeting held in Goiânia, Brazil, 2022. Insightful comments emerged in a conference at UFSC Philosophy Meeting in 2022. This chapter has benefited considerably from class discussion in the graduate course Ethics during Pandemic Time: Some Guidelines. We are especially grateful for detailed comments from Gigi, Warren, Lan, Massa, Catalina, and Vicki for helpful feedback on earlier drafts.

Notes

1 An institutional agent is any individual performing institutionally designated activities or exercising institutionally delegated authority or responsibility (https://www.lawinsider.com/dictionary/institutional-agent).
2 For example, the story of the pharmacy industry Ravkoo, which reinvented itself as an ivermectin supplier, seizing on misinformation and medical distrust to peddle unproven and potentially dangerous prescription drugs to treat COVID-19 (Content, H. F. Found 15715 Result (s)).
3 Social agents as interactants are "ones who are interdependent, vulnerable, intermittently reflexive, possessors of capacities that can only be practiced in joint actions, and capable of sensitive responses to others and to the situations of interaction" (Burkitt 2016, 322–339).
4 Broadly speaking, individual agents are understood as autonomous, independent, and reflexive individuals (Burkitt 2016).
5 This representative list summarizes these duties, but there are other possible lists. Perhaps the discussion that best summarizes this debate comes from the WHO itself in its "Pandemic Influenza Preparedness and Response: A WHO Guidance Document" (2009) in which it summarizes the role of agents (governments, health sectors, and others sectors, civil society) and the duty to prepare and respond. See https://www.ncbi.nlm.nih.gov/books/NBK143067/ and https://www.who.int/publications/who-guidelines. Still, the discussion is more extensive in terms of responsibility. Zack (2009) discusses what she calls disaster preparation and disaster-response planning from a moral point of view for extreme contexts, such as a pandemic. Selgelid (2009, 225) discusses what he considers the main duties in the face of pandemic scenarios, using influenza as a parameter: "the obligation of individuals to avoid infecting others, healthcare workers *duty to treat*, allocation of scarce resources, and coercive social distancing measures." Araujo (2021) establishes some pandemic responsibilities before the onset, during, and in the aftermath of a pandemic. Davies and Savulescu (2022) establish "two sites of responsibility": institutional and personal to define responsibilities. From this, they also distinguish between prospective and retrospective claims of responsibility levels of speech in prospective responsibility and retrospective responsibility of individuals in the face of a pandemic.
6 The WHO declared on January 30, 2020, that the new coronavirus was a type of Public Health Emergency of International Concern – the organization's highest alert level as provided for in the International Health Regulations. The same year, on March 11, WHO declared the novel coronavirus (COVID-19) outbreak a pandemic – the term "pandemic" refers to the geographic distribution of a disease, not its severity.
7 Madhav et al. (2017) mentions other strategies for carrying out this type of activity, which include a strict animal zoonosis control system, monitoring of populations with a greater likelihood of risk, biosecurity, and others. For more details, see Paez-Espino et al. (2016), Jonas (2013), Pike (2010), and Wolfe et al. (2007).

8 An indirect consequence of this discussion is to indicate what Davies and Savulescu call retrospective and prospective claims of responsibility (see 2022, Section 2). Retrospective responsibility concerns the possibility of attributing blame to the states concerning past events. Consider insufficient preparedness for the latest pandemic. A series of studies done to test how much we are prepared for a pandemic indicates that the states had relevant scientific information about the risk of a pandemic and lack of preparedness to face it. If this is true, states have retroactive responsibility for the consequences of the COVID-19 pandemic. On the other hand, we can assume that agents at all levels have enough scientific evidence to understand the dangers of a new pandemic. In that case, there is a prospective liability with respect to future pandemic occurrences.

9 Vallor (2022) warns of the media's impact by making it difficult for the authorities to alert the population about the dangers of SARS-CoV-2 and the ongoing pandemic.

10 Studies (Achonu, Laporte, and Gardam 2005; Burns et al. 2006) indicate that pandemics are followed by a long period of reduced investments. This kind of consideration matters because individual agents carry a more significant pandemic burden if their economic condition is more vulnerable – mainly the working class.

11 This makes room for a parallel debate. We can imagine a different situation when the level of pandemic severity is under control, creating a softer phase during which obligations and responsibilities can be reduced or relaxed. In these conditions, although it is advisable to follow basic security measures, it may not be mandatory.

12 Even punishment-style incentives are an incentive to perform the morally expected action. Take Brazil as a detailed case. In Brazil, disseminating or the possibility of disseminating coronavirus is a crime under the country's penal code. At least four articles punish attitudes related to disrespect for the determination of isolation and measures applied to patients diagnosed with coronavirus (COVID-19). (Brasil 2022) Article 267 states that disseminating the pathogenic agent (viruses, germs, bacteria, among others) is considered a criminal violation, with a penalty of 10 to 15 years of imprisonment (in intentional attitude). Without intention, the penalty is one to two years in prison or two to four if this action results in death. In Article 268, the conduct considered unlawful is the violation of a determination by the public authority, which aims to prevent the entry or spread of a contagious disease, such as isolation or quarantine. Anyone disrespecting the imposed health measures can be sentenced from one month to a year of imprisonment and a fine. Article 131 provides for the crime of danger of severe disease contagion, with a penalty of one to four years imprisonment and a fine. In Article 132, the conduct recriminated is the exposure of the life or health of another person to danger. Something that can happen if those infected with COVID-19, aware of their condition, fail to comply with the isolation order or other measures imposed to prevent the spread of the disease. The penalty is increased by one-third if the agent is a public health official or works as a doctor, pharmacist, dentist, or nurse (Criminal Code – Decree-Law No. 2,848, of December 7, 1940 – Included by Law No. 9,777, of 1998 and Law No. 8,072, of 7.25.1990). (https://www.tjdft.jus.br/institucional/imprensa/campanhas-e-produtos/direito-facil/edicao-semanal/disseminar-o-corona-virus-e-crime).

13 See https://understanding.herefordshire.gov.uk/inequalities/index-of-multiple-deprivation-imd/.

References

Abou Ghayda, R., et al. 2022. "The global case fatality rate of coronavirus disease 2019 by continents and national income: A meta-analysis." *Journal of Medical Virology*, 94(6): 2402–2413. https://doi.org/10.1002/jmv.27610

Achaiah, N. C., and Subbarajasetty, S. B. 2020. "R0 and re of Covid-19: Can we predict when the pandemic outbreak will be contained?" *Indian Journal of Critical Care Medicine*, 24(11): 1125–1127. https://doi.org/10.5005/jp-journals-10071-23649

Achonu, C., Laporte, A., and Gardam, M. A. 2005. "The financial impact of controlling a respiratory virus outbreak in a teaching hospital: Lessons learned from SARS." *Canadian Journal of Public Health*, 96(1): 52–54.

Araujo, Marcelo de. 2021. "The nascent field of pandemic ethics: Prevention, mitigation, responsibility, and adaptation." *SSRN*. https://doi.org/10.2139/ssrn.3984756

Ball, Philip. 2021, December. What the COVID-19 Pandemic Reveals about Science, Policy and Society. *Interface Focus* 11(6): 20210022. https://doi.org/10.1098/rsfs.2021.0022.

Barbosa, Evandro. 2022. "The COVID-19 pandemic as a severe scarcity condition: Testing the tenacity of ideal theories of justice." In: Schweiger, Gottfried (Org.). *The Global and Social Consequences of the COVID-19 Pandemic: An Ethical and Philosophical Reflection*, 1st ed. Cham: Springer, v. 1, pp. 19–34. https://doi.org/10.1007/978-3-030-97982-9_2

Brasil. 2022. *Código Penal: Decreto Lei: No. 2,848, of December 7, 1940.* Included by Law No. 9.777/1998 and Law No. 8.072/7.25.1990). Available at: https://www.tjdft.jus.br/institucional/imprensa/campanhas-e-produtos/direito-facil/edicao-semanal/disseminar-o-corona-virus-e-crime. (Accessed: November 25, 2022).

Burkitt, Ian. 2016, August. "Relational agency: Relational sociology, agency and interaction." *European Journal of Social Theory* 19(3): 322–339. https://doi.org/10.1177/1368431015591426.

Burns, A., Van der Mensbrugghe, D., and Timmer, H. 2006. "Evaluating the economic consequences of avian influenza." *Working Paper 47417*, World Bank, Washington, DC.

Chan, E. H., et al. 2010. "Global capacity for emerging infectious disease detection." *Proceedings of the National Academy of Sciences of the United States of America*, 107(50), 21701–21706.

Davies, Ben, e Julian Savulescu. "Institutional responsibility is prior to personal responsibility in a pandemic." *The Journal of Value Inquiry* janeiro de 2022. https://doi.org/10.1007/s10790-021-09876-0

de Arruda, Rodrigo Gomes et al. The Effect of Politician Denialist Approach on COVID-19 Cases and Deaths. *EconomiA*. 22(3) dezembro de 2021: 214–224. https://doi.org/10.1016/j.econ.2021.11.007

Gage, K. L., and Kosoy, M. Y. 2005. "Natural history of plague: Perspectives from more than a century of research." *Annual Review of Entomology*, 50(1): 505–528. https://doi.org/10.1146/annurev.ento.50.071803.130337

Galang, J. R. F. 2021. "Science and religion for COVID-19 vaccine promotion." *Journal of Public Health*, 43(3): e513–e514. https://doi.org/10.1093/pubmed/fdab128

Gopez, J. M. W. 2021. "Building public trust in COVID-19 vaccines through the Catholic Church in the Philippines." *Journal of Public Health*, 43(2): e330–e331. https://doi.org/10.1093/pubmed/fdab036

Grennan, D. 2019. "What is a pandemic?" *JAMA* 321: 910. https://doi.org/10.1001/jama.2019.0700

Han, Q. (2020). "Introduction: The COVID-19 pandemic calls for the strengthening of scientific culture." *Cultures of Science* 3(4): 223–226. https://doi.org/10.1177/20966083211003343

Hegarty, S. 2022. "'The Gospel truth?' Covid-19 vaccines and the danger of religious misinformation." *BBC News*. Available at: https://www.bbc.com/news/av/health-56416683 (Accessed: November 24, 2022).

Hern, Alex. Kylie Jenner helps to wipe $1bn from Snapchat with tweet over redesign woes. 2018. *The Guardian*. Available at: https://www.theguardian.com/technology/2018/feb/22/snapchat-redesign-12m-signature-petition-social-media-app-kylie-jenner-celebrities.

Huijsmans, I. L. et al. 2019. "A scarcity mindset alters neural processing underlying consumer decision making." *Proceedings of the National Academy of Sciences*, 116, 1699–11704.

Izmirlieva, Milena. 2020. "COVID-19 pandemic: Health system surge capacity." *Pharmaceutical Technology*. Available at: https://www.pharmaceutical-technology.com/pricing-and-market-access/covid19-pandemic-health-system-surge-capacity-html/

Johnson, N. P., and Mueller, J. 2002. "Updating the accounts: Global mortality of the 1918–1920 'Spanish' influenza pandemic." *Bulletin of the History of Medicine* 76: 105–115. https://doi.org/10.1353/bhm.2002.0022

Jonas, O. B. 2013. Pandemic risk. Background paper for *World Development Report 2014: Risk and Opportunity; Managing Risk for Development*, World Bank, Washington, DC.

Kim, S., and Grady, C. 2020. "Ethics in the time of COVID: What remains the same and what is different?" *Neurology* 94: 1007–1008. https://doi.org/10.1212/WNL.0000000000009520

Lavazza, Andrea and Farina, Mirko. 2020 The role of experts in the Covid-19 Pandemic and the limits of their epistemic authority in democracy. *Frontiers in Public Health* 8: 356. doi: 10.3389/fpubh.2020.00356

Madhav, et al. 2017. "Pandemics: Risks, impacts, and mitigation." In Jamison, D. T., Gelband, H., Horton, S., Jha, P., Laxminarayan, R., Mock, C. N., and Nugent, R. (Orgs.). *Disease Control Priorities, Third Edition (Volume 9): Improving Health And Reducing Poverty*. The World Bank. https://doi.org/10.1596/978-1-4648-0527-1

Malekpour, Mohammad-Reza, et al. 2021, September 30. How the scientific community responded to the COVID-19 pandemic: A subject-level time-trend bibliometric analysis. *PLoS One* 16(9): e0258064. doi: 10.1371/journal.pone.0258064

Mani, A., et al. 2013. "Poverty impedes cognitive function." *Science* 341(6149): 976–980.

Marshall, M. 2020. "How COVID-19 can damage the brain." *Nature* 585: 342–343. https://doi.org/10.1038/d41586-020-02599-5

McElwee, J. 2021. "Pope Francis suggests people have moral obligation to take coronavirus vaccine." *National Catholic Reporter*. Available at: https://www.

ncronline.org/news/vatican/pope-francis-suggests-people-have-moral-obliga-tion-take-coronavirus-vaccine (Accessed: March 24, 2021).

Mill, J. S. 1965–1991. [1859]. *On Liberty*. Collected Works of John Stuart Mill, 33 volumes, ed. Robson, J.. Toronto: University of Toronto Press.

Morton, J. 2017. "Reasoning under scarcity." *Australasian Journal of Philosophy* 95: 543–559.

Nassif-Pires, L., et al. 2020a. "Pandemic of inequality." *Economics Public Policy Brief Archive* 149, Levy Economics Institute.

Nassif-Pires, L., Barbosa de Carvalho, L., and Lederman Rawet, E. 2020b. "Multi-dimensional inequality and Covid-19 in Brazil." *Investigación Económica* 80(315): 33. https://doi.org/10.22201/fe.01851667p.2021.315.77390

OECD. n.d. *The pandemic has triggered an unprecedented mobilisation of the scientific community – OECD*. Available at: https://www.oecd.org/sti/science-technology-innovation-outlook/crisis-and-opportunity/thepandemichastrig geredanunprecedentedmobilisationofthescientificcommunity.htm

Okello, A. L., et al. 2011. "One health and the neglected zoonoses: Turning rheto-ric into reality." *Veterinary Record* 169: 281–285. https://doi.org/10.1136/vr.d5378

One Health Commission [OHC]. 2020. *One health joint plan of action, 2022–2026*. 2022. FAO; UNEP; WHO; World Organisation for Animal Health (WOAH) (founded as OIE). https://doi.org/10.4060/cc2289en

Paez-Espino, D., et al. 2016. "Uncovering Earth's virome." *Nature* 536(7617): 425–430.

Pike, et al. 2010. "The origin and prevention of pandemics." *Clinical Infectious Diseases* 50(12): 1636–1640.

Piret, J., and Boivin, G. 2021. "Pandemics throughout history." *Frontiers in Microbiology* 11: 631736. https://doi.org/10.3389/fmicb.2020.631736

Porter, R. 1997. *The Greatest Benefit to Mankind: A Medical History of Humanity from Antiquity to the Present*. London: Fontana Press.

Rabozzi, G., et al. 2012. "Emerging zoonoses: The 'one health approach'" *Saf. Health Work* 3: 77–83. https://doi.org/10.5491/SHAW.2012.3.1.77

Reid, A. H., et al. 1999. "Origin and evolution of the 1918 'Spanish' influenza virus hemagglutinin gene." *Proc. Natl. Acad. Sci. U.S.A.* 96: 1651–1656. https://doi.org/10.1073/pnas.96.4.1651

Rinaldi, G., and Paradisi, M. 2020. "An empirical estimate of the infection fatal-ity rate of COVID-19 from the first Italian outbreak." *Infectious Diseases (except HIV/AIDS)*. https://doi.org/10.1101/2020.04.18.20070912

Rosen, G. 1993. *A History of Public Health* (exp. ed.). Baltimore: The Johns Hopkins University Press.

Selgelid, M. J. 2009, March. "Pandethics." *Public Health* 123(3): 255–259. https://doi.org/10.1016/j.puhe.2008.12.005

Sidik, S.M. 2022. "How COVID has deepened inequality—in six stark graphics." *Nature*. Available at: https://www.nature.com/immersive/d41586-022-01647-6/index.html (Accessed: November 30, 2022)

Silva, G. A. B. e, et al. 2020. "Healthcare system capacity of the municipalities in the State of Rio de Janeiro: Infrastructure to confront COVID-19." *Revista de Administração Pública* 54(4): 578–594. https://doi.org/10.1590/0034-761220200128x

Snitow, S., and Brennan, L. 2011. Reducing drunk driving-caused road deaths: Integrating communication and social policy enforcement in Australia. In H.

Cheng, P. Kotler, and N. Lee (eds.), *Social Marketing for Public Health*. Burlington, MA: Jones & Bartlett Learning.

Strategic preparedness, readiness and response plan to end the global COVID-19 emergency in 2022. 2022. Geneva: *World Health Organization*; (WHO/WHE/SPP/2022.01). Licence: CC BY-NC-SA 3.0 IGO.

The Independent Panel for Pandemic Preparedness and Response. 2020. COVID-19: *Make it the last pandemic*. Available at: https://theindependentpanel.org/wp-content/uploads/2021/05/COVID-19-Make-it-the-Last-Pandemic_final.pdf.

The World Bank. 2023. *Labor force, total*. Available at: https://data.worldbank.org/indicator/SL.TLF.TOTL.IN

Vallor, S. 2022. "Social networking and ethics." In Zalta, E. N. and Nodelman, U. (Orgs.), *The Stanford Encyclopedia of Philosophy* (Fall 2022). Metaphysics Research Lab, Stanford University. Available at: https://plato.stanford.edu/archives/fall2022/entries/ethics-social-networking/

Wilson, N., et al. 2020. "Case-fatality risk estimates for COVID-19 calculated by using a lag time for fatality." *Emerging Infectious Diseases* 26(6): 1339–1441.

Wolfe, N. D., Dunavan, C. P., and Diamond, J. 2007. "Origins of major human infectious diseases." *Nature* 447(7142): 279–283.

World Health Organization. [WHO] Regional Office for the Western Pacific. 2020. Indicators to monitor health-care capacity and utilization for decision-making on COVID-19(WPR/DSE/2021/026). *WHO Regional Office for the Western Pacific*. Available at: https://apps.who.int/iris/handle/10665/333754.

Zack, N. 2009. *Ethics for Disaster*. Lanham: Rowman & Littlefield Publisher.

15 Community, care, and social recognition in a post-COVID world of work

Joshua Preiss

15.1 Introduction

The COVID-19 pandemic ushered in dramatic changes to the world of work and the moral relations between individual managers, workers, customers, and their families. For a period, the economy ground to a halt. Restaurants and shops closed. Theaters and stadiums sat empty. Global centers of commerce like Manhattan, London, and Shanghai looked like ghost towns. The result was widespread unemployment and economic contraction, which (perhaps surprisingly) in many ways hit workers in wealthier countries the hardest (Deaton 2021). In addition, the pandemic accelerated, often quite dramatically, existing trends toward greater work from home (WFH), ecommerce, and automation. Even as day-to-day life has recently returned to relative normalcy, it is clear that some of these changes are here to stay. Gigantic investments in technological infrastructure have been and continue to be made. While displaced workers have significantly (though not fully) returned to full-time work, many have done so in new firms and with different job descriptions. The preferences of workers and employers evolved along with these changes.

This chapter considers the ways in which the transformation of work during the pandemic hinders or furthers the ability to enjoy important *relational goods*. By relational goods, I mean nonsubstitutable goods we enjoy in relationship(s) with other human beings. For our purposes here, it is not necessary to distinguish between valuing these goods as an essential component of human flourishing and treating them as indispensable resources to our efforts to be successful according to other standards or measures. It is enough to simply recognize that for most people, these goods are important, intrinsically or instrumentally, to their well-being. The focus is on three relational goods impacted by changes to the content, location, and valuation of work: community, care, and social recognition. In the course of my analysis, I consider recent work in moral, political, and legal philosophy that treats the opportunity to enjoy these goods as an issue of distributive justice. This analysis points to the ways in which a "bad" of work, domination,[1] threatens the enjoyment of the

DOI: 10.4324/9781003310129-19

goods at work. Finally, I highlight labor market policies that not only further the enjoyment of these relational goods but also help to create a more just post-COVID world of work.

15.2 Community

Citing work from philosophy, psychology, and sociology, Anca Gheaus and Lisa Herzog identify four goods of work (other than money): (1) attaining excellence, (2) making a social contribution, (3) experiencing community, and (4) social recognition. Similarly, Pablo Gilabert argues that in modern societies, work "plays a crucial role" in delivering goods that reflect important human interests, including (1) compensation, (2) self-development, (3) socializing (4) contribution (contributing to the well-being of others), and (5) self-esteem and self-respect (Gilabert 2018, 2019). In this section, our focus is on *socializing* or *experiencing community*. The pandemic itself undermined the ability to experience community with sustained and widespread social isolation impacting individual quality of life in ways that may only be fully recognized over time. In order to keep their economic and social lives going, people around the world turned to technology. As a result, the pandemic accelerated the ongoing trend toward WFH.

The impact has been dramatic. Comparing pre-COVID data from the American Time Use Survey to surveys from more than 60,000 workers (from more than 1,000 firms) economist Nicholas Bloom claims that whereas WFH days had doubled every 12 years prior to the pandemic, they increased twelvefold in March 2020 (Bloom 2017). Firms and individuals made sizable investments in physical and human capital resources to make WFH feasible and effective, investments which tend to stick (Barrero et al. 2021). A significant portion of work remains at home. Utilizing data from the monthly Survey of Working Arrangements and Attitudes (SWAA) Bloom, Jose Maria Barerro, and Stephen J. Davis conclude that the number of paid hours worked from home in the United States has stabilized around 30% for workers in general and 50% for workers able to WFH at least one day a week. As of June 2022, approximately 55% of full-time workers work fully in person, with 15% wholly online and 30% in a hybrid work arrangement. While the "amenity value"[2] of remote work has dropped substantially from the height of the pandemic, the gap between worker preferences and employer expectations has also narrowed significantly. Of workers able to WFH, the average worker preference (2.8 remote days) and employer plan (2.4) are separated by less than half a day (Barrero et al. 2021, 2022). The SWAA data fits well with other studies of the post-COVID economy (Robinson 2022). Research points to a similar increase in WFH in many countries around the world (Owl Labs 2022; Askoy et al. 2022; Van Dam 2022). While the available data is preliminary by necessity, it is safe to conclude that a sizable portion of WFH is here to stay.

Gheaus and Herzog argue not only that people identify goods as valuable but also that the opportunity to experience these goods at work is an issue of justice.[3] Central to their case is the fact that work occupies such a large portion of our waking lives. "If it is true that the goods of work are central to individuals' flourishing lives," they write, "and as long as we live in societies in which their realization is closely tied to the nature of paid employment, the equal concern owed to individual implies that their distribution is a matter of justice" (Gheaus and Herzog 2016, 80). With respect to community, as Cynthia Estland notes, "the workplace is the single most important site of cooperative interaction and sociability among individuals outside the family" (Estlund 2003, 7). It's an element most workers value. For those in what might be considered less rewarding or personally meaningful work, including "dirty work," these bonds with colleagues play a vital role in the self-esteem and social identity of workers (Ashworth and Kreiner 1999). Even workers who prefer to spend a portion of the work week WFH list face-to-face collaboration and socializing with colleagues as the two main benefits of working in person. WFH workers report significantly less interaction with colleagues than those who work in person, even when we include electronic interaction. They are more likely to feel disconnected from their colleagues and that they have less say in decisions that affect the firm (Barrero et al. 2021, 2022). Something seemingly as insignificant as in-person small talk appears to have important benefits (Methot et al. 2021). WFH involves the loss of an important good of work.

Nonetheless, there are reasons to think that the loss of community or socializing is neither unjust nor too devastating to human flourishing. First, recall that despite the rapid rise in WFH hours, the percentage of workers who work exclusively remotely is just 15%, with high concentrations in information and technology, finance, and business services. A hybrid approach, with two to three days at home and two to three days in the office, has quickly settled in as the preferred option. Second, as the risk of catastrophic infection recedes, WFH is perhaps more accurately characterized as "remote work," as people work at cafes and other "shared" workspaces that themselves offer opportunities for community (Amador de San Jose 2021). WFH is particularly popular in large urban areas where long commute times are common. Employees list the lack of commute and more time with friends/family as two of the top benefits of WFH, perhaps substituting time with locals for time with coworkers (Barrero et al. 2021, 2022). Third, while we shouldn't dismiss the ways in which fully remote and hybrid work models change the qualitative experience of collaborative work, it does not prevent such work. More than that, the rapid development and adoption of technology to WFH also eases collaboration with colleagues very far away from the office (from virtually anywhere in the world).

Finally, the opportunity to WFH is sharply divided by class, with college graduates more than twice as likely to do so as those without a college degree. The 55% of those who work fully in person includes the vast majority of lower-paid service workers. If, following Gheaus, Herzog, and Gilabert, we understand the goods of work as a matter of justice rather than (merely) human flourishing, then those who experience the greatest loss of community as a result of WFH generally fare much better in terms of wages, power, and status than the average worker.[4] Depending on the relevant theory of justice, including views that consider relational goods or *relational resources* on par with more economic metrics of distributive justice, this feature of WFH may not be regressive. WFH is a clear preference among many of these workers, one they are able to satisfy in part to their comparatively strong bargaining power.[5]

15.3 Care

A central relational good is the ability to care for and be cared for by other humans. This good is the subject of immense literature in the ethics and politics of care following landmark work by psychologist Carol Gilligan (Gilligan 1982; Held 1993; Tronto 1993; Noddings 1984). This literature posits care as a universal human value, reflecting the basic fact that all humans need care throughout their lives, not only to flourish but also in many cases – infancy, old age, and during periods of illness or disability – to simply survive (Kittay 1999; Ruddick 1998). The subject of much of this literature is the ways in which a changing world of work facilitates or hinders relations of care. One of the possible bads of work is that it makes it harder to develop and maintain relationships with those we care for. For many theorists, the ability to do so is a basic feature of justice. For example, Daniel Engster argues that a just economic system enables workers to earn adequate pay to support themselves and their dependents without making it difficult for them to realize close and caring relationships with them (Engster 2007). WFH, in this way, may make it easier to meet a demand of justice by mitigating the trade-off between providing for and realizing close relationships with their kids. Indeed, a central reason that workers continue to push for WFH is that it allows them to spend more time with, and better care for, their children (Barrero et al. 2021, 2022; Owl Labs 2022; Askoy et al. 2022).

Though they don't expressly frame their arguments in terms of care, one of the central bads of work that Gheaus and Herzog identify is a lack of discretionary time. Their point is not that we treat work as fundamentally a dis-utility, something we merely understand as a means to an end, a source of alienation, or something that ideally machines would do for us (Spencer 2014; Marx 1844; Keynes 1930/1963; Russell 1932). Rather, it reflects the basic concern, present in centuries of labor politics,[6] that a large portion of workers' waking lives should be their own, to do with as they please. We might think of greater time for care as a particularly important example of a more general concern for "free time" or "work/life balance." Assuming the same amount of time working, the flexibility afforded by WFH, combined with the time saved from commuting and getting ready for work, means more time for family, civic engagement, joining a club, exercise, sleep, and leisure.

In the process, however, WFH tends to further blur boundaries between work life and personal or family life. As such, it may exacerbate a tendency of modern work life to *always be working*. The same technologies that enable WFH also enable employers and managers to not only contact workers at any time but also expect that they respond to emails, address proposal demands, attend unscheduled meetings with colleagues or clients, and so on. Erin Kelley and Phyllis Moen describe the phenomenon in their pre-pandemic work *Overload*. "Professionals and managers," they write,

> [f]ind that what had been good jobs have morphed into something more intense and less secure. New communications technologies foster an always-on, always-working culture. Managers and coworkers know that they can contact employees at any time, anywhere, and they often do reach out before and after official workdays. Moreover, globalization, automation, and artificial intelligence make it clear to even the most educated, experienced, and skilled workers in a variety of occupations and industries that their jobs are changing radically, and may even disappear. Earnings and benefits are still relatively generous, but there is an increasing price to pay. Good jobs, previously characterized by relative autonomy and security, have become bad, with rising workloads, a sped-up pace, and escalating expectations that seem impossible to meet.
>
> (Kelly and Moen 2020, 4–5)

Kelly and Moen emphasize the conflict between "old rules" and "new realities," as workers are expected to *both* be in the office nine to five (or eight to six) *and* always be available to work after hours. WFH breaks down some of the old rules. That's part of what workers like about it. The new realities, however, represent a qualitative change in how we think about family or leisure time. Even if WFH makes it possible for workers to spend more time physically in the presence of family, there is a sense in which that time is not fully *discretionary*, not completely their own.

Being available at home, in turn, can sometimes make it extremely difficult to focus on work, providing little respite from the growing and overlapping demands that led to unprecedented burnout across the professions during the pandemic (Abramson 2022). Perhaps for this reason, workers list clarity of work/personal life boundaries as one of the two main benefits of working in person, right up there with time with colleagues (Barrero et al. 2022).

Of course, relations of care are not only valuable between immediate family members, and developing care relations with those outside your family, and from a young age, can itself be valuable (Gheaus 2011). What matters most is that everyone's care needs are well met. The pandemic itself reveals the importance of care work. For care workers and theorists, it also rekindled hope that governments would take action to address long-lamented crises of care. Michael Fine and Joan Tronto write that in the pandemic, we witnessed care work "emerging from the shadows as a taken-for-granted afterthought in public life. Through spontaneous (and nearly spontaneous) events around the world, healthcare workers were rapidly cheered as heroes" as were, "less visible care workers who are often forgotten," including supermarket shelf stockers, cleaners, transport workers and delivery drivers, and childcare and eldercare providers (Fine and Tronto 2020, 302). Despite such recognition, workers in health care, childcare, senior care, and education confronted massive burnout during the pandemic. The result is that long-term shortages in the United States and elsewhere have gotten worse (Murthy 2022; Natanson 2022; Jack and Cocco 2022).

These shortages are an extension of pre-pandemic "care deficits" (Heymann 2001; Tronto 2013; Robeyns 2013; de Vries 2022). For generations, gender inequality of opportunity functioned to subsidize paid care work. Talented women, who might otherwise have found their place in more lucrative or prestigious professions, were crowded into care work, particularly in occupations such as teachers and nurses (Goldin 2021). The inevitable effect is to drive down the wages for these workers. Absent such subsidies, filling these occupations with talented workers requires a substantial increase in pay and status. Care work, which does not generally admit of economies of scale, should get more expensive over time. These increases in pay and status have not been sufficiently forthcoming. In the United States, pay for child and home health-care workers is around half that of the average worker (Banerjee et al. 2021). In many contexts, the pandemic issued in a fresh wave of teacher vilification, even harassment.[7]

The pandemic also interacted with the gendered division of labor to create sudden and dramatic increases in gender wage and employment disparities, which many feared would seriously impact women's relative career advancement long-term (Preiss 2021a, Ch 5). These impacts were by no means limited to the United States, as the pandemic threatens to undermine decades of progress in women's income, employment, and education (Tang et al. 2021). Throughout the world, the costs borne by people who provide essential care work often include lower pay, power, and prestige (Folbre 2001, 2006; Folbre et al. 2020; Barron and West 2013; ILO 2018). COVID-19 raises the costs to those who provide essential care work. Given other opportunities, fewer and fewer people are willing to accept these costs. In aging societies throughout the world (in particular), providing the basic good of care depends upon collective efforts to raise the pay and status of care workers.

WFH can only do so much to alleviate this systemic problem. In addition, it does so in ways that threaten to exacerbate injustice. During the pandemic, people able to WFH provided much-needed support to their kids who were learning from home or regularly had to miss in-person school due to exposure, infection, or rising local incidence of COVID. The negative impacts of pandemic education were disproportionately borne by the children of poorer and less educated workers (Mohan et al. 2021; Saavedra 2022) who generally had less access to technology, and whose parents were less likely to be able to WFH. In this way, COVID magnifies pre-pandemic inequalities. Consider something as simple as being able to make teacher-parent conferences or volunteer in your child's classroom. A parent's willingness and ability to do so is frequently understood, by educators and by fellow parents, as illustrative of their interest in their child's learning and success. A parent whose job (even when it involves more hours in total) allows them to WFH will be much more likely to come in than a wage worker who, in order to make it, would have to take a day off of work and lose that full day's pay (even if their employer granted them time off). Insofar as WFH helps to address care deficits in general, it likely does so by widening existing inequalities in access to care (Heymann 2001).

15.4 Social recognition

Gheaus and Herzog identify *social recognition* as a central good whose realization is shaped by the nature and conditions of our work. Similarly, Gilabert recognizes that part of the importance of the other goods is their instrumental significance in achieving self-esteem and self-respect. While the "self" frame may suggest something more first personal, Gilabert quickly clarifies that "we are social creatures for whom relationships with others are central to our well-being" (Gilabert 2018, 71). These goods are central to his understanding of dignity at work. While the ends and terminology differ, on both of these accounts, the essential goods of work involve the status of workers, in ways they as individual workers internalize, but which are fundamentally shaped by their relations with other human beings. Their relational understanding of the goods of work, in turn, serves as a foundation for claims of justice or rights.

Treating social recognition as a good of work is not new. Indeed, this relational good is central to Adam Smith's moral argument for markets.[8] Human beings, as Smith understood, desire to be worthy of praise. This desire to be worthy, however, is difficult to distinguish from the desire to be praised. The two motivations, he reasons, are often "blended together," with the former not subsisting long without the latter. "Very few men," Smith writes, "can be satisfied with their own private sense that their qualities and conduct are the kinds the admire and think praiseworthy in other people, unless they *actually* receive praise for those qualities and that conduct" (Smith 2009, 151, emphasis added). A person's place in society, and the value that other members of society give them and their work, is central to their sense of self. A great virtue of a market economy, relative to feudalist and mercantilist alternatives, is that it better recognizes and rewards the contributions of workers. This "liberal reward of labor," in turn, encourages "industry of the common people…which, like every other human quality, improves in proportion to the encouragement it receives" (Smith 1999, 184). For Smith, this desire to be thought well of by others, and to be seen as an important contributor to society, is essential for both societies and markets to flourish over time (Herzog 2011, 2013; Gintis et al. 2005; Bowles 2011, 2016; Schliesser 2017).

While analytically distinct, Gheaus and Herzog note that social recognition is *mediated* by the other goods of work, including compensation (Gheaus and Herzog 2016, 78). Few recognized this link better than Martin Luther King Jr. Addressing striking sanitation workers in Memphis, King declares,

> You are demanding that this city will respect the dignity of labor. So often we overlook the work and the significance of those who are not in professional jobs, of those who are not in the so-called big jobs. But let me say to you tonight that whenever you are engaged in work that serves humanity and is for the building of humanity, it has dignity and it has worth.
>
> (King 2011, 157–158)

If we reconstruct King's argument according to Gilabert's framework, the claim is that though all workers who make a social contribution (one good of work) can justifiably claim the *basis of* dignity, the *circumstances of dignity*, the structural foundation for satisfying that claim, often go unmet due to insufficient compensation (another good) for that contribution. On Gheaus and Herzog's schema, the good of social recognition depends in no small part on workers' relative compensation. Tommie Shelby describes this distributional aspect of King's relational understanding of economic justice,

> King thought persons who are poor can't maintain their *dignity*, that is, their sense of intrinsic worth and equal civic standing, in the presence of great wealth. … In what is supposed to be a society of equals – where each has the same moral standing and no one has natural authority over anyone else – it is a public expression of contempt to act in a way that suggests others' urgent needs have less moral weight than one's own access to extravagant objects of desire. The poor naturally, and appropriately, see such attitudes as an attack on their status as equal citizens.
>
> (Shelby 2018, 196)

While King and Shelby invoke poverty and urgent needs, it is clear that King does not understand these terms in a context-independent way. Justice, on his view, means more than surviving or not living in poverty, even as he recognizes that a society where no one lived in poverty would be more just than the one he is living in.

In *Just Work for All*, I argue that this social recognition is central to thinking about justice for workers. Drawing insight from Smith and King, the book provides an account of the economics of *relational egalitarianism* for workers in the post-COVID economy.[9] Even if modern economies do not produce enough jobs where workers have the opportunity to fully realize human excellence or develop their productive and creative capabilities, market societies that enable all citizens to claim their share of the fruits of economic growth and recognize the value of workers who make such contributions better reflect that dignity than those that do not. By contrast, a market society clearly fails to respect the dignity of workers when the gains or losses are so inequitable that people watch a segment of the population leave them behind, economically insecure,[10] and with little hope that through hard work they can achieve a middle-class life for themselves and their families (Preiss 2021a, Ch 3–4). COVID threatens the social recognition of ordinary workers by exacerbating trends that erode their wages and bargaining power. Our discussion of WFH foreshadowed one source of this erosion: for several decades, technological change has led to labor market *polarization*, as skill-biased technological change drives an economy with high-education, high-wage jobs for some and low-wage jobs for most everyone else (Autor et al. 2006; Goldin and Katz 2010).[11] In addition, Acemoglu and Restrepo argue that a central driving force is the adoption of task displacing-technology – in particular, the automation of routine tasks – which accounts for approximately 50% of observed wage changes (and 80% of the increase in the college premium) in the United States from 1981 to 2016, while only resulting in a 3.8% gain in total factor productivity[12] (Acemoglu and Restrepo 2021). The adoption and development of such technology play a central role in the collapse of middle-class[13] employment, particularly among male workers without a college degree. In part because the gains in total factor productivity are marginal, however, it is far from clear that these displaced good jobs will be reinstated any time soon, if at all (Acemoglu and Restrepo 2017, 2019a, 2019b, 2021).

Economists Angus Deaton and Anne Case don't offer a philosophical analysis of social recognition and dignity for workers. Nonetheless, it is clear that the decline in these goods of work is a significant source of the rise in what they call *deaths of despair*. Case and Deaton document the dramatic rise in death from suicide and drug and alcohol abuse in parts of the United States most hit by winner-take-all political and economic trends.[14] As formerly middle-class workers are pushed into competition with one another in a burgeoning low-productivity service sector, productivity gains are increasingly captured by those at the top, including the highly concentrated ownership of corporate stock. Even as unemployment rates rise and fall over time in many parts of the country, for many workers, what is happening is that a worse job – with lower pay (particularly in the sense of a lower share of the fruits of economic growth), less security, less autonomy or opportunity for initiative, little opportunity for promotion – is replacing a better one (Case and Deaton 2017, 2020).[15] Unwilling to accept such a step down in status, security, and compensation, many workers drop out of the labor force altogether.

More often than not, both between countries and within countries, COVID made inequality worse (Narayan et al. 2022; Stiglitz 2022; Filipini and Yeyati 2022).[16] The issue is not only one of distributive injustice. Nor is it sufficient to respond that workers are not materially worse off than their ancestors in an absolute sense (as measured, for example, in terms of purchasing power parity). Instead, distributive inequalities matter to workers because of the way in which they *work through* people's enjoyment of the relational goods of work. The loss of middle-class jobs, combined with declining hope for a better future for individuals, their families, and communities, can be devastating to the self-esteem and self-respect of workers. The diminishing social recognition for their labor infects the home life, making working-class men and women less "marriageable" and contributing to greater conflict within the home (Case and Deaton 2020, Ch 12). The pandemic, including the ongoing risk of future variants, threatens to make things worse by incentivizing the adoption of labor-replacing technologies. Automated firms are far better insulated from potential shutdowns or delays due to illness. Robots don't call in sick, transmit viruses to coworkers and clients, or demand safety equipment or procedures in the workplace. While highly skilled workers in technology, banking, and business services are able to transition with relative ease from in-person work to WFH, service workers are not. The pandemic, as a result, led to widespread job displacement, particularly for low-income workers.

The segregation of WFH by class points to an important link between workplace community and social recognition. Consider the growing reliance on "contract workers." Many workers – including cleaners, security, food service workers, delivery drivers, and so on – who ostensibly work in the same firm now are no longer admitted to the corporate community, as Robert Solomon would put it (Solomon 1992). They live in separate worlds, with little contact between them or hope for advancement from one world to the next. Case and Deaton describe this evolution:

> [W]orkers who once would have worked for the firms they are supplied to and would have claimed relatively high wages there but are today not employed in the place that they work...everything looks the same, people are doing similar jobs, but the working conditions

of those who are outsourced – sometimes ex-employees – are often worse, with lower wages, fewer benefits, and limited opportunities for promotion...the outsourced workers are no longer part of the main company, they don't identify with it, and, in the evocative words of the economist Nicholas Bloom, they are no longer invited to the holiday party.

(Case and Deaton 2020, 165–166)

The status of workers suffers from the lack of connection to fellow citizens "above" their class. Many workers state that business reorganization removes a central source of pride, community, and hope for advancement for workers contracted, but not technically employed by, powerful firms such as Alphabet (Google), Meta (Facebook), and Amazon (Cherlin 2014; Bloodworth 2018; Irwin 2017; Bloom 2017). The distinction between those able to WFH and those who clearly cannot, makes this division even starker.

For Gheaus and Herzog, a central bad of work, which permeates their discussion of the goods of work, is being subject to domination on the job. Authority relations based on "sheer power" rather than expertise, they continue, "are a serious threat to the experience of community at work" (Gheaus and Herzog 2016, 77). That said, it is clearly possible for workers to develop community among themselves, even as they are all subject to domination. What isn't possible is community between classes of employees, where workers are able to speak honestly and freely with their bosses. Dominated workers, borrow from Philip Pettit, are unable to "act on a basis that such speech might justify" but instead "must always have an eye out for what will please the powerful and keep them sweet" (Pettit 2001, 78). As Anderson notes in *Private Government*, workers accept all sorts of intrusions into their personal liberty from employers – limitations on their bodily movement (even asking permission to go to the bathroom), regulation of their speech, forced to submit to random drug tests, restrictions on who they date or have sex with, how they cut their hair, which political candidates they support, and so on – including many a free person would never accept from their government (Anderson 2017).

The decline in the social recognition and workplace domination are two sides of the same coin. They are part and parcel of the eroding power and security of workers who do not possess high-end human capital (Graetz and Shapiro 2020). As technological change has pushed employment from domestic life, then to factories, then to consumer-oriented service and "knowledge" work, work itself has become increasingly *public*. "From the perspective of the worker's lived experience," as Isabelle Ferreras writes, "the client's presence in the workplace has caused a fundamental shift in the actual fabric – and conceptual location – of the workplace, pushing it away from the familiar space it once occupied in the margins of the private sphere" (Ferreras 2017, 86). Technological change, in turn, expands the ability of employers to monitor and control even their remote workers, while expecting them to be "available to work" at all hours of the day. When work becomes public and pervasive, it is inevitable that worker freedom and autonomy, including their ability (or lack thereof) to say no to unreasonable demands by employers and customers, plays a central role in their dignity and sense of self. While domination is not inconsistent with workers being recognized for the contributions of their labor, it undermines their dignity.[17]

15.5 Relational goods, relational justice, and public policy

Policy reform is urgently needed to secure important relational goods. The specifics of reform, of course, depend upon the relevant institutional context, and any path dependencies that have developed. What I want to emphasize here are policies that target multiple goods of work. To address the loss of social recognition in the United States, I suggest modernizing labor law (including sectoral bargaining or co-determination) and developing sovereign wealth funds to increase the bargaining power of workers and give citizens more say in the productive process (Preiss 2021a, Ch 7). Such reforms better enable workers to "stand tall in their negotiations with various agents that might significantly effect their labor conditions" (Gilabert 2018, 78). In addition, they make it more likely that firms will focus on labor-augmenting productivity (Acemoglu 2019, 2021) and bring workers together to bargain for wages, both of which enable them to claim better recognition for their labor (Rosenfeld 2014).

Perhaps even more important are reforms that raise demand for workers, including those most harmed by winner-take-all trends. These policies include public investment in physical and digital infrastructure and, more radically, a federal jobs guarantee. With growing demand comes better wages through increased bargaining power. With workers able to reclaim a larger share of the rents in monopsonist[18] labor markets, a tight labor market may actually be more effective at both incentivizing productivity growth and securing a larger worker share of that growth than proposals that focus on anti-trust legislation (Manning 2021; Naidu and Posner 2022). It also encourages workers, in particular those toward the bottom of the income and security ladders, to move to better jobs (Okun 1973). For all workers, a tight labor market provides greater freedom to say no to unreasonable demands by employers and customers (Tcherneva 2020). By eliminating corrosive forms of domination, these reforms provide the structural foundation for a more rewarding, more egalitarian, workplace community. Over time, the impact on the social recognition and self-respect of workers can be enormous (Preiss 2021a, Ch 3, 7; Friedman 2005).[19]

One policy that not only furthers the social recognition of workers but does so in a way that enables citizens to better (and more equally) experience the relational good of care, is public support for child care and early childhood education. While investment in early childhood education provides substantial benefits, in the United States, such investment depends upon those who can least afford it (and can't borrow to pay for it). As a result, Americans experience widespread care deficits, even as the pandemic underlines the importance of care work to the day-to-day lives of workers and the overall productivity of the economy. The availability of publicly provided child care, by contrast, allows workers to stay in full-time positions that provide better compensation, community, social recognition, and the possibility of development and advancement. It also makes it easier for people, in particular lower-wage workers, to move in search of better employment in a rapidly changing post-COVID marketplace, a move which often involves losing access to trusted family and friends who could help care for children. In addition, by raising the demand (and with it the pay, security, and status) of care workers, it lowers the costs that such workers pay for providing essential work while combating inequalities from what remains of our gendered division of labor (Preiss 2021a, Ch 5). Publicly provided childcare and early childhood education, in sum, offers tremendous payoff to both justice and the ability of workers to enjoy important relational goods.

15.6 Conclusion

The pandemic triggered (or accelerated) a number of transformations in the nature of work and the ability of workers and their families to enjoy three important relational goods: community, care, and social recognition. The rapid rise of WFH undermines their enjoyment of community at work and the rewards they get through in-person socializing and collaboration. Despite this cost, many workers express a clear preference for remote or hybrid work. Indeed, the ability to WFH is highly segregated by pay and education, with comparatively powerful workers more able to secure the benefits of remote work. Worker preference for WFH, in no small part, reflects the perceived gain in the ability to enjoy another important relational good: care. While WFH provides greater opportunity to provide in-person care for family members, it further blurs the lines between work and family life for overloaded professional workers, for whom the expectation is that in some ways they will always be working. In part for this reason, worker burnout across the professions is on the rise. Moreover, since WFH is so segregated by class, its ability to address care deficits may also widen existing gaps in access to care. In the process, it exacerbates ongoing polarization within the economy and within modern firms, a changing workplace community that denies "lower-skilled" workers (who are no longer invited to the holiday party) opportunities for advancement and recognition for their contributions to the firm.

COVID also threatens to make matters worse by amplifying political and economic trends that erode the wages and bargaining power of workers. This erosion leads to what Gheaus, Herzog, and Gilabert all identify as significant bad of work, one that undermines the dignity of workers and their ability to enjoy other goods of work: domination. As work becomes public and pervasive, it is inevitable that worker wages, freedom, and autonomy, including their ability to say no to unreasonable demands by employers and customers, is central to their self-respect. Policy reform, I argue, is urgently needed in order to further the welfare, power, and status of ordinary workers (Preiss 2021a). In this chapter, I highlight policies that target multiple relational goods, including a federal jobs guarantee and public investment in child care and early childhood education. The goal is not only to further the ability of workers and their families to enjoy essential relational goods but also to create a more free and just post-COVID world of work.

Notes

1 Domination, most basically, is a kind of unconstrained or unaccountable imbalance of power that enables some agents to control other agents or the conditions of their actions. For a discussion of workplace domination in global value chains, see Preiss (2014, 2019).
2 The amount of pay workers state they would be willing to forgo for the option of working from home.
3 While it is reasonably intuitive to argue that relational goods matter from the perspective of welfarist or perfectionist understandings of justice – where the metric of justice is well-being or human flourishing – Chiara Cordelli also argues that "the just distribution of relational resources – resources that either distinctively exist within interpersonal relationships or are themselves constitutive of those relationships – across society should be regarded as a legitimate concern for resourcist theories of distributive justice, no different from the distribution of economic resources" (Cordelli 2015, 86).
4 Which does not mean, of course, that the state of affairs is perfectly just or good.
5 This segregation of WFH by class does raise an additional concern for workplace community, amplfying the negative impact on social recognition of the growing reliance on "contract workers." I discuss this impact in Section 15.4.
6 Perhaps most iconically in the 19th-century slogan "Eight hours for work, eight hours for rest, and eight hours for what we will."
7 According to a recent survey, six in ten workers in American primary and secondary education have experienced violence, threats, and harassment since the start of the pandemic (McMahon et al. 2022).
8 Herzog herself has written a good deal about Smith, including an excellent book contrasting Smith and Hegel's vision of the market (Herzog 2013).
9 Relational egalitarians, including Elizabeth Anderson, Samuel Scheffler, and Jonathan Wolff, distinguish their conceptions of justice from accounts that focus on just distribution; in particular, the just distribution of material goods or resources (Anderson 1999, 2010; Scheffler 2003, 2010; Wolff 1998, 2010,

2015a, 2015b; Wolff and de-Shalit 2007). "The goal of equality" as Wolff puts it, "is not so much to achieve an egalitarian distribution of material goods, but to create a society in which each individual can think of themselves as valued as an equal" (Wolff 2010, 337).

10 Even before COVID-19, nearly half of American families did not possess the liquid assets necessary to support even a poverty-level existence for three months (Wolff 2017, 675). As a result, the debt of middle-income workers exploded. This explosion reflects income insecurity and the rapidly rising cost of higher education, health care, and housing relative to stagnating wages (Wolff 2017, Ch 3, 15).

11 Such labor market polarization through growing rate of return on human capital parallels the rising rate of return on what Erik Brynjolfsson and Andrew McAfee call "digital capital" (Brynjolfsson and McAfee 2014).

12 What remains after the contributions of education and capital deepening. By this measure, productivity growth in the mid-century American economy is nearly triple the periods from 1890 to 1920 and 1970 to 2014 (Gordon 2016, 16).

13 By contrast with middle income, *middle class* is a context-relative normative standard that includes people's status, security, and share of the benefits of economic growth (Preiss 2021a).

14 These trends include supply chain globalization, the rise of mass markets through advances in communication, the decline of organized labor, the use of task displacing automation and AI, the way in which slow growth contributes greater inequality by raising the importance of capital (which is highly concentrated) the role and expansion of intellectual property in an increasingly "intangibles" economy, and the rise of finance. For an overview or these trends, see Preiss (2021a, Ch 1, 7).

15 For further normative analysis of deaths of despair, including the disconnect between the concerns of workers and prominent philosophical accounts of justice (including luck egalitarian and libertarian theories) see Preiss (2021a, Ch 2).

16 Though, initially, wealthier countries experienced greater losses (Deaton 2021).

17 Gilabert identifies domination as a central threat to dignity at work (Gilabert 2018, 81). A *dignitarian* approach to labor law, he argues, strengthens the justification of labor rights, including collective bargaining rights, while providing a useful framework for understanding the scope of those rights.

18 An asymmetry of bargaining power between workers and employers such that, to use the terminology of economics, the labor supply curve of a given employer not infinitely elastic (that is, where cuts to wages do not lead to expected loss of workers).

19 Very recent analysis by David Autor and Arindrajit Dube suggests that American workers witnessed significant compression in wages in the past year, breaking decades long trends of widening inequality (Autor and Dube 2022). Unfortunately, tight labor markets in the United States and elsewhere are in no small part the product of declines in immigration, labor market participation and, most tragically, the number of workers available due to pandemic related disability and death (Bauer et al. 2022, da Silva et al. 2022). As such, they raise significant concerns for future growth, even as the rapid unleashing of consumer demand exacerbates inflation due to disruptions in global supply chains and global commodity shortage. There is real danger that these efforts will culminate in a global economic recession that stops progress to worker wages and power in its tracks (real wages in many contexts are already in rapid decline). In this scenario, workers in developing and emerging markets are likely to suffer the most, as capital flows out of their countries (Behsudi 2022).

Bibliography

Abramson, Ashley. 2022. "Burnout and stress are everywhere." *American Psychological Association* 53(1): 72.

Acemoglu, Daron. 2019. "Where do good jobs come from?" *Project Syndicate*. April 26. https://www.project-syndicate.org/commentary/automation-vs-job-creation-by-daron-acemoglu-2019-04

Acemoglu, Daron. 2021. "Redesigning AI." In Joshua Cohen and Deborah Chasman (eds.) *Redesigning AI: Work, Democracy, and Justice in the Age of Automation*. Cambridge: MIT Press.

Acemoglu, Daron and Pascual Restrepo. 2017. Robots and jobs: Evidence from U.S. labor markets. NBER Working Paper No. 232285. March.

Acemoglu, Daron and Pascual Restrepo. 2019a. The wrong kind of AI? artificial intelligence and the future of labor demand. Working Paper. https://economics.mit.edu/files/16819

Acemoglu, Daron and Pascual Restrepo. 2019b. "Automation and new tasks: How technology displaces and reinstates labor." *Journal of Economic Perspectives* 33(2): 3–30.

Acemoglu, Daron and Pascual Restrepo. 2021. Tasks, automation, and the rise in US wage inequality. *NBER Working Paper* 28920.

Adams, James Truslow. 1931. *The Epic of America*. Boston: Little, Brown, & Company.

Amador de San Jose, Cecilia. 2021. Coworking is the new normal, and these stats prove it. *Allwork: The Future of Work*. March 8. https://allwork.space/2021/03/coworking-is-the-new-normal-and-these-stats-prove-itt/

Anderson, Elizabeth. 1999. "What is the point of equality?" *Ethics* 109: 287–337.

Anderson, Elizabeth. 2010. "The fundamental disagreement between luck egalitarians and relational egalitarians." *Canadian Journal of Philosophy* 40(1): 1–23.

Anderson, Elizabeth. 2017. *Private Government: How Employers Rule Our Lives (And Why We Don't Talk About It)*. Princeton: Princeton University Press.

Ashworth, Blake E. and Glen E. Kreiner. 1999. "How can you do it? Dirty work and the challenge of constructing a positive identity." *Academy of Management Review* 99(24): 413–434.

Askoy, Cevat Giray, Jose Maria Barrero, Nicholas Bloom, Steven J. Davis, Mathias Dolls and Pablo Zarate. 2022. Working from home around the world. NBER Working Paper, September.

Autor, David, Lawrence Katz and Melissa Kearney. 2006. "The polarization of the U.S. labor market." *American Economic Review* 96(2): 189–194.

Autor, David and Arindrajit Dube. 2022. The unexpected compression: Employment and wage trends before and after the pandemic. Presentation to the *CBO Advisory Board Meeting*, June.

Banerjee, Asha, Elise Gould and Marowky Sawo, 2021. Setting higher wages for child and home health care workers is long overdue. *Economic Policy Institute*. November 18.https://www.epi.org/publication/higher-wages-for-child-care-and-home-health-care-workers/

Barrero, Jose Maria, Nicholas Bloom and Steven J. Davis. 2021. Why working from home will stick. NBER Working Paper 28731.

Barrero, Jose Maria, Nicholas Bloom and Steven J. Davis. 2022. Survey of working arrangements and attitudes. https://wfhresearch.com/

Barron, David N. and Elizabeth West. 2013. "The financial costs of caring in the British labor market: Is there a wage penalty for workers in caring occupations?" *British Journal of Industrial Relations* 51(1): 104–123.

Bauer, Lauren, Aiden Creeron, Wendy Edelberg and Sara Estep. 2022. Can a hot but smaller labor market keep making gains in participation? *Brookings Institution.* August 4. https://www.brookings.edu/2022/08/03/can-a-hot-but-smaller-labor-market-keep-making-gains-in-participation/

Behsudi, Adam. 2022. "Where the fed's inflation-crushing campaign may hurt the most." *Politico.* August 3. https://www.politico.com/news/2022/08/03/the-feds-global-problem-00048745

Bloodworth, James. 2018. *Hired: Six Months Undercover in Low-Wage Britain.* London: Atlantic Books.

Bloom, Nicholas. 2017. "Corporations in the age of inequality." *Harvard Business Review.* https://hbr.org/2017/03/corporations-in-the-age-of-inequality

Blyth, Mark and Eric Lonergan. 2020. *Angrynomics.* New York: Agenda Publishing.

Bowles, Samuel. 2011. Is Liberal Society a Parasite on Tradition? *Philosophy& Public Affairs* 39(1): p. 46–81.

Bowles, Samuel. 2016. *The Moral Economy: Why Good Incentives are No Substitute for Good Citizens.* New Haven: Yale University Press.

Breen, Keith. 2007. "Work and emancipatory practice: Towards a recovery of human beings' productive capacities." *Res Publica* 13: 381–414.

Brynjolfsson, Erik and Andrew McAfee. 2014. *The Second Machine Age: Work, Progress, and Prosperity in a Time of Brilliant Technologies.* New York: W. W. Norton.

Case, Anne and Angus Deaton. 2017. Mortality and morbidity in the 21st century. *Brookings Papers on Economic Activity.* https://www.brookings.edu/bpea-articles/mortality-and-morbidity-in-the-21st-century/

Case, Anne and Angus Deaton. 2020. *Deaths of Despair and the Future of Capitalism.* Princeton: Princeton University Press.

Cherlin, Andrew. 2014. *Labor's Love Lost: The Rise and Fall of the Working Class in America.* New York: Russell Sage Foundation.

Cordelli, Chiara. 2015. "Justice as fairness and relational resources." *Journal of Political Philosophy* 23(1): 86–110.

da Silva, António Dias, Desislava Rusinova, and Marco Weißler. 2022. "The labor market recovery in the euro area through the lens of the ECB consumer expectations survey." *ECB Economic Bulletin,* Issue 2. https://www.ecb.europa.eu/pub/economic-bulletin/focus/2022/html/ecb.ebbox202202_06~d69e287c16.en.html

De Vries, Bouke. 2022. "Care deficits and polarization: Why the time is right for universal care conscription." *Nursing Ethics* 29(3): 709–718.

Deaton, Angus. 2021. Covid-19 and global income inequality. NBER Working Paper 28292.

Engster, Daniel. 2007. *The Heart of Justice: Care Ethics and Political Theory.* Oxford: Oxford University Press.

Estlund, Cynthia. 2003. *Working Together: How Workplace Bonds Strengthen a Diverse Democracy.* New York: Oxford University Press.

Ferreras, Isabelle. 2017. *Firms as Political Entities: Saving Democracy through Economic Bicameralism.* Cambridge: Cambridge University Press.

Fine, Michael and Joan Tronto. 2020. "Care goes viral: Care theory and research confront the global Covid-19 pandemic." *International Journal of Care and Caring* 4(3): 301–309.

Filipini, Federico and Eduardo Levy Yeyati. 2022. Pandemic divergence: A short note on Covid-19 and global income inequality. Brookings Working Paper 168. March.

Folbre, Nancy. 2001. *The Invisible Heart: Economics and Family Values*. New York: New Press.

Folbre, Nancy. 2006. "Measuring care: Gender, empowerment, and the care economy." *Journal of Human Development* 7(2): 183–199.

Folbre, Nancy, Leila Gautham and Kristin Smith. 2020. "Essential workers and care penalties in the United States." *Feminist Economics* 27(2): 173–187.

Friedman, Benjamin. 2005. *The Moral Consequences of Economic Growth*. New York: Knopf.

Friedman, Marilyn. 1993. *What Are Friends For? Feminist Perspectives on Personal Relationships and Moral Theory*. Ithaca, NY: Cornell University Press.

Gheaus, Anca. 2011. "Arguments for non-parental care for children." *Social Theory & Practice* 37(3): 483–509.

Gheaus, Anca and Lisa Herzog. 2016. "The goods of work (other than Monay!)." *Journal of Social Philosophy* 47: 70–89.

Gilabert, Pablo. 2018. "Dignity at work." In Hugh Collins, Gillian Lester and Virginia Mantouvalou (eds.) *Philosophical Foundations of Labor Law*. Oxford: Oxford University Press.

Gilabert, Pablo. 2019. *Human Dignity and Human Rights*. Oxford: Oxford University Press.

Gilligan, Carol. 1982. *In a Different Voice: Psychological Theory and Women's Development*. Cambridge: Harvard University Press.

Gintis, Herbert, Samuel Bowles, Robert Boyd, and Ernst Fehr, E. 2005. *Moral Sentiments and Material Interests: The Foundations of Cooperation in Economic Life*. Cambridge: MIT Press.

Goldin, Claudia and Lawrence Katz. 2010. *The Race Between Education and Technology: The Evolution of U.S. Educational Wage Differentials, 1890–2005*. Cambridge, MA: Belknap Press of Harvard University Press.

Goldin, Claudia. 2021. *Career & Family: Women's Century-Long Journey Toward Equity*. Princeton: Princeton University Press.

Gordon, Robert. 2016. *The Rise and Fall of American Growth*. Princeton: Princeton University Press.

Gourevitch, Alex. 2015. *From Slavery to the Cooperative Commonwealth: Labor and Republican Liberty in the Nineteenth Century*. Cambridge: Cambridge University Press.

Graetz, Michael J. and Ian Shapiro. 2020. *The Wolf at the Door: The Menace of Economic Security and What to Do About It*. Cambridge, MA: Harvard University Press.

Held, Virginia. 1993. *Feminist Morality: Transforming Culture, Society, and Politics*. Chicago: University of Chicago Press.

Herzog, Lisa. 2011. Higher and Lower Virtues in Commercial Society: Adam Smith and Motivation Crowding Out. *Politics, Philosophy, & Economics* 10(4): 270–295.

Herzog, Lisa. 2013. *Inventing the Market*. Oxford University Press.

Heymann, Jody. 2001. *Widening the Gap: Why America's Working Families Are in Jeopardy – and What Can Be Done About It*. New York: Basic Books.

International Labor Organization (ILO). 2018. *Care Work and Care Jobs for a Future of Decent Work*. Geneva. https://www.ilo.org/global/publications/books/WCMS_633135/lang--en/index.htm

Irwin, Neil. 2017. "To understand rising inequality, consider the janitors at two top companies, then and now." *New York Times*, September 3. https://www.nytimes.com/2017/09/03/upshot/to-understand-rising-inequality-consider-the-janitors-at-two-top-companies-then-and-now.html

Jack, Andrew and Federica Cocco. 2022. "Wanted: Tens of thousands of teachers to staff europe's schools." *Financial Times*. September 2. https://www.ft.com/content/116d8c88-aa3f-426f-aeb8-c0a0325c43bb

Keynes, John Maynard. 1930/1963 "Economic possibilities for our grandchildren." In *Essays in Persuasion*. New York: W.W. Norton and Co.

Kelly, Erin L. and Phyllis Moen. 2020. *Overload: How Good Jobs Went Bad and What to Do About It*. Princeton University Press.

King, Martin Luther, Jr. 2011. *All Labor Has Dignity*. Edited and Introduced by Michael K. Honey. Boston: Beacon Press.

Kittay, Eva F. 1999. *Love's Labor: Essays on Women, Equality, and Dependency*. New York: Routledge.

Kurer, Thomas and Bruno Palier. 2019. "Shrinking and shouting: The declining middle in times of employment polarization." *Research and Politics* 6(1): 1–6.

Leonhardt, David. 2022. "Covid and race: The death rate for white Americans has recently exceeded the rates of Black, Latino, and Asian Americans." *New York Times*. August 9. https://www.nytimes.com/2022/06/09/briefing/covid-race-deaths-america.html

Lippert-Rasmussen, Kaspar. 2018. *Relational Egalitarianism: Living as Equals*. Cambridge University Press.

MacIntyre, Alasdair, 1984. *After Virtue: A Study in Moral Theory*, 2nd edition. Notre Dame: University of Notre Dame Press.

Manning, Alan. 2021. "Monopsony in labor markets: A review." *ILR Review* 74(1): 3–26.

Marx, Karl. 1844. "Economic and philosophical manuscripts." In Lawrence N. Simon (ed.) 1994. *Karl Marx: Selected Writings*. New York: Hackett Publishing.

McMahon, S.D., Anderman, E.M., Astor, R.A., Espelage, D.L., Martinez, A., Reddy, L.A. and Worrell, F.C. 2022. Violence against educators and school personnel: Crisis during COVID. Policy brief. *American Psychological Association*. March 17. https://www.apa.org/news/press/releases/2022/03/school-staff-violence-pandemic

Methot, Jessica R., Emily H. Rosado-Soloman, Patrick E. Downs and Allison S. Gabriel. 2021. "Office chitchat as a social ritual: The uplifting yet distracting effects of daily small talk at work." *Academy of Management Journal* 64(5): 1445–1471.

Milanovic, Branko. 2016. *Global Inequality: A New Approach for the Age of Globalization*. Cambridge: Belknap Press of Harvard University Press.

Mohan, Gretta, Eamon Carroll, Selina McCoy, Ciarán Mac Domhnaill and Georgiania Mihut. 2021. "Magnifying inequality? Home learning environment and social reproduction during school closures in Ireland." *Irisah Educational Studies* 40(2): 265–274.

Murthy, Vivek H. 2022. "Confronting health worker burnout and well-being." *New England Journal of Medicine* 387: 577–579.

Narayan, Ambar, Alexandru Cojocaru, Sarthak Agrawal, Tom Bundevoet, Maria Davalos, Natalia Garcia, Christoph Lakner, Danierl Gerszon Mahler, Veronica Montalva Talledo, Andrey Ten and Nishant Yonzan. 2022. "Covid-19 and economic inequality: Short-term impacts with long-term consequences." World Bank: Policy Research Working Paper 9902.

Naidu, Suresh and Eric A. Posner. 2022. "Labor monopsony and the limits of law." *Journal of Human Resources* 57(3): S284–S323.

Natanson, Hannah. 2022. "'Never seen it this bad': America faces catastrophic teacher shortage." *Washington Post.* August 4. https://www.washingtonpost.com/education/2022/08/03/school-teacher-shortage/

Noddings, Nei. 1984. *Caring: A Feminine Approach to Ethics & Moral Education.* London: University of California Press.

Okun, Arthur M. 1973. Upward mobility in a high-pressure economy. *Brookings Papers on Economic Activity.*

Owl Labs. 2022. State of hybrid work 2022: Europe. https://owllabs.eu/state-of-hybrid-work-emea/2022

Pettit, Philip. 1997. *Republicanism: A Theory of Freedom and Government.* Oxford: Oxford University Press.

Pettit, Philip. 2001. *A Theory of Freedom: From the Psychology to the Politics of Agency.* Oxford: Oxford University Press.

Pettit, Philip. 2012. *On the People's Terms: A Republican Theory and Model of Democracy.* Cambridge: Cambridge University Press.

Preiss, Joshua. 2014. "Global labor justice and the limits of economic analysis." *Business Ethics Quarterly* 24(1): 55–83.

Preiss, Joshua. 2019. "Freedom, autonomy, and harm in global supply chains." *Journal of Business Ethics* 160: 881–891.

Preiss, Joshua. 2021a. *Just Work for All: The American Dream in the 21st Century.* New York: Routledge.

Preiss, Joshua. 2021b. "Did we trade freedom for credit? Finance, domination, and the political economy of freedom." *European Journal of Political Theory* 20(3): 486–509.

Rawls, John. 1971. *A Theory of Justice.* Cambridge: Belknap Press of Harvard University Press.

Rawls, John. 2001. *Justice as Fairness: A Restatement,* edited by Erin Kelly, Cambridge: Belknap Press of Harvard University Press.

Robeyns, Ingrid. 2013. "A universal duty to care." In Axel Gosseries and Philippe Vanderborght (ed.) *Arguing About Justice: Essays for Philippe van Parijs.* Louvain-la-Neuve: Presses Universitaires de Louvain, 283–290.

Robinson, Bryan. 2022. "Remote work is here to stay and will increase into 2023." *Forbes.* February 1. https://www.forbes.com/sites/bryanrobinson/2022/02/01/remote-work-is-here-to-stay-and-will-increase-into-2023-experts-say/?sh=7c07e47220a6

Rosenfeld, Jake. 2014. *What Unions No Longer Do.* Harvard University Press.

Ruddick, Sara. 1998. "Care as labor and relationship." In Joram G. Haber and Mark S. Halfon (eds.) *Norms and Values: Essays on the Work of Virginia Held.* Lanham, MD: Rowman & Littlefield Publishers, 3–25.

Russell, Bertrand, 1932. "In praise of idleness." *Harper's Magazine*. October 1932.

Saavedra, Jaime. 2022. A silent and unequal education crisis. And the seeds for its solution. *World Bank*. January 5. https://blogs.worldbank.org/education/silent-and-unequal-education-crisis-and-seeds-its-solution

Sandbu, Martin. 2020. *The Economics of Belonging: A Radical Plan to Win Back the Left Behind and Achieve Prosperity for All*. Princeton: Princeton University Press.

Schliesser, Eric. 2017. *Adam Smith: Systematic Philosopher and Public Thinker*. Oxford: Oxford University Press.

Shelby, Tommie. 2018. "Prisons and the forgotten: Ghettos and economic justice." In Tommie Shelby and Brandon M. Terry (eds.) *To Shape a New World: Essays on the Political Philosophy of Martin Luther King Jr*. Cambridge, MA: Belknap Press of Harvard University Press, 187–204.

Smith, Adam. 1999. *The Wealth of Nations Books I-III*. Penguin Classics.

Smith, Adam. 2009. *The Theory of Moral Sentiments*. New York: Penguin Classics.

Solomon, Robert. 1992. *Ethics and Excellence: Cooperation and Integrity in Business*. New York: Oxford University Press.

Spencer, David A. 2014. "Conceptualizing work in economics: Negating a disutility." *Kyklos: International Review of Social Sciences* 67(2): 280–294.

Stiglitz, Joseph. 2022. "COVID has made global inequality much worse." *Scientific American*. March 1. https://www.scientificamerican.com/article/covid-has-made-global-inequality-much-worse/

Tang, Vincent, Aroa Santiago, Zohra Kahn, David Anaglobeli, Esuna Dugarova, Katherine Gifford, Laura Gomes, Jiro Honda, Alexander Klemm, Carolina Renteria, Alberto Soler, Siike Staab, Carolina Osorio-Buitron, Qianqian Zhang. 2021. Gender equality and Covid-19: Policies and institutions for mitigating the crisis. *International Monetary Fund*. https://blog-pfm.imf.org/en/pfmblog/2021/07/gender-equality-and-covid-19-policies-and-institutions-for-mitigating-the-crisis

Tcherneva, Pavlina R. 2020. *The Case for a Job Guarantee*. New York: Polity.

Tronto, Joan C. 1993. *Moral Boundaries: A Political Argument for an Ethic of Care*, New York: Routledge.

Tronto, Joan C. 2013. *Caring Democracy: Markets, Equality, and Justice*. New York University Press.

Van Dam, Andrew. 2022. "The remote work revolution is already reshaping America." *Washington Post*, August 22, https://www.washingtonpost.com/business/2022/08/19/remote-work-hybrid-employment-revolution/

Walzer, Michael, 1983. *Spheres of Justice: A Defense of Pluralism and Equality*, New York: Basic Books.

Wolff, Edward N. 2017. *A Century of American Wealth*. Cambridge: Belknap Press of Harvard University Press.

Wolff, Jonathan. 1998. "Fairness, respect, and the egalitarian ethos." *Philosophy & Public Affairs* 27(2): 97–122.

Wolff, Jonathan. 2010. "Fairness, respect, and the egalitarian ethos revisted." *Journal of Ethics* 14(3/4): 335–359.

Wolff, Jonathan. 2015a. "Social equality and social inequality." In Carina Fourie, Fabian Schuppert and Ivo Wallimann-Helmer (ed.) *Social Equality: On What it Means to be Equals*. Oxford University Press.

Wolff, Jonathan. 2015b. "Social equality, relative poverty, and marginalised groups." In George Hull (ed.) *The Equal Society: Essays on Equality in Theory and Practice*. New York: Lexington Books.
Wolff, Jonathan and Avner De-Shalit, 2007. *Disadvantage*. Oxford: Oxford University Press.

16 The emerging field of pandemic ethics

Marcelo de Araujo

16.1 Introduction

Human beings can have varying degrees of responsibility – both moral and causal responsibility – for the material and non-material consequences of a pandemic. There are pandemics for which human beings have little or no moral responsibility at all, and pandemics for which human beings are from moderately to highly responsible. At one extreme of the spectrum of responsibilities, we can think, for example, of pandemics that emerged in previous centuries due to precarious sanitation, poor knowledge about the causes of diseases, and lack of expertise as to how to fight infectious diseases with pharmaceutical or non-pharmaceutical interventions. In this case, nobody can be held morally responsible for the outbreak of a new disease and the emergence of a pandemic, even if, at a causal level, different actors may have had varying degrees of responsibility. At the other extreme, we can think of a pandemic that originates from the actions of bioengineers and bioterrorists, spreading rapidly throughout the world due to lack of coordination among states, poor leadership among political authorities, lack of engagement of the private sector, and reckless behaviours among individual citizens. Whether or not an outbreak – deliberate or unintentional – develops into a pandemic depends on the decisions and attitudes of multiple actors, in different parts of the world.

The more human beings learn about pandemics – their history, their causes and consequences, and the strategies to prevent and fight them – the more human beings become morally responsible for the human and economic costs of a pandemic. The problem, however, is that no single actor can be held morally responsible for the emergence of a pandemic, for a pandemic can only arise through the actions (and omissions) of a multitude of actors, scattered across different legal, cultural, political, and geopolitical contexts. It does not follow from this, of course, that no one can be held responsible for the consequences of a pandemic, but only that it is difficult to identify the relevant actors, to assess their respective degrees of responsibility, and to make them morally and, as the case may

DOI: 10.4324/9781003310129-20

be, legally accountable for the human and economic costs of a global health crisis. Pandemics, though, are not the only kind of threat that may represent an "existential risk" to humanity in the future (Ord 2020, 124–138; Nouri and Chyba 2008). Climate change, too, is a major threat that raises important questions of responsibility and that has drawn the attention of many philosophers over the last decades. The analogy with "the young field of climate ethics" (Gardiner and Obst 2023, xx) – or "the growing field of climate ethics" (Markowitz, Grasso, and Jamieson 2015, 467) – may thus prove fruitful for elucidation of some the theoretical issues that the still younger, but already growing, field of pandemic ethics has to address. In what follows, I intend to explore the relevance, but also the limits of this analogy.

16.2 Dimensions of justice in the climate ethics debate

As climate ethics gradually emerged as a broad field of philosophical inquiry, some authors realized that our traditional moral and political theories – utilitarianism, Kantian moral theory, virtue ethics, and classical social contract theories – were not entirely adequate to address questions of climate responsibility (Jamieson 1992, 149; 2014, 144; Gardiner 2011, 41–48).[1] Influential and compelling as these theories may still be, they were originally proposed at a time when anthropogenic climate change was unheard of. The assumption that human activities might one day disrupt our planet's climate system, with devastating consequences for humanity, had not been taken into account, not even as a mere hypothetical testing ground for the tenability of moral and political ideas. Writing in 1992, Dale Jamieson, for instance, suggested, "I believe that our dominant value system is inadequate and inappropriate for guiding our thinking about global environmental problems, such as those entailed by climate changes caused by human activity" (Jamieson 1992, 148). Nearly twenty years later, Stephen Gardiner defended a similar position in his influential book *A Perfect Moral Storm: The Ethical Tragedy of Climate Change*:

> We are extremely ill-equipped to deal with many problems characteristic of the long-term future. Even our best moral and political theories face fundamental and often severe difficulties addressing basic issues such as intergenerational equity, international justice, scientific uncertainty, contingent persons, and the human relationship to animals and nature more generally. But climate change involves all of these matters and more. Given this, our theories are poorly placed to respond. Theoretically, we are currently 'inept,' in the (nonpejorative) sense of lacking the skills and basic competence for the task.
>
> (Gardiner 2011, 41)

Over the last years, though, our moral and political theories have become less "inept" (or less "inadequate"), partially thanks to the contributions of Gardiner and Jamieson themselves, along with the efforts of other leading philosophers working in the field of climate ethics. Some recent approaches have taken into account, for instance, the unequal contribution to past emissions in the course of the 20th century (richer countries have emitted more than poorer countries); they have also taken into account the excusable-ignorance argument (richer countries could not have known from the beginning that their emissions would have such a huge impact on the climate system); and criticism of the excusable-ignorance argument (poorer countries increased their own emissions in a time when scientific evidence for anthropogenic climate change had already become overwhelming). Recent approaches have also taken into account the benefits that people living in richer countries today have gained from past emissions, even if they have not themselves contributed to those emissions; or the demand poorer countries make for compensation for loss and damage caused by climate change; or the role of individual responsibility as opposed to state and corporate responsibility; or the moral responsibility human beings have towards non-human animals, which cannot adapt to the climate change in the same ways human beings can. Many philosophers have addressed these and other normatively relevant questions with increasing acuity in the recent literature on climate ethics (Cripps 2013; Birnbacher 2016; Serdeczny, Waters, and Chan 2016; Meyer and Sanklecha 2017; Van der Geest and Schindler 2017; Wallimann-Helmer et al. 2019; Gesang 2020; Moellendorf 2022). However, I do not intend to provide a historical account of the evolution of climate ethics as a philosophical field of investigation over the last few years. My intention is simply to point out that until recently many scholars have argued that traditional moral theories could not be deployed in the climate change debate without further qualification, for climate change has implications that concern simultaneously different dimensions of justice. Climate change concerns the relationship between richer and poorer states (it involves therefore issues of *international justice*), it also concerns the relationship between the current and future generations (it involves therefore issues of *intergenerational justice*), the relationship between richer and poorer people living within the same state (*social justice*), and the relationship between humans and non-human animals (*animal justice*). In the climate ethics debate, it is thus methodologically difficult to examine one dimension of justice without also having to examine the others.

Now, these theoretical and methodological difficulties also affect the debate on the attribution of responsibilities when we have specifically in mind the threats posed by pandemics, rather than climate change. I do not mean to suggest, though, that recent theoretical advances in the young field of climate ethics can be applied in the debate on pandemic ethics without further qualification. My point is, rather, that pandemic ethics needs to address issues related to the attribution of responsibility in a more systematic way, as the new field of climate ethics has done in our recent past, if it aspires to grow into a distinctive field of investigation, rather than remaining as an unsystematized aggregate of moral issues loosely related to one another. And one reason to recognize that recent developments in climate ethics cannot be integrated into the nascent field of pandemic ethics without further qualification is the realization that pandemics raise questions of responsibility in ways that do not have clear counterparts in the climate ethics debate. While *anthropogenic* climate change is a one-off phenomenon in the history of human civilization, pandemics have been cyclical events, visiting upon humanity at different historical stages. Pandemics have also become increasingly more frequent than they used to be in the past. The cyclical nature of pandemics, as I intend to show, has important implications for our understanding of pandemic ethics as a field of investigation in its own rights.

16.3 Pandemic cycles

Questions of pandemic responsibility relate to actions (and omissions) performed by different types of agents within three specific time frames – namely, actions (and omissions) that occur *before*, *during*, or in the *aftermath* of a pandemic. Seen in this light, it is clear that climate ethics and pandemic ethics differ in some important ways. I would like to explain this point further and draw attention to some particular moral issues that stand out in each of these three time frames.

16.3.1 *Responsibility for actions and omissions before the emergence of a pandemic*

One might perhaps think of the COVID pandemic as a quite unpredictable event, which has taken governments and civil society by surprise. But that would be a mistake. For more than two decades preceding the rapid emergence of the COVID pandemic, several researchers, government agencies, intergovernmental bodies, and journalists had been calling attention to the increasing occurrences of new diseases outbreaks, which had the potential to grow into a major global health crisis, and to the lack of corresponding policies to mitigate pandemic risks and to promote pandemic preparedness.[2] Some studies compared, for instance, the economic costs of fighting a pandemic to the much lower costs of preventing pandemics in the first place (Osterholm 2007; Pike et al. 2014).

In order to promote pandemic preparedness, the United Nations issued in February 2016 a document with recommendations for the development of "pandemic plans," including plans for the implementation of "simulation exercises" among all states party to the International Health

Regulations (United Nations General Assembly (UNGA) 2016, 12, 14, 36, 42). One such simulation, named "Exercise Cygnus", took place in the United Kingdom in October 2016 (United Kingdom [Public Health England] 2017; Dyer 2020; Pegg 2020). And between 2018 and 2019, three further simulations were carried out in the United States. One simulation, named the "Clade X," was conducted by the Johns Hopkins Center for Health Security in 2018 (Myers 2018; The Johns Hopkins Center for Health Security 2018; Twilley 2018; Watson et al. 2019; Maxmen and Tollefson 2020). A second one, called "Crimson Contagion," was conducted by the Department of Health and Human Services in 2019 (Bramble 2020, 32–33; Maxmen and Tollefson 2020). And a third simulation, named "Event 201: A Global Pandemic Exercise," was carried out by the Johns Hopkins Center for Health Security, also in 2019 (The Johns Hopkins Center for Health Security 2019; Maxmen and Tollefson 2020). Previous pandemic exercises had focused mainly on threats posed by bioterrorism. These include, for instance, the "Dark Winter" exercise, from 2001 (O'Toole, Mair, and Inglesby 2002; Lakoff 2008; 2017, 52–58; Maxmen and Tollefson 2020; Perry 2020), and the "Atlantic Storm" simulation, carried out in 2005 (Smith et al. 2005; Maxmen and Tollefson 2020; Perry 2020).

The reports resulting from these simulations, whether they focused on bioterrorism or on non-intentional disease outbreaks, showed that the United States and the United Kingdom – and the world at large – were unprepared for a pandemic. One passage from the 2017 "Exercise Cygnus," for instance, states that "the exercise did show that the UK's capability to respond to a worst case pandemic influenza should be critically reviewed" (United Kingdom [Public Health England] 2017, 6, 28). Yet, these findings have neither been translated into public policies to mitigate pandemic risks nor to prepare health workers and the population in general for a major health crisis. Given the abundance of early warnings, issued before 2020, there is really no reason to assume, as it has sometimes been suggested, that the new coronavirus caught the world by surprise. The only surprising thing, indeed, is that neither risk mitigation nor pandemic preparedness efforts had been considered issues of paramount importance among policymakers. Although lack of appreciation for evidence-based health policies may have prompted many politicians to make disastrous decisions during the COVID pandemic, it is clear that the mismanagement of the global health crisis started even before the first new coronavirus case was confirmed. As we can see, questions of pandemic responsibility should not focus solely on actions and omissions that unfold in the course of a pandemic, but also on actions and omissions that take place even *before* a pandemic strikes. The problem, however, as Nita Madhav and colleagues put it, is that "accountability for preparedness is diffuse" (Madhav et al. 2017, 338). One can blame political leaders for failing to deploy effective health policies based on scientific evidence during a pandemic, but it is a much harder task to make them accountable for actions and omissions before a pandemic arises.

Questions of pandemic responsibility before a pandemic strikes concern not only the actions (and omissions) performed by policymakers and politicians within their own jurisdictions, but also within the community of states as a whole. Some studies suggest, for instance, that the probability of new disease outbreaks increases towards the Equator (Jones et al. 2008; Olival et al. 2017; Ellwanger and Chies 2018; Allen et al. 2017). Does it mean, then, that countries that are more susceptible to new outbreaks bear more responsibility for the emergence of pandemics than other countries or, rather, that they are more vulnerable and that, for this reason, other countries have a *prima facie* duty to help them to enhance their mitigation capabilities and pandemic preparedness infrastructure? It seems plausible to assume that just in the same way wealthier states have a duty to help poorer states to adapt to climate change, as the most vulnerable countries are also those that are least responsible for the increase of greenhouse gas emissions over the last decades, wealthier states have a duty, too, to help poorer states to mitigate pandemic risks, as being more vulnerable to new disease outbreaks solely on the grounds of being closer to the Equator is not something a country is responsible for, even considering that a country can – and indeed should – be held accountable for lack of willingness to promote pandemic mitigation within its own territory.

16.3.2 Responsibility for actions and omissions during a pandemic

Questions of pandemic responsibility in the course of a pandemic differ, in some important respects, from questions of responsibility in the context of the ongoing climate crisis. One citizen alone cannot compromise climate mitigation efforts significantly, even considering that individual citizens do also share a degree of responsibility for the threats posed by climate change and for the promotion of climate mitigation (Cripps 2013; Sinnott-Armstrong and Howarth 2005; Schwenkenbecher 2014). On the other hand, individual citizens can significantly compromise the efforts to fight an ongoing pandemic. An individual can, for instance, forge a vaccine certificate and, then, board an airplane to enjoy holidays in a country with a poor public health infrastructure. This can have devastating consequences for people in that country. During the COVID pandemic, some countries took legal measures against individual spreaders of the coronavirus, or against individuals who promoted super-spreading events (France-Presse 2021; Rambo et al. 2021; Robertson and Oliver 2021). Some politicians, too, have been accused of mismanaging the health crisis in their respective countries and, for this reason, there has been some discussion on the feasibility of procedures to hold them legally accountable for the premature death of countless victims of COVID

(Giuffrida 2020; Phillips 2021; Chin et al. 2021). Former Brazilian president Jair Bolsonaro, for instance, faced accusations of crimes against humanity (The Economist 2021b; Williams 2021). However, it is not clear whether most domestic jurisdictions, or the provisions of international law, can address these issues appropriately.

During the pandemic, there was some discussion for the enactment of a pandemic treaty so as to minimize the chances of another pandemic through the enforcement of concerted international cooperation in areas such as pandemic risk mitigation and pandemic preparedness (Fukuda-Parr, Buss, and Ely Yamin 2021; Labonté et al. 2021; Nikogosian and Kickbusch 2021; Vinuales et al. 2021; Wenham et al. 2021; Zarocostas 2021; Taylor 2021; Council of the European Union 2020; Clark and Sirleaf 2021; World Health Organization (WHO) 2021). It quickly became clear, though, that national interest would stand in the way of such a treaty as states would be required to make concessions that might be perceived as encroachment on their sovereignty, such as for instance granting international health authorities unrestrained access to market places or research facilities that might be traced back to the origin of a new disease outbreak (Araujo and Meyer 2022, 58).

In the course of a pandemic, as people feel the effects of the health crisis in their everyday lives, the demand for accountability is, understandably, greater than in the period that precedes its emergence. But the urge to find culprits can also easily lead to the misattribution of responsibility, which is a moral issue in its own right. During the COVID pandemic, several cases of xenophobia and racism were reported, as some groups were considered carriers of the disease, or even held responsible for the original outbreak (Addo 2020; Bieber 2020; Human Rights Watch 2020; Chou and Gaysynsky 2021). Discrimination against foreigners occurred mostly at an individual level, but patterns of discrimination at the state level have also been found. Krystlelynn Caraballo, for instance, argues, "[T]he pandemic is another example of how governments use crises to accelerate nativist policies and preexisting, anti-immigrant agendas" (Caraballo 2020, 455). Similar patterns of discrimination were seen in the 1980s, as gay men were seen not so much as victims of the AIDS pandemic but as the main culprits for the emergence and rapid spread of a heretofore unknown infectious disease (Winston and Beckwith 2011; Snowden 2019, 433–435; Christakis 2020, 318). It was not until 2010 that the American Government lifted a 22-year law that prevented HIV seropositive people from traveling into the United States. According to Susanna Winston and Curt Beckwith, it was anti-immigration feelings, rather than scientific evidence, that had contributed to the creation of that law in the first place (Winston and Beckwith 2011).

Another important question of moral responsibility that arises during a pandemic concerns the establishment of triage protocols for an ethically acceptable allocation of life-saving and life-supporting equipment, including ventilators, medication, and vaccines. During the COVID pandemic, some of these protocols had to be established rapidly – if established at all – and without previous debate or public consultation. It also became apparent that some ethnic groups were more vulnerable than others. In Brazil, for instance, indigenous populations and *quilombo* people, inhabitants of still-existing old settlements of 19th-century runaway slaves (Florentino and Amantino 2011), were reported to be more likely to die from COVID than other ethnic groups (Charlier and Varison 2020; Palamim, Ortega, and Marson 2020; Polidoro et al. 2020). Governments, therefore, have the responsibility to address racial and ethnic health disparities in order to render triage protocols more sensitive to the vulnerabilities and needs of specific social groups. In the course of a pandemic, though, it is understandably more difficult to engage the population in the attempt to elaborate more inclusive triage protocols, especially if most people are under lockdown or quarantine, or taking care of family members, or if they are ill themselves. As a pandemic rages on, policymakers will also be under pressure to implement triage protocols quickly, which in turn may either compromise the quality of public consultation or make public consultation practically impossible. Public consultation for the establishment of fair triage protocols should therefore preferably occur before the onset of a pandemic. As John Barry aptly put the problem as early as 2005, "Questions about who will have the authority to make and enforce such decisions, and under what circumstances, must be settled in advance. Neither an epidemic nor an attack will leave time for debate" (Barry 2005, 459). On the other hand, Barry also argues that even if these decisions are taken in advance, it may not be immediately clear which moral principles should inform them (Barry 2005, 460).

During the COVID pandemic, there was much debate on the moral principles that should underlie the establishment of triage protocols. Some authors have suggested that when life-saving and life-preserving resources become critically scarce, the health authority's goal should be to save the greatest number of lives, or the greatest predicted number of years to live (White 2009; Jerry 2020; Savulescu, Persson, and Wilkinson 2020; White and Lo 2020; Altman 2021; Goozen 2021; Wilkinson 2021). The idea here is not to abandon an egalitarian approach for the sake of utilitarian principles but to recognize that pandemics may put severe strains on a country's health system and that, for this reason, utilitarian principles might be called for. Depending on how severe the pandemic is, health workers, for instance, will have to strive to save human lives while also trying to prevent the health system itself from collapsing. It is as though the health system itself became a patient whose life must be preserved at all costs in order to save the lives of real patients. Granting medical treatment to all patients on purely equalitarian grounds, then, may fail to be an option. At some point, hard choices will have to be made as to who is granted treatment, and who is not. Writing on the ethics of triage protocols at the beginning of the COVID pandemic, Dominic Wilkinson has put the problem as follows:

> Decisions about who to admit can either aim to secure the greatest benefit from allocation of ICU beds, or they can aim to prioritise fairness, responding as equally as possible to patient claims or need for treatment. Plausibly, the approach to ICU triage decisions attempts to balance these two values.
>
> (Wilkinson 2020, 287)

Depending on how overwhelmed a country's health system is, the "balance" may tip to the utilitarian side. This means that a triage protocol may determine, for instance, that older persons, or persons without the prospect of quicker recovery, should be given less priority than younger people, or people who have greater chances of surviving (White and Lo 2020, 1773; Emanuel, Phillips, and Persad 2020). This does not mean, of course, that the inclusion of utilitarian principles in triage protocols is uncontroversial. Some authors have recently argued that this approach might aggravate social injustice, as patients who have slim prospects of recovery are usually those who also have limited access to health care, sanitation, or healthy diet (Supady et al. 2021).

As the COVID pandemic recedes and more data on the efficacy of different triage protocols start to emerge, ethicists and policymakers will have the opportunity to further assess the balance of different ethical principles. But in this case, it would be perhaps more accurate to refer to the establishment of new protocols as something that happens in the aftermath of a pandemic, and not as something that happens during a pandemic.

16.4 Responsibility for actions and omissions after a pandemic

As of December 2022, more than six million people are reported to have been killed by the COVID pandemic.[3] The estimates for the economic costs vary, but they are equally dismaying. The consequences of the COVID pandemic are likely to be felt for many years to come. In this subsection, I intend to examine two morally relevant questions that arise in the period following a pandemic – the COVID pandemic for that matter. The first question concerns the impact of the COVID pandemic on climate policies (Subsection 16.4.1.1). The second relates to hitherto widespread attitudes towards other infectious diseases at both domestic and international levels (Subsection 16.4.1.2).

16.4.1.1 Climate change, pandemics, and the costs for future generations

I have referred earlier to Stephen Gardiner's 2011 book *A Perfect Moral Storm: The Ethical Tragedy of Climate Change*. Gardiner's understanding of a "perfect storm" may prove fruitful for elucidation of questions of responsibility in the aftermath of a pandemic. According to Gardiner, the "perfect storm" in the book title refers to a convergence of pressing issues that makes climate change an especially difficult problem to tackle. Climate change involves questions related to (*i*) international politics, with all the imbalance of power that characterizes the relation among states; (*ii*) intergenerational relations, with the obvious asymmetry of power between the present and future generations; and (*iii*) "ineptitude" of our traditional moral and political theories, to which I have referred earlier. As he puts it, "In my metaphor of the perfect moral storm, the three problems (or 'storms') are all obstacles to our ability to behave ethically" (Gardiner 2011, 7). Back in 2011, it may not have occurred to Gardiner that no storm is too bad that it cannot get any worse, not even a "perfect storm."

The COVID pandemic clearly imposes a further strain on the pursuit of effective climate mitigation and adaptation efforts. It counts now as another "storm," with the potential to prompt both individuals and decision-makers to eschew their duty to "behave ethically."[4] Yet, the COVID pandemic clearly should not be used as an excuse to slow down the pursuit of mitigation and adaptation policies. For unmitigated climate change, along with inaction as regards climate adaptation, will not only aggravate the consequences of the COVID pandemic, but also further aggravate the danger of new disease outbreaks in the future (Jones et al. 2008; Lindahl and Grace 2015; Quick and Fryer 2018, chap. 2; United Nations 2018, sec. 6; United Nations Environment Programme 2020; Beyer, Manica, and Mora 2021; Lemieux et al. 2022). This means that policymakers, at both domestic and international levels, have a responsibility to mitigate the long-term consequences of the COVID pandemic while further pursuing strategies to achieve climate goals.

Alternatively, the threat posed by pandemics – both the COVID pandemic and other pandemics that are likely to emerge in the future – can be seen as a "perfect storm" in its own right. It is not just another "storm" in the pursuit of climate goals because the threats posed by pandemics contain, indeed, all the ingredients to which Gardiner alludes in his depiction of a "perfect storm." Pandemics spread across borders, being, therefore, a matter of international politics; they affect different generations unequally, and they also lay bare the shortcomings of our traditional normative theories. And to compound the problem, the threats posed by pandemics will have to be addressed amidst the ongoing climate crisis.

Pandemics may not give rise to questions of intergenerational justice as regards *non-overlapping* generations. This is a pressing problem in the climate ethics debate, for the current generation does not overlap with the generation that is going to live, say, in a hundred years' time from now. This means that the current generation will have to bear the costs of climate adaptation and especially climate mitigation without enjoying *all* the corresponding benefits (Gardiner 2011, 36, 147; Moellendorf 2022, 98–99). This in turn may render the current generation less motivated to act for the benefit of (non-overlapping) future generations. This problem, apparently, does not arise in the pandemic ethics debate, for the current generation, having endured the hardships imposed by the COVID pandemic, may be strongly motivated to support pandemic risk mitigation and pandemic preparedness in the expectation to benefit from these efforts, whether or not the efforts also promote the interest of (non-overlapping) future generations. Thus, the effective pursuit of long-term pandemic mitigation strategies and pandemic preparedness efforts does not have to face the same kind of motivational constraints that affect the long-term pursuit of climate adaptation and, especially, climate mitigation policies (Meyer and Araujo 2020, 2021, 225; Araujo and Meyer 2022, 50).

On the other hand, when it comes to questions of intergenerational justice as regards *overlapping* generations – younger and older people, from different generations, but living in the same time frame – pandemics, too, pose pressing issues of intergenerational justice. The COVID pandemic affected the interests of younger and older generations differently. The older generation was more likely to die from COVID than the younger generation. This means, among other things, that members of the younger generation might feel less motivated to wear masks and practice social distancing, or to self-isolate if they become infected, than the older generation. This kind of inconsiderate behaviour is certainly unfair towards older people. On the other hand, the economic costs of the COVID pandemic are likely to be a much heavier burden for the younger generation. As David Yarrow has recently put the problem,

> COVID-19 presents a distinctive problem for intergenerational justice: *the costs of fighting the pandemic have fallen disproportionally on those least at risk from it.* This has informed calls for post-COVID fiscal and welfare policy to have the explicit aim of intergenerational redistribution.[5]
>
> (Yarrow 2021, 80)

As the pandemic recedes and new evidence emerges, it has also become apparent that the long periods of social isolation have been more severely detrimental to the mental health of the younger generation than to the older (Lykkeskov and Di Nucci 2022; Woolston 2022).

In the longer run, the costs to promote the mitigation of pandemic risks and pandemic preparedness could be comparable to the costs to promote climate mitigation and climate adaptation. And this may represent a further burden on the currently living generation. The implementation of effective climate mitigation policies could in principle lead to carbon neutrality by 2050. Then, as long as humanity does not emit more greenhouse gases than it can remove from the atmosphere (or maybe humanity will have given up fossil fuels entirely), concerns over anthropogenic climate change will be (hopefully) a thing of the past. If one generation, for whatever reasons, relapses into past patterns of behaviour towards the environment, it may take some time, maybe decades or centuries, until greenhouse gases build up in the atmosphere in such a way as to disrupt the climate system again. This might give the next generation time to adapt to the new environment and, once more, to promote climate mitigation in order to compensate for past emissions. But it is unclear whether humanity might ever achieve a similar stage in the future as regards the threats posed by pandemics. The deployment of strategies for pandemic prevention and preparedness may help humanity to avert another major health crisis, but sooner or later a new pandemic may still arise as a result, for instance, of virus mutation and lack of expertise as to how to make our immune system able to fight an entirely new pathogen, or due to some laboratory accident (United States Department of Health and Human Services 2022, 6), or to the further development of affordable and easy-to-use gene-editing technologies such as CRISPR, which may pave the way to bioterrorism (Longini et al. 2007; Nouri and Chyba 2008, 460, 470, 473–474; Dando 2016; Clapper 2016, 9; Kupferschmidt 2017; Noyce and Evans 2018; Coats 2019, 16; Rourke, Phelan, and Lawson 2020). To compound the problem, terrorists could also learn from previous pandemics – including the COVID pandemic – how a pandemic unfolds, which countries are particularly vulnerable, or how to disrupt the otherwise effective supply chain for the rapid development of vaccines. In this regard, there is no clear counterpart to the threat posed by bioterrorism in the climate ethics debate.[6]

Thus, although pandemics – unlike climate change – do not give rise to pressing questions of intergenerational justice as regards non-overlapping generations, the whole infrastructure created to promote pandemic risk mitigation and pandemic preparedness will have to be kept in place indefinitely into the future, one generation after the next.

16.4.1.2 *Pandemics and neglected diseases*

During the COVID pandemic, research centres, governments, and the private sector cooperated in a variety of ways to develop, manufacture, and roll out billions of doses of at least three different kinds of vaccines against the new coronavirus. This is an unprecedented achievement in the history of global health, comparable only to the eradication of the smallpox virus in the 1970s, which took anyway about ten years to complete. But this success has come at a price – namely, funds and efforts to fight tropical neglected diseases, and diseases that typically affect poorer countries, have been diverted to accelerate research on the new virus and on the development of vaccines (Ntoumi 2020; Roberts 2021). The Global Fund to Fight AIDS, Tuberculosis and Malaria released a report in 2021 in which they state, for instance, the following:

> COVID-19 has been the most significant setback in the fight against HIV, TB and malaria, that we have encountered in the two decades since the Global Fund was established, exacerbating existing inequalities, diverting critical resources, stopping or slowing access to treatment and prevention activities, and putting vulnerable people further at risk.
>
> (The Global Fund to Fight AIDS, Tuberculosis and
> Malaria 2021, 7)

Whether or not it is morally acceptable to divert funds from research on diseases that together kill yearly more people than the new coronavirus and its variants have killed thus far is not a question I intend to address here.[7] It might be correctly argued that failure to deploy intense and coordinated efforts to combat the COVID pandemic would have led to a much higher number of premature deaths. However, individuals and communities that have benefited from international efforts to combat the COVID pandemic have now a *prima facie* duty to compensate people, in poorer parts of the world, for the harm that has been inflicted on them. They have been allotted a smaller share of vaccines and deprived of precious resources to fight treatable diseases, which had already been afflicting them for a much longer time. Francine Ntoumi, a researcher in the Republic of Congo, expressed her position on this problem as follows:

> What if the world had tackled malaria with the energy now dedicated to the coronavirus? Might malaria have been defeated? [...] this is how I see the COVID-19 pandemic: as an opportunity to build structures that will reduce the burden of all tropical diseases.[8]
>
> (Ntoumi 2020)

Inequality in the distribution of health resources affects also the treatment of diseases such as influenza, tuberculosis, and cancer, which affect different segments of the world population in both rich and poorer countries.[9] According to Neil Levy and Julian Savulescu, influenza has a much greater "cumulative toll" than COVID. However, the number of cumulative annual deaths from influenza has received less attention than the number of deaths resulting from the COVID pandemic. The question arises then as to whether, starting in the post-pandemic period, governments would not have a duty to promote policies for the prevention and preparation for influenza epidemics with the same energy with which they fought the COVID pandemic. As Levy and Savulescu put the problem,

[T]he new knowledge we have, of what kinds of interventions are possible and what their effects are likely to be, transforms our responsibilities. Once we know that we have the power to prevent significant harms, we acquire the responsibility to do so.[10]

(Levy and Savulescu, 2021, 130)

The same question can be asked with regard to the domain of individual responsibility: if people agreed, for example, to self-isolate and wear masks after contracting (or after suspecting having contracted) COVID, should not they for the same reasons adopt these measures when contracting (or after suspecting having contracted) influenza? As our knowledge of the prevention and treatment of new diseases increases, so does the scope of our responsibilities, whether at an individual or institutional level.

In this section, I have examined some questions of responsibility concerning actions and omissions that occur *before*, *during*, and in the *aftermath* of a pandemic. I have adopted this *before-during-after* temporal framework in order to characterize the unique character of threats posed by pandemics, especially if compared to the threats posed by climate change. Yet a clear-cut line between one time frame and the other cannot be drawn, for what counts as "after a pandemic" from one policy's point of view may also count as "before a pandemic" from another policy's point of view. Given the cyclical nature of pandemics, policymakers have to fight a pandemic and deal with the hardships of a post-pandemic period while also deploying resources to minimize the risks of another pandemic and preparing for the next pandemic. This is a further reason to think of pandemic ethics as a unified field of investigation, and not as a simple cluster of unrelated moral questions.

16.5 Conclusion

Pandemics are not one-off events: they are cyclical. And humanity, at all levels of agency, has the moral responsibility to break the cycle of pandemics. This means that many of the societal changes and technological breakthroughs that emerge *during* a pandemic can become instrumental for the development of capabilities that may enable us to avert *future* pandemics; and if another pandemic does strike again, we have a duty to employ lessons from *past* pandemics in order to better address the *current* one. At a more theoretical level, the implication is clear: the normative theories we deploy to address issues that arise in one time frame should not be taken as unrelated to the moral reasons we articulate in another time frame. In this regard, pandemics differ significantly from *anthropogenic* climate change, for there is nothing we can learn from previous patterns of anthropogenic climate change. Anthropogenic climate change, as we know it, is a one-off event.[11] On the other hand, there is much we can and should learn from past pandemics. And this, in turn, gives rise to kinds of responsibility that can only be properly addressed within the nascent field of pandemic ethics.

Although we do not have to live indefinitely under the shadow of dangerous climate change, humanity will probably have to live under the shadow of pandemics. Thus, pandemics may represent an even greater existential risk to humanity than climate change. In this chapter, I have presented the outlines of what I call the emerging field of pandemic ethics. Just in the same way climate ethics emerged some 20 years ago as a philosophical field of investigation, systematizing ethical questions that had been heretofore treated as only loosely related to each other, I have argued throughout this chapter that several ethical questions posed by the COVID pandemic, or relative to other pandemics in the past, or to the threats posed by future pandemics, and which have hitherto been largely discussed as unrelated to each other, should be addressed now as part of a unified whole – the field of pandemic ethics.

Acknowledgements

The author benefited from extensive discussions with Lukas Meyer (University of Graz, Austria). The author also benefited from financial support provided by FAPERJ (Research Support Foundation of the State of Rio de Janeiro, Brazil, Grant Nr. 26/200.432/2023) and CNPq (National Council for Scientific and Technological Development, Brazil, Grant No. 304635/2022-7).

Notes

1 Hans Jonas' 1979 influential book *The Imperative of Responsibility: In Search of an Ethics for the Technological Age* is worth mentioning as well. Although Jonas did not have climate change in mind, he recognized that traditional moral theories were not adequate to address a whole new range of problems humanity would have to face in the future: "No previous ethics had to consider the global condition of human life and the far-off future, even existence, of the race. These now being an issue demands, in brief, a new conception of duties and rights, for which previous ethics and metaphysics provide not even principles, let alone a ready doctrine" (Jonas 1984, 28–29; 1985, 8). Another pioneering author worth mentioning in this regard is John Herz. As early as 1957, Herz argued for a more comprehensive ethics, which would account for both the global and intergenerational dimensions of human existence: "Ethics thus becomes comprehensive in two ways – latitudinally or geographically, so to speak, because it turns global, and longitudinally, in its time dimension, in that it turns futuristic, taking into account the future of mankind, the generations that (hopefully) will come after us. [...] As for he second, or temporal, dimension, it means that, for the first time, we are compelled to take the futuristic view if we want to make sure that there will be future generations at all" (Herz 1957, 108–109). Herz also argued for the emergence of a new interdisciplinary field, which he named "survival studies" (Herz 2003; Seidel 2003; Stevens 2020).

298 *Marcelo de Araujo*

2 For an extensive list of pandemic early warnings, see Araujo and Costa (2023). Araujo, Marcelo de, and Daniel de Vasconcelos Costa (2023). "A Survey of Pandemic Early Warnings (1999–2019)." *SSRN (Social Science Research Network)*. https://doi.org/10.2139/ssrn.4357126.

3 See Worldometer (website): https://www.worldometers.info/coronavirus/.

4 For the impact of the COVID pandemic on individuals' willingness to support climate mitigation policies, see Klösch, Wardana, and Hadler (2021); Wardana, Klösch, and Hadler (2022).

5 See, e.g., Jörg Tremmel: "In almost every country of the world, supplementary budgets or economic stimulus packages were adopted in the first half of 2020 to cushion the economic slump. As a result, the national debt, in principle a burden shifted from today's to future generations, reached astronomical levels" (Tremmel 2021, 9).

6 There is a caveat here, though: If at some point in the future governments decide to fight climate change unilaterally by means of geoengineering, *climate terrorism* might indeed become an issue of major concern, or perhaps even an existential risk in its own right (C. Hamilton 2013, 113; Hulme 2014, 78; Parker and Irvine 2018). For it is at least imaginable that the whole infrastructure that keeps the global temperature below some agreed upon threshold might be destroyed single-handedly by a group of terrorists. This might prompt, then, a "termination shock," that is an abrupt increase of the global temperature, leaving most populations with no time to adapt. Successful geoengineering might also trigger *climate wars*, as more powerful states might try to adjust the global temperature in such a way as to promote their own interests (The Economist 2021a).

7 For the number of COVID deaths in comparison to the number of deaths resulting from other infectious diseases, see, e.g., Nature Index (2021).

8 See also the proceedings of a workshop at the National Academies of Sciences, Engineering, and Medicine in 2022: "Unfortunately, COVID-19 and its mitigation efforts have taken a destructive toll on countries with the highest burden of TB disease and have diverted attention and resources from the global TB response, threatening to reverse years of progress toward eliminating the disease" (Biffl, Liao, and Nicholson 2022, 1). See also Msomi et al. (2021).

9 For research on the impact of COVID on cancer research and cancer treatment, see Lawler et al. (2022); Maringe et al. (2020); W. Hamilton (2020). For the impact of COVID on tuberculosis treatment, see (Biffl, Liao, and Nicholson 2022).

10 See also Jörg Tremmel: "Careless handling of influenza viruses should be a thing of the past after the current corona pandemic" (Tremmel 2021, 12).

11 For a recent account of previous patterns of non-anthropogenic climate change, see Fagan and Durrani (2021).

References

Addo, Isaac Yeboah. 2020. "Double pandemic: Racial discrimination amid coronavirus disease 2019." *Social Sciences & Humanities Open* 2 (1): 100074. https://doi.org/10.1016/j.ssaho.2020.100074.

Allen, Toph, Kris A. Murray, Carlos Zambrana-Torrelio, Stephen S. Morse, Carlo Rondinini, Moreno Di Marco, Nathan Breit, Kevin J. Olival, and Peter Daszak. 2017. "Global hotspots and correlates of emerging zoonotic diseases." *Nature Communications* 8 (1): 1124. https://doi.org/10.1038/s41467-017-00923-8.

Altman, Matthew C. 2021. "A consequentialist argument for considering age in triage decisions during the coronavirus pandemic." *Bioethics* 35 (4): 356–365. https://doi.org/10.1111/bioe.12864.

Araujo, Marcelo de. 2021. "The nascent field of pandemic ethics: Prevention, mitigation, responsibility, and adaptation." *SSRN Electronic Journal.* https://doi.org/10.2139/ssrn.3984756.

Araujo, Marcelo de, and Lukas H. Meyer. 2022. "Climate change and pandemics: Feasibility constraints on mitigation and adaptation." In *Climate Change, Responsibility and Liability*, ed. Eva Schulev-Steindl, Monika Hinteregger, Gottfried Kirchengast, Lukas Meyer, Oliver C. Ruppel, Gerhard Schnedl, and Karl W. Steininger, 41–74. volume 1. Baden-Baden: Nomos.

Araujo, Marcelo de, and Daniel de Vasconcelos Costa. 2023. "A Survey of Pandemic Early Warnings (1999–2019)". *SSRN Electronic Journal.* https://doi.org/10.2139/ssrn.4357126.

Barry, John M. 2005. *The Great Influenza: The Epic Story of the Deadliest Plague in History.* New York: Viking.

Beyer, Robert M., Andrea Manica, and Camilo Mora. 2021. "Shifts in global bat diversity suggest a possible role of climate change in the emergence of SARS-CoV-1 and SARS-CoV-2." *Science of the Total Environment* 767 (May): 145413. https://doi.org/10.1016/j.scitotenv.2021.145413.

Bieber, Florian. 2020. Global nationalism in times of the COVID-19 pandemic. *Nationalities Papers*, April, 1–13. https://doi.org/10.1017/nps.2020.35.

Biffl, Claire, Julie Liao, and Anna Nicholson. 2022. *Innovations for Tackling Tuberculosis in the Time of COVID-19: Proceedings of a Workshop.* Washington, D.C.: National Academies Press.

Birnbacher, Dieter. 2016. *Klimaethik: Nach Uns Die Sintflut?* Stuttgart: Reclam.

Bramble, Ben. 2020. *Pandemic Ethics: 8 Big Questions of COVID-19.* Sydney: Bartleby Books.

Caraballo, Krystlelynn. 2020. "Immigration, law, and (in)justice: Coronavirus and its impact on immigration." *International Criminal Justice Review* 30 (4): 448–457. https://doi.org/10.1177/1057567720951848.

Charlier, Philippe, and Leandro Varison. 2020. "Is COVID-19 being used as a weapon against indigenous peoples in Brazil?" *The Lancet* 396 (10257): 1069–1070. https://doi.org/10.1016/S0140-6736(20)32068-7.

Chin, Dorothy, Elizabeth J. King, Elize Massard da Fonseca, Salvador Vázquez del Mercado, Scott L. Greer, and Sumit Ganguly. 2021. "World's worst pandemic leaders: 5 Presidents and Prime Ministers who badly mishandled COVID-19." *The Conversation.* May 18, 2021. http://theconversation.com/worlds-worst-pandemic-leaders-5-presidents-and-prime-ministers-who-badly-mishandled-covid-19-159787.

Chou, Wen-Ying Sylvia, and Anna Gaysynsky. 2021. "Racism and xenophobia in a Pandemic: Interactions of online and offline worlds." *American Journal of Public Health* 111 (5): 773–775. https://doi.org/10.2105/AJPH.2021.306230.

Christakis, Nicholas. 2020. *Apollo's Arrow: The Profound and Enduring Impact of Coronavirus on the Way We Live.* New York: Little, Brown and Company.

Clapper, James R. 2016. Statement for the Record Worldwide Threat Assessment of the US Intelligence Community, February 9. *US Intelligence Community.* https://www.armed-services.senate.gov/imo/media/doc/Clapper_02-09-16.pdf.

Clark, Helen, and Ellen Johnson Sirleaf. 2021. "Ending this pandemic and securing the future." *BMJ*, November, n2914. https://doi.org/10.1136/bmj.n2914.

Coats, Daniel R. 2019. Statement for the Record Worldwide Threat Assessment of the US Intelligence Community. *US Intelligence Community.* https://www.dni.gov/files/ODNI/documents/2019-ATA-SFR---SSCI.pdf.

Council of the European Union. 2020. Press release by President Charles Michel on an international treaty on pandemics. *European Council.* December 3, 2020.https://www.consilium.europa.eu/en/press/press-releases/2020/12/03/press-release-by-president-charles-michel-on-an-international-treaty-on-pandemics/.

Cripps, Elizabeth. 2013. *Climate Change and the Moral Agent: Individual Duties in an Interdependent World.* Oxford: Oxford University Press.

Dando, Malcolm. 2016. "Find the time to discuss new bioweapons." *Nature* 535 (7610): 9. https://doi.org/10.1038/535009a.

Dyer, Clare. 2020. "Report of UK's pandemic preparedness leaves questions unanswered, says doctor." *BMJ.* November, m4499. https://doi.org/10.1136/bmj.m4499.

Ellwanger, Joel Henrique, and José Artur Bogo Chies. 2018. "Zoonotic spillover and emerging viral diseases – time to intensify zoonoses surveillance in Brazil." *The Brazilian Journal of Infectious Diseases* 22 (1): 76–78. https://doi.org/10.1016/j.bjid.2017.11.003.

Emanuel, Ezekiel J., James Phillips, and Govind Persad. 2020. "Opinion. How the coronavirus may force doctors to decide who can live and who dies." *The New York Times*, March 12, 2020, sec. Opinion. https://www.nytimes.com/2020/03/12/opinion/coronavirus-hospital-shortage.html.

Fagan, Brian M., and Nadia Durrani. 2021. *Climate Chaos: Lessons on Survival from Our Ancestors.* New York: PublicAffairs.

Florentino, Manolo, and Márcia Amantino. 2011. "Runaways and *quilombolas* in the Americas." In *The Cambridge World History of Slavery*, ed. David Eltis and Stanley L. Engerman, 708–740. Cambridge: Cambridge University Press.

France-Presse, Agence. 2021. "Mallorca man arrested for infecting 22 people with COVID." *The Guardian*, April 24, 2021, sec. World news. https://www.theguardian.com/world/2021/apr/24/mallorca-man-arrested-for-infecting-22-people-with-covid.

Fukuda-Parr, Sakiko, Paulo Buss, and Alicia Ely Yamin. 2021. "Pandemic treaty needs to start with rethinking the paradigm of global health security." *BMJ Global Health* 6 (6): e006392. https://doi.org/10.1136/bmjgh-2021-006392.

Gardiner, Stephen. 2011. *A Perfect Moral Storm: The Ethical Tragedy of Climate Change.* Oxford: Oxford University Press.

Gardiner, Stephen, and Arthur R. Obst. 2023. *Dialogues on Climate Justice.* New York: Routledge.

Gesang, Bernward. 2020. *Mit kühlem Kopf: Vom Nutzen der Philosophie für die Klimadebatte.* München: Carl Hanser Verlag.

Giuffrida, Angela. 2020. "Relatives of Italian COVID victims to file lawsuit against leading politicians." *The Guardian*, December 22, 2020, sec. World news.https://www.theguardian.com/world/2020/dec/22/relatives-of-italian-covid-victims-to-file-lawsuit-against-leading-politicians.

Goozen, Sara Vav. 2021. "How should we distribute scarce medical resources in a pandemic?" In *Political Philosophy in a Pandemic: Routes to a More Just Future*, ed. Fay Niker and Aveek Bhattacharya, 29–41. London, New York: Bloomsbury Academic.

Hamilton, Clive. 2013. *Earthmasters: The Dawn of the Age of Climate Engineering*. New Haven: Yale University Press.

Hamilton, William. 2020. "Cancer diagnostic delay in the COVID-19 era: What happens next?" *The Lancet Oncology* 21 (8): 1000–1002. https://doi.org/10.1016/S1470-2045(20)30391-0.

Herz, John. 1957. "Rise and demise of the territorial state." *World Politics* 9 (4): 473–493. https://doi.org/10.2307/2009421.

———. 2003. "On human survival: Reflections on survival research and survival policies." *World Futures* 59 (3–4): 135–143. https://doi.org/10.1080/02604020310123.

Hulme, Mike. 2014. *Can Science Fix Climate Change? A Case Against Climate Engineering*. Cambridge: Polity Press.

Human Rights Watch. 2020. "COVID-19 fueling anti-Asian racism and xenophobia worldwide." *Human Rights Watch* (blog). May 12, 2020. https://www.hrw.org/news/2020/05/12/covid-19-fueling-anti-asian-racism-and-xenophobia-worldwide.

Jamieson, Dale. 1992. "Ethics, public policy, and global warming." *Science, Technology, & Human Values* 17 (2): 139–153.

———. 2014. *Reason in a Dark Time: Why the Struggle Against Climate Change Failed – And What It Means for Our Future*. Oxford; New York: Oxford University Press.

Jerry, Robert H. 2020. "COVID-19: Responsibility and accountability in a world of rationing." *Journal of Law and the Biosciences* 7 (1): lsaa076. https://doi.org/10.1093/jlb/lsaa076.

Jonas, Hans. 1984. *Das Prinzip Verantwortung: Versuch einer Ethik für die technologische Zivilisation*. Frankfurt am Main: Suhrkamp.

———. 1985. *The Imperative of Responsibility: In Search of an Ethics for the Technological Age*. Chicago: University of Chicago Press.

Jones, Kate E., Nikkita G. Patel, Marc A. Levy, Adam Storeygard, Deborah Balk, John L. Gittleman, and Peter Daszak. 2008. "Global trends in emerging infectious diseases." *Nature* 451 (7181): 990–993. https://doi.org/10.1038/nature06536.

Klösch, Beate, Rebecca Wardana, and Markus Hadler. 2021. "Impact of the COVID-19 pandemic on the willingness to sacrifice for the environment: The Austrian case." *Österreichische Zeitschrift Für Soziologie* 46 (4): 457–469. https://doi.org/10.1007/s11614-021-00464-x.

Kupferschmidt, Kai. 2017. "How Canadian researchers reconstituted an extinct poxvirus for $100,000 using mail-order DNA." *Science*, July. https://doi.org/10.1126/science.aan7069.

Labonté, Ronald, Mary Wiktorowicz, Corinne Packer, Arne Ruckert, Kumanan Wilson, and Sam Halabi. 2021. "A pandemic treaty, revised international health regulations, or both?" *Globalization and Health* 17 (1): 128. https://doi.org/10.1186/s12992-021-00779-0.

Lakoff, Andrew. 2008. "The generic biothreat, or, how we became unprepared." *Cultural Anthropology* 23 (3): 399–428.

———. 2017. *Unprepared: Global Health in a Time of Emergency*. Oakland, California: University of California Press.

Lawler, Mark, Lynne Davies, Simon Oberst, Kathy Oliver, Alexander Eggermont, Anna Schmutz, Carlo La Vecchia, et al. 2022. "European groundshot – addressing Europe's cancer research challenges: A *Lancet* Oncology Commission." *The*

Lancet Oncology, November, S147020452200540X. https://doi.org/10.1016/S1470-2045(22)00540-X.

Lemieux, Audrée, Graham A. Colby, Alexandre J. Poulain, and Stéphane Aris-Brosou. 2022. Viral spillover risk increases with climate change in high Arctic Lake sediments. *Proceedings of the Royal Society B: Biological Sciences* 289 (1985): 20221073. https://doi.org/10.1098/rspb.2022.1073.

Lindahl, Johanna F., and Delia Grace. 2015. "The consequences of human actions on risks for infectious diseases: A review." *Infection Ecology & Epidemiology* 5 (1): 30048. https://doi.org/10.3402/iee.v5.30048.

Longini, Ira M., M. Elizabeth Halloran, Azhar Nizam, Yang Yang, Shufu Xu, Donald S. Burke, Derek A.T. Cummings, and Joshua M. Epstein. 2007. "Containing a large bioterrorist smallpox attack: A computer simulation approach." *International Journal of Infectious Diseases* 11 (2): 98–108. https://doi.org/10.1016/j.ijid.2006.03.002.

Lykkeskov, Anne, and Ezio Di Nucci. 2022. "COVID-19 and intergenerational justice: The case of Denmark." In *The Global and Social Consequences of the COVID-19 Pandemic*, ed. Gottfried Schweiger, 1212: 51–63. Studies in Global Justice. Cham: Springer. https://doi.org/10.1007/978-3-030-97982-9_4.

Madhav, Nita, Ben Oppenheim, Mark Gallivan, Prime Mulembakani, Edward Rubin, and Nathan Wolfe. 2017. "Pandemics: Risks, impacts, and mitigation." In *Disease Control Priorities, Third Edition (Volume 9): Improving Health and Reducing Poverty*, ed. Dean T. Jamison, Hellen Gelband, Susan Horton, Prabhat Jha, Ramanan Laxminarayan, Charles N. Mock, and Rachel Nugent, 315–345. Washington, DC: World Bank. https://doi.org/10.1596/978-1-4648-0527-1.

Maringe, Camille, James Spicer, Melanie Morris, Arnie Purushotham, Ellen Nolte, Richard Sullivan, Bernard Rachet, and Ajay Aggarwal. 2020. "The impact of the COVID-19 Pandemic on cancer deaths due to delays in diagnosis in England, UK: A National, population-based, modelling study." *The Lancet Oncology* 21 (8): 1023–1034. https://doi.org/10.1016/S1470-2045(20)30388-0

Markowitz, Ezra M., Marco Grasso, and Dale Jamieson. 2015. "Climate ethics at a multidisciplinary crossroads: Four directions for future scholarship." *Climatic Change* 130 (3): 465–474. https://doi.org/10.1007/s10584-015-1404-4

Maxmen, Amy, and Jeff Tollefson. 2020. "Two decades of pandemic war games failed to account for Donald Trump." *Nature* 584 (7819): 26–29. https://doi.org/10.1038/d41586-020-02277-6

Meyer, Lukas H., and Araujo, Marcelo de. 2020. "The COVID-19 pandemic and climate change: Why have responses been so different?" *E-International Relations*, April, 1–6.

———. 2021. "Soft constraints on the feasibility of climate goals: An analysis in the light of the 2020 pandemic." In *Climate Justice and Feasibility: Normative Theorizing, Normative Principles, and Climate Action*, ed. Sarah Kenehan and Corey Katz, 213–238. Lanham: Rowman & Littlefield.

Meyer, Lukas H., and Pranay Sanklecha, eds. 2017. *Climate Justice and Historical Emissions*. Cambridge, United Kingdom, New York: Cambridge University Press.

Moellendorf, Darrel. 2022. *Mobilizing Hope: Climate Change and Global Poverty*. New York: Oxford University Press.

Msomi, Nokukhanya, Richard Lessells, Koleka Mlisana, and Tulio de Oliveira. 2021. "Africa: Tackle HIV and COVID-19 together." *Nature* 600 (7887): 33–36. https://doi.org/10.1038/d41586-021-03546-8.

Myers, Nathan. 2018. "Global health security is global security: The lessons of Clade X." *World Affairs* 181 (4): 403–412. https://doi.org/10.1177/0043820018811495.

Nature Index. 2021. "By the numbers: Counting the costs of infectious illness." *Nature* 598 (7882): S18–19. https://doi.org/10.1038/d41586-021-02911-x

Nikogosian, Haik, and Ilona Kickbusch. 2021. "The case for an international pandemic treaty." *BMJ*, February, n527. https://doi.org/10.1136/bmj.n527.

Nouri, Ali, and Christopher F. Chyba. 2008. "Biotechnology and biosecurity." In *Global Catastrophic Risks*, ed. Nick Bostrom and Milan M. Cirkovic, 450–480. Oxford: Oxford University Press.

Noyce, Ryan S., and David H. Evans. 2018. "Synthetic horsepox viruses and the continuing debate about dual use research." *PLOS Pathogens* 14 (10): e1007025. https://doi.org/10.1371/journal.ppat.1007025.

Ntoumi, Francine. 2020. "What if tropical diseases had as much attention as COVID?" *Nature* 587 (7834): 331–331. https://doi.org/10.1038/d41586-020-03220-5.

Olival, Kevin J., Parviez R. Hosseini, Carlos Zambrana-Torrelio, Noam Ross, Tiffany L. Bogich, and Peter Daszak. 2017. "Host and viral traits predict zoonotic spillover from mammals." *Nature* 546 (7660): 646–650. https://doi.org/10.1038/nature22975.

Ord, Toby. 2020. *The Precipice: Existential Risk and the Future of Humanity*. New York: Hachette Books.

Osterholm, Michael. 2007. "Unprepared for a pandemic, sounding the alarm, again." *Foreign Affairs* 86 (2): 47–57.

O'Toole, Tara, Michael Mair, and Thomas V. Inglesby. 2002. "Shining light on 'Dark Winter'" *Clinical Infectious Diseases* 34 (7): 972–983. https://doi.org/10.1086/339909.

Palamim, Camila Vantini Capasso, Manoela Marques Ortega, and Fernando Augusto Lima Marson. 2020. "COVID-19 in the indigenous population of Brazil." *Journal of Racial and Ethnic Health Disparities* 7 (6): 1053–1058. https://doi.org/10.1007/s40615-020-00885-6.

Parker, Andy, and Peter J. Irvine. 2018. "The risk of termination shock from solar geoengineering." *Earth's Future* 6 (3): 456–467. https://doi.org/10.1002/2017EF000735.

Pegg, David. 2020. "Official report that said UK was not prepared for pandemic is published." *The Guardian*, October 22, 2020. https://www.theguardian.com/world/2020/oct/22/official-report-exercise-cygnus-uk-was-not-prepared-for-pandemic-is-published.

Perry, Mark. 2020. "America's pandemic war games don't end well." *Foreign Policy*, April 1, 2020. https://foreignpolicy.com/2020/04/01/coronavirus-pandemic-war-games-simulation-dark-winter/.

Phillips, Tom. 2021. "Charge Bolsonaro with murder over COVID toll, draft Brazil Senate report says." *The Guardian*, October 19, 2021, sec. World News. https://www.theguardian.com/world/2021/oct/19/bolsonaro-coronavirus-brazil-murder-charges-senate-report.

Pike, Jamison, Tiffany Bogich, Sarah Elwood, David C. Finnoff, and Peter Daszak. 2014. "Economic optimization of a global strategy to address the pandemic threat." *Proceedings of the National Academy of Sciences* 111 (52): 18519–18523. https://doi.org/10.1073/pnas.1412661112.

Polidoro, Maurício, Francisco de Assis Mendonça, Stela Nazareth Meneghel, Alan Alves-Brito, Marcelo Gonçalves, Fernanda Bairros, and Daniel Canavese. 2020. "Territories under siege: Risks of the decimation of indigenous and *quilombolas* peoples in the context of COVID-19 in South Brazil." *Journal of Racial and Ethnic Health Disparities*, September. https://doi.org/10.1007/s40615-020-00868-7.

Quick, Jonathan D., and Bronwyn Fryer. 2018. *The End of Epidemics: The Looming Threat to Humanity and How to Stop It*. New York: St. Martin's Press.

Rambo, Ana Paula Schmitz, Laura Faustino Gonçalves, Ana Inês Gonzáles, Cassiano Ricardo Rech, Karina Mary de Paiva, and Patrícia Haas. 2021. "Impact of super-spreaders on COVID-19: Systematic review." *São Paulo Medical Journal* 139 (2): 163–169. https://doi.org/10.1590/1516-3180.2020.0618.r1.10122020.

Roberts, Leslie. 2021. "How COVID is derailing the fight against HIV, TB and malaria." *Nature* 597 (7876): 314–314. https://doi.org/10.1038/d41586-021-02469-8.

Robertson, Christopher, and Wesley Oliver. 2021. "Is it a crime to forge a vaccine card? And what's the penalty for using a fake?" *The Conversation*. August 30, 2021.http://theconversation.com/is-it-a-crime-to-forge-a-vaccine-card-and-whats-the-penalty-for-using-a-fake-166788.

Rourke, Michelle F., Alexandra Phelan, and Charles Lawson. 2020. "Access and benefit-sharing following the synthesis of horsepox virus." *Nature Biotechnology* 38 (5): 537–539. https://doi.org/10.1038/s41587-020-0518-z.

Savulescu, Julian, Ingmar Persson, and Dominic Wilkinson. 2020. "Utilitarianism and the pandemic." *Bioethics* 34 (6): 620–632. https://doi.org/10.1111/bioe.12771.

Schwenkenbecher, Anne. 2014. "Is there an obligation to reduce one's individual carbon footprint?" *Critical Review of International Social and Political Philosophy* 17 (2): 168–188. https://doi.org/10.1080/13698230.2012.692984.

Seidel, Peter. 2003. "'Survival research': A new discipline needed now." *World Futures* 59 (3–4): 129–133. https://doi.org/10.1080/02604020310134.

Serdeczny, Olivia, Eleanor Waters, and Sander Chan. 2016. *Non-Economic Loss and Damage in the Context of Climate Change: Understanding the Challenges*. Discussion Paper / Deutsches Institut Für Entwicklungspolitik 2016/3. Bonn: Deutsches Institut für Entwicklungspolitik.

Sinnott-Armstrong, Walter, and Richard B. Howarth, eds. 2005. "It is not my fault: Global warming and individual moral obligations." *Perspectives on Climate Change: Science, Economics, Politics, Ethics*, 221–253. New York: Elsevier.

Smith, Bradley T., Thomas V. Inglesby, Esther Brimmer, Luciana Borio, Crystal Franco, Gigi Kwik Gronvall, Bradley Kramer, et al. 2005. "Navigating the storm: Report and recommendations from the *Atlantic Storm* Exercise." *Biosecurity and Bioterrorism: Biodefense Strategy, Practice, and Science* 3 (3): 256–267. https://doi.org/10.1089/bsp.2005.3.256.

Snowden, Frank M. 2019. *Epidemics and Society: From the Black Death to the Present*. New Haven: Yale University Press.

Stevens, Tim. 2020. "Productive pessimism: Rehabilitating John Herz's Survival Research for the anthropocene." In *Pessimism in International Relations: Provocations, Possibilities, Politics*, ed. Tim Stevens and Nicholas Michelsen, 83–98. Cham, Switzerland: Palgrave Macmillan, Springer Nature.

Supady, Alexander, J Randall Curtis, Darryl Abrams, Roberto Lorusso, Thomas Bein, Joachim Boldt, Crystal E Brown, Daniel Duerschmied, Victoria Metaxa, and Daniel Brodie. 2021. "Allocating scarce intensive care resources during the COVID-19 pandemic: Practical challenges to theoretical frameworks." *The Lancet Respiratory Medicine* 9 (4): 430–434. https://doi.org/10.1016/S2213-2600(20)30580-4.

Taylor, Luke. 2021. "World Health Organization to begin negotiating international pandemic treaty." *BMJ*, December, n2991. https://doi.org/10.1136/bmj.n2991.

The Economist. 2021a. "Governing the atmosphere. technologies which might stabilise the climate could do the reverse to international relations." *The Economist*, October 20, 2021. https://www.economist.com/science-and-technology/2022/11/02/americas-defence-department-is-looking-for-rogue-geoengineers.

———. 2021b. "Jair Bolsonaro is accused of crimes against humanity in Brazil." *The Economist*, October 23, 2021. https://www.economist.com/the-americas/2021/10/23/jair-bolsonaro-is-accused-of-crimes-against-humanity-in-brazil.

The Global Fund to Fight AIDS, Tuberculosis and Malaria. 2021. *Results Report 2021*. Geneva: The Global Fund to Fight AIDS, Tuberculosis and Malaria. https://www.theglobalfund.org/en/results/.

The Johns Hopkins Center for Health Security. 2018. Clade X. A pandemic exercise. Johns Hopkins Center for Health Security. https://www.centerforhealthsecurity.org/our-work/events/2018_clade_x_exercise/index.html.

———. 2019. Event 201, a pandemic exercise to illustrate preparedness efforts. *Even 201*. 2019. https://www.centerforhealthsecurity.org/event201/.

Tremmel, Jörg. 2021. "Pandemics and intergenerational justice: Vaccination and the wellbeing of future societies." *Intergenerational Justice Review*, FRFG policy paper, 7 (1): 4–19.

Twilley, Nicola. 2018. "The terrifying lessons of a pandemic simulation." *The New Yorker*, 1 June 2018. https://www.newyorker.com/science/elements/the-terrifying-lessons-of-a-pandemic-simulation.

United Kingdom [Department of Health]. 2007. Exercise winter willow: Lessons identified. https://data.parliament.uk/DepositedPapers/Files/DEP2007-0334/DEP2007-0334.pdf.

United Kingdom [Public Health England]. 2017. *Exercise cygnus report*, October 18–20, 2016. https://assets.publishing.service.gov.uk/government/uploads/system/uploads/attachment_data/file/927770/exercise-cygnus-report.pdf.

United Nations. 2018. Sendai framework for disaster risk reduction 2015–2030. United Nations Office for Disaster Risk Reduction. https://www.undrr.org/publication/sendai-framework-disaster-risk-reduction-2015-2030.

United Nations Environment Programme. 2020. *Preventing the Next Pandemic. Zoonotic Diseases and How to Break the Chain of Transmission*. New York. https://www.preventionweb.net/publication/preventing-next-pandemic-zoonotic-diseases-and-how-break-chain-transmission.

United Nations General Assembly (UNGA). 2016. Protecting humanity from future health crises. Report of the high level panel on the global response to health crises. https://digitallibrary.un.org/record/822489?ln=en.

United States Department of Health and Human Services (HHS). 2022. 'National Biodefense Strategy and Implementation Plan for Countering Biological Threats, Enhancing Pandemic Preparedness, and Achieving Global Health

Security'. Washington, D.C. https://www.whitehouse.gov/wp-content/uploads/2022/10/National-Biodefense-Strategy-and-Implementation-Plan-Final.pdf.

Van der Geest, Kees, and Markus Schindler. 2017. *Report: Handbook for assessing loss and damage in vulnerable communities.* Bonn: United Nations University Institute for Environment and Human Security. https://collections.unu.edu/eserv/UNU:6032/Online_No_21_Handbook_180430.pdf.

Vinuales, Jorge, Suerie Moon, Ginevra Le Moli, and Gian-Luca Burci. 2021. "A global pandemic treaty should aim for deep prevention." *The Lancet* 397 (10287): 1791–1792. https://doi.org/10.1016/S0140-6736(21)00948-X.

Wallimann-Helmer, Ivo, Lukas Meyer, Kian Mintz-Woo, Thomas Schinko, and Olivia Serdeczny. 2019. "The ethical challenges in the context of climate loss and damage." In *Loss and Damage from Climate Change*, ed. Reinhard Mechler, Laurens M. Bouwer, Thomas Schinko, Swenja Surminski, and JoAnne Linnerooth-Bayer, 39–62. Climate Risk Management, Policy and Governance. Cham: Springer. https://doi.org/10.1007/978-3-319-72026-5_2.

Wardana, Rebecca, Beate Klösch, and Markus Hadler. 2022. "Umwelt in der Krise. Einstellungen zu Klimawandel und Umweltbesorgnis sowie Bereitschaft zu umweltbewusstem Verhalten in Krisenzeiten." In *Die österreichische Gesellschaft während der Corona-Pandemie*, ed. Wolfgang Aschauer, Christoph Glatz, and Dimitri Prandner, 241–267. Wiesbaden: Springer. https://doi.org/10.1007/978-3-658-34491-7_9.

Watson, Crystal, Eric S. Toner, Matthew P. Shearer, Caitlin Rivers, Diane Meyer, Christopher Hurtado, Matthew Watson, et al. 2019. "Clade X: A pandemic exercise." *Health Security* 17 (5): 410–417. https://doi.org/10.1089/hs.2019.0097.

Wenham, Clare, Matthew Kavanagh, Irene Torres, and Gavin Yamey. 2021. "Preparing for the next pandemic." *BMJ*, May, n1295. https://doi.org/10.1136/bmj.n1295.

White, Douglas B. 2009. "Who should receive life support during a public health emergency? Using ethical principles to improve allocation decisions." *Annals of Internal Medicine* 150 (2): 132. https://doi.org/10.7326/0003-4819-150-2-200901200-00011.

White, Douglas B., and Bernard Lo. 2020. "A framework for rationing ventilators and critical care beds during the COVID-19 pandemic." *JAMA* 323 (18): 1773–1774. https://doi.org/10.1001/jama.2020.5046.

Wilkinson, Dominic. 2020. "ICU triage in an impending crisis: Uncertainty, pre-emption and preparation." *Journal of Medical Ethics* 46 (5): 287–288. https://doi.org/10.1136/medethics-2020-106226.

———. 2021. "Ethics and evidence: Learning lessons from pandemic triage." *The Lancet Respiratory Medicine* 9 (4): 328–330. https://doi.org/10.1016/S2213-2600(21)00132-6.

Williams, Matt. 2021. "Bolsonaro faces 'crimes against humanity' charge over COVID-19 mishandling: 5 essential reads." *The Conversation*, October 21, 2021. http://theconversation.com/bolsonaro-faces-crimes-against-humanity-charge-over-covid-19-mishandling-5-essential-reads-170332.

Winston, Susanna E., and Curt G. Beckwith. 2011. "The impact of removing the immigration ban on HIV-infected persons". *AIDS Patient Care and STDs* 25 (12): 709–711. https://doi.org/10.1089/apc.2011.0121.

Woolston, Chris. 2022. "Stress and uncertainty drag down graduate students' satisfaction." *Nature* 610 (7933): 805–808. https://doi.org/10.1038/d41586-022-03394-0.

World Health Organization (WHO). 2021. Global leaders unite in urgent call for international pandemic treaty. March 30, 2021. https://www.who.int/news/item/30-03-2021-global-leaders-unite-in-urgent-call-for-international-pandemic-treaty.

Yarrow, David. 2021. "Should the older generation pay more of the COVID-19 debt?" In *Political Philosophy in a Pandemic: Routes to a More Just Future*, ed. Fay Niker and Aveek Bhattacharya, 71–83. London; New York: Bloomsbury Academic.

Zarocostas, John. 2021. "Countries prepare for pandemic treaty decision." *The Lancet* 398 (10315): 1951. https://doi.org/10.1016/S0140-6736(21)02651-9.

Index

Pages followed by "n" refer to notes.